Pearls in Biological and Molecular Tissue Repair Pathways
http://dx.doi.org/10.5772/intechopen.1001709
Edited by Peter A. Everts and Robert W. Alexander

Contributors
Ane Miren Bilbao, Beatriz Aizpurua, Carla S. Soares, Diego Delgado, Febe Antoinette Bruwer, Felix A. Pyatakovich, Inessa A. Minenko, Jonathan Kaj, Jon Mercader Ruiz, Juan Azofra, Luga Podesta, Mahmud Amin, Maider Beitia, Maria dos Anjos Pires, Mikel Sánchez, Mikhail Yu. Artamonov, Min Zhang, Moiz Khan, Nicolas Fiz, Nimisha Rawat, Pedro P. Carvalho, Pello Sánchez, Peter A. Everts, Praveen Arany, Ridham Varsani, Robert W. Alexander, Rodrigo Crespo Mosca, Rohan Rajaram, Sally Kiu-Huen Ng, Smitha Segu, Tyler W. LeBaron, Victoria Oliveira, Vita Boyar

First published in London, United Kingdom, 2024 by IntechOpen
IntechOpen is the global imprint of INTECHOPEN LIMITED, registered in England and Wales, registration number: 11086078, 167-169 Great Portland Street, London, W1W 5PF, United Kingdom

British Library Cataloguing-in-Publication Data
A catalogue record for this book is available from the British Library

Additional hard and PDF copies can be obtained from orders@intechopen.com

Pearls in Biological and Molecular Tissue Repair Pathways
Edited by Peter A. Everts and Robert W. Alexander
p. cm.
Print ISBN 978-0-85466-704-8
Online ISBN 978-0-85466-703-1
eBook (PDF) ISBN 978-0-85466-705-5

For EU product safety concerns:
IN TECH d.o.o., Prolaz Marije Krucifikse Kozulić 3, 51000 Rijeka, Croatia,
info@intechopen.com or visit our website at intechopen.com.

Meet the editors

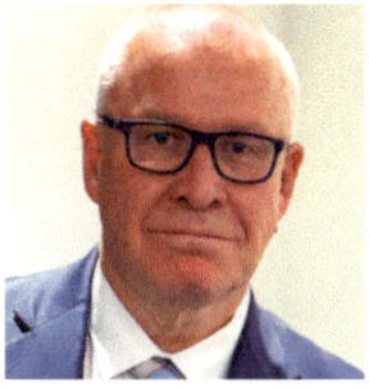

Prof. Dr. Peter A. Everts, Ph.D., FRSM, received his Ph.D. from the prestigious University of Utrecht, The Netherlands. He is an international professor at the Frontiers Health Program of the Faculty of Medicine and OrthoRegen International of the Max Planck University Center, and Medical School in Indaiatuba, São Paulo Brazil, and is the chief scientific officer for Gulf Coast Biologics, Fort Myers, Florida, USA, a nonprofit organization specializing in autologous biological education and research. Dr. Everts dedicated his career to many clinical regenerative applications, including chronic wound care treatments, and research in autologous biological preparations for tissue repair, regeneration, and wound healing. Dr. Everts is an international educator, lecturer, and scientist with over 100 published articles and book chapters, and his work has been cited more than 5,000 times. Dr. Everts is a reviewer for respected international journals and serves as a board member of several international organizations with a focus on autologous orthobiological and regenerative therapies.

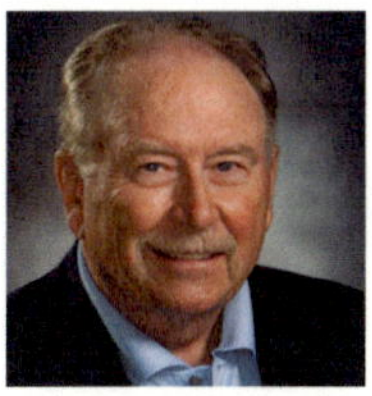

Prof. Dr. Robert W. Alexander, MD, FICS is a dual board-certified, internationally recognized aesthetic reconstructive surgeon, author, teacher, and pioneer in the use of stem/stromal cells in research and clinical practices. He is acknowledged for his leadership in the fields of cellular and biocellular regenerative medicine, with an emphasis on uses in aesthetic and musculoskeletal applications, wound healing, and systemic cellular therapies. He is recognized as one of the "Top 10 Innovators in the Field of Stem Cell Innovation" by the Academy of Regenerative Practices. Dr. Alexander graduated with advanced standing from the University of Florida School of Medicine and was inducted into the International College of Surgeons. He has numerous peer-reviewed publications and book contributions, in aesthetic journals, regenerative medicine, wound healing in trauma, pathology, and degenerative changes, with an emphasis on autologous biocellular therapies including nanofats and blood derivatives in wound healing and orthobiologics. Dr. Alexander is a recognized international lecturer.

Contents

Preface

The biological and biomolecular pathways that are involved in tissue repair, regeneration, and wound healing are fascinating. Tissue repair and regeneration of tissues are complex processes involving well-defined multicellular pathways that encompass the regulation of a variety of cells and molecules, including growth factors, proteins, mesenchymal cells, cytokines, chemokines, local resident cells, matrix components, and inflammatory cells. As pathophysiological aspects of damaged tissues, chronic wounds, and degenerative tissues become better understood, the interest in and clinical application of biological and molecular stimulatory technologies is growing rapidly.

Pearls in Biological and Molecular Tissue Repair Pathways is a book on tissue repair from a biological perspective. It presents the latest developments in autologous and non-autologous tissue repair treatments. A growing understanding of the pathophysiology of damaged tissues, chronic wounds, and degenerative tissues has led to the development of novel instruments and technologies to stimulate cell function so that tissue repair can ultimately be achieved.

An international group of authors has assembled this book to discuss the new frontiers and strategies for wound healing. There will be various chapters that will discuss the research and clinical application of a variety of biological preparations, as well as the tissue molecular effects following the use of medical devices to induce tissue repair. Additionally, some tissue reparative pathways are presented in reconstructive surgery, neonatal and pediatric wound management, and veterinary medicine.

This book begins with a chapter by Drs. Everts, Podesta, and Alexander entitled "A Comprehensive Guide of Cellular Blood-Derived and Mesenchymal Stem Cell-Based Autologous Biological Preparations for Tissue Repair, Regeneration, and Wound Healing". This first chapter provides a comprehensive and updated overview of currently available autologous biological preparations, such as platelet-rich plasma (PRP), bone marrow-derived mesenchymal stem cell products, adipose tissue stromal vascular fraction, and concentrated protein and fibrin matrixes. Additionally, these biological preparations are described both as stand-alone products and as combined preparations. Moreover, this chapter discusses the position that autologous preparations hold in the realm of healthcare treatment options compared to surgical procedures and medications.

The next chapter, "New Formulations of Platelet-Rich Plasma: The Relevance of Extraplatelet Molecules" by Mercader Ruiz et al., from the group of Dr. Mikel Sanchez, reviews some nontraditional preparation methods for platelet-rich plasma and describes the main components of platelets.

The authors place a particular emphasis on extra platelet biomolecules and growth factors, such as insulin-like growth factor and hepatocyte growth factor, as these growth factors are not found in platelet alpha granules but have important roles in tissue regeneration and can enhance some cellular modulatory effects of PRP.

In Chapter 3 of the book, "Regenerative Medicine in the Treatment of Traumatic Skin Wounds in Dogs and Cats Using Platelet-Rich Fibrin (PRF) Therapy", authored by Soares and coauthors, several hemoderivative platelet-derived products are discussed, such as platelet-rich fibrin (PRF). In this chapter, the authors describe the structural and biochemical characteristics of PRF and describe its use in the repair of veterinary wounds, as well as several clinical cases supported by photographic evidence.

In the following chapter, "Amniotic Membrane in the Treatment of Hard-to-Heal Wounds", Dr. Bruwer examines the utilization of amniotic membranes in chronic wounds. In this chapter, the author discusses the definition of chronic wounds, as well as the process of wound bed preparation, including debridement. Several wound care treatments are reviewed, with a particular emphasis on the use of amniotic membranes (AMs). An in-depth analysis of the structural and functional characteristics of various types of AM is presented, as well as their mechanisms of action. Furthermore, the application of non-autologous AMs is discussed in several patient cases.

"Molecular Hydrogen and Its Effect on Wound Healing and Tissue Regeneration", the book chapter by the group of Artamonov et al., explains how molecular hydrogen may be used as a therapeutic gas for patients with chronic, nonhealing wounds. This chapter reviews the various phases of the classical healing cascade and discusses the factors that contribute to wound healing impairment.

The authors elaborate on how molecular hydrogen is applied to chronic wounds and emphasize how radical scavenging mechanisms, the activation of antioxidant enzymes, and the anti-inflammatory effects of molecular oxygen have a positive effect on cell signaling and wound healing.

"Rationale for Discrete Light Treatment Approaches in Wound Care" by Varsani and associates is the next chapter in the book. In this chapter, they outline the fundamentals of laser therapy in patients with chronic wounds as well as the laser–biological tissue interactions of various photothermal, photodynamic, and photobiomodulation therapies for wound healing. The biological and molecular cellular significance of light treatments is discussed, such as immunomodulation and antimicrobial potential. A description of clinical applications of these unique light therapies is provided, for instance in patients suffering from oral wounds, burns, venous leg ulcers, and pressure ulcers.

Chapter 7, "The Evolving Role of Dermal Matrices in Reconstructive Surgery", authored by Rajaram et al., presents the use of biological, biosynthetic, and fully synthetic dermal matrixes as a viable and advanced technology in reconstructive surgical procedures.

In this comprehensive overview, the heterogeneity and diversity of dermal matrices, the multifaceted origins of matrices, biological consequences, and mechanisms of action are described in great detail. In this chapter, several patient case series are presented and illustrated, as well as several commercially available matrixes have been evaluated in an objective manner.

In the last chapter, titled "Innovative Biologic Dressings for Neonatal and Pediatric Wounds", produced by Dr. Vita Boyar, the challenges, complexities, and pathophysiology of wound conditions in neonates and pediatrics are discussed.

As part of the chapter, the author discusses common neonatal and pediatric wounds, the differences between neonatal and adult skin characteristics, their typical healing stages, and methods for managing wounds in a safe and effective manner, as well as the application of AM, umbilical cord dressings, collagen preparations, and xenograft technology using intact acellular fish skin grafts. The chapter illustrates several wound types treated with a variety of dressings and therapies in addition to describing typical characteristics of those treatments.

Summa Summarum

This book is an attempt to inform you about state-of-the-art developments in the growing field of tissue repair, regeneration, and wound healing.

Even though there are many publications and textbooks available to ensure that you are well informed, there continues to be an unmet need when it comes to new treatment options for treating wound/tissue healing issues, both in our youngest patients as well as in adults.

There is not a single therapeutic option or treatment strategy that will deliver a 100% success rate in the treatment of the many pathological tissue conditions. As a result, we must identify new technologies, continue our research efforts, and develop and search for multidisciplinary collaborations, the goal being to improve the quality of life of patients by providing effective and consistent functional tissue repair outcomes.

It is our sincere pleasure to thank all the authors who contributed to this book and congratulate them on all the excellent contributions they have made in sharing their perspectives with us. We hope that you will find this book to be a useful and valuable addition to your practice.

Some personal notes: It is with great pleasure that I acknowledge the support of my dear friend and coeditor, Dr. Robert Alexander. Bob, thank you very much for all the help, as always. It is a great pleasure to collaborate with you. Your vast experience and commitment to sharing your knowledge in an open and transparent manner are commendable.

I'm grateful for the support of the staff of IntechOpen to realize this informative textbook! As well, I would like to take this opportunity to thank Dr. Luga Podesta, my long-term friend and valued "tag-team colleague", for his support and contributions in this challenging field of innovative medicine, and I am thankful for the many close collaborations we had, and still have, over the years.

I wish to express my gratitude to my dear friend Dr. José Fabio Lana, with whom I also share many similar thoughts on how regenerative medicine can be advanced with adequate data, training, and education to improve patient care. He is one of the main driving forces behind OrthoRegen International at Max Planck University in Brazil.

Also, I would like to extend my gratitude to my good friend Professor André van Zundert, chair of anesthesia at the University of Queensland Australia, for believing in me so early on in my career (2004) that he convinced me to pursue a Ph.D. career in order to explore and research the possibilities of biological preparations in orthobiological and regenerative medicine applications.

Last but not least, a big thanks goes out to my wife Joan Everts-Koning for all the support she has given me during my career.

Dr. Peter A. Everts, Ph.D., FRSM
Professor,
Gulf Coast Biologics,
A Non-Profit Organization,
Fort Myers, FL, USA

Max-Planck University (UniMAX),
OrthoRegen International Course,
Indaiatuba, São Paulo, Brazil

Medical School,
Max-Planck University Center (UniMAX),
Indaiatuba, São Paulo, Brazil

Dr. Robert W. Alexander, MD, FICS
Professor,
School of Medicine and Dentistry,
Department of Surgery and Maxillofacial Surgery,
Seattle, WA, USA

Chapter 1

A Comprehensive Guide of Cellular Blood-Derived and Mesenchymal Stem Cell-Based Autologous Biological Preparations for Tissue Repair, Regeneration, and Wound Healing

Peter A. Everts, Luga Podesta and Robert W. Alexander

Abstract

The use of autologous biological preparations (ABPs) and their combinations fills a void in health care treatment options that exists between surgical procedures and current pharmaceutical treatments. *There is a wide range of ABPs that can safely and effectively be prepared at point of care using tissues from the patient such as peripheral blood, bone marrow, and adipose tissue to treat a wide range of clinical conditions.* The use of blood-derived and mesenchymal stem cell cellular preparations plays important roles in the modulation of tissue repair processes in complex biological settings. Biological products derived from autologous tissues are advantageous because of their autologous nature and their safety profiles. ABPs include platelet-rich plasma (PRP), bone marrow concentrates (BMCs), and adipose tissue complex (ATC) with its unique stromal vascular fractions (SVFs). In addition, ABPs can be combined to create biological preparations that are more diverse and possess a high degree of regenerative activity and potential. Likewise, concentrated acellular plasma proteins can generate a temporary fibrin matrix to interact with the bioactive molecules of various ABPs. Practitioners reason that the application of ABPs can mimic the classical healing and angiogenesis cascades to initiate tissue repair, regeneration, and wound healing during non-surgical interventions, aiming to restore the integrity and function of damaged tissues.

Keywords: autologous, biological preparations, tissue repair, tissue regeneration, wound healing, platelet-rich plasma, bone marrow aspirate concentrate, mesenchymal stem cell, adipose tissue stromal vascular fraction, protein rich platelet concentrate

IntechOpen

1. Introduction

Various pathological conditions, chronic recalcitrant wounds, damaged tissue structures, or degenerative tissues may cause wound healing and tissue repair to be highly complex and dynamic processes. These conditions dependent upon local and systemic multicellular biological processes including cell signaling [1–4]. The application of autologous biological preparations, prepared at point-of-care, hold the promise of promoting tissue healing, regeneration, and repair in a natural fashion [5]. Blood-derived and mesenchymal stem cell-based preparations play key roles in tissue repair mechanisms and the modulation of wound healing processes in complex biological microenvironments. Moreover, plasma and concentrated proteins in a provisional fibrin matrix can interact with bioactive molecules and cells and controlling the spatial-temporal distribution of these molecules and cells [6]. There is an unmet need in treatment options of degenerative and traumatized tissues, difficult-to-heal acute and chronic wounds. Regenerative medicine is an area of specialized, interventional, and non-surgical medicine, often not achievable via surgery of medications. In general, ABPs for therapeutic interventions are increasingly being utilized to support the healing of chronic wounds and the repair and regeneration of tissues by delivering allogeneic or autologously prepared biological cells.

The purpose of this chapter is to provide a comprehensive overview of the most widely used cellular autologous blood-derived, bone marrow-derived, and adipose-derived mesenchymal stem cell-based biological therapies, as well as some combinations of these therapies in tissue repair, regeneration, and wound healing treatment strategies.

2. Positioning ABPs

Traditionally, health care treatment options consist of a variety of surgical procedures and techniques and the use of medicinal treatment protocols and formulations. Alternatively, regenerative medicine therapies have been introduced, using biological treatment strategies to enhance healing and improve symptoms in many tissues in a large variety of medical conditions [7]. These non-surgical treatment options are referred to as interventional autologous biologically based procedures. In many instances, regenerative medicine procedures result in adequate patient outcomes that are often not achievable via surgeries or the use of medications, as shown in **Figure 1**.

ABPs can be safely derived from several freshly acquired biologically derived materials, originating from human blood, bone marrow, or adipose tissue, at point of care [8].

2.1 The biology of tissue repair, tissue regeneration, and wound healing using ABPs

ABPs are live cellular and stromal biomaterials that include a wide variety of platelet-rich plasma (PRP), bone marrow concentrate (BMC), and adipose tissue-derived tissue SVF (tSVF) bioformulations. The foremost advantages of autologous biological products (ABPs) are their autologous nature and their safety profile [9].

Within these specific ABPs, a diversity of bioformulations can be prepared to treat different tissue types and pathologies. An overview of the most cited cells, stroma, bioactive matrix and molecules that play significant roles in non-surgical

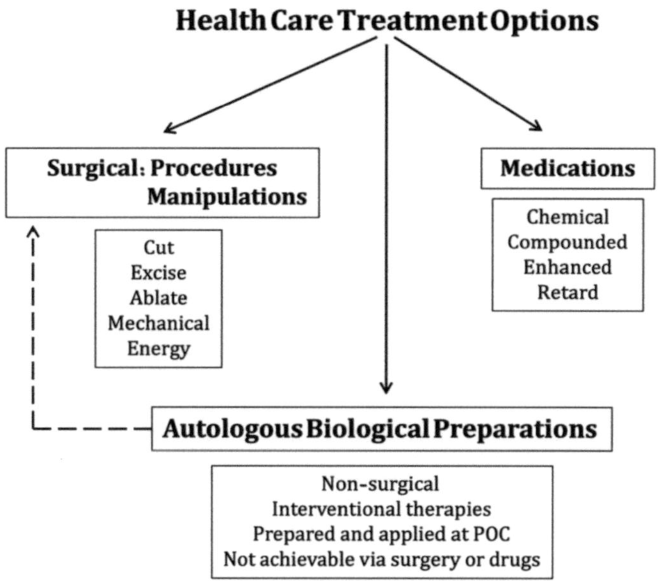

Figure 1.
Schematic representation of some characteristics and options of current health care treatment options, including the use of ABPs for tissue repair, regeneration, and wound healing as non-surgical interventions therapies. Additionally, ABPs are also used in combination with surgical procedures (Biosurgery) to achieve improved patient outcomes.

biological interventional procedures to induce cell-cell communication, cellular and molecular signaling in a treated pathological microenvironment has been published extensively by us [10]. Once precisely delivered, biologics will locally initiate and regulate biological mechanisms and pathways, to interact with the local niche resident cells that potentially lead to tissue repair, tissue regeneration, and wound healing. For these reasons, these multi-cellular heterogeneous cell concentrates have become a valuable biological instrument to treat non-surgically complex pathologies. Furthermore, these preparations are often used to enhance the results of bio-surgical procedures [2, 11].

2.2 The role of ABPs in tissue healing

Autologous biological technologies are designed to mimic the initiation of the classical and angiogenesis healing cascades in a wide-ranging field of medical applications [12]. Ultimately, tissue repair, tissue regeneration, and wound healing are complex biological processes aimed at restoring the integrity and function of damaged tissues. These processes follow well-defined cascades of events, with a magnitude of systemic and local cellular activities taking place in a sequential manner.

The traditional healing cascade can be categorized into distinct phases, each characterized by specific cellular activities. The initial phase involves hemostasis, which is achieved by the aggregation of platelets at the site of tissue injury, promoting blood clotting while forming a fibrinous network. Thereafter, platelets play a crucial role in regulating the healing process by secreting their granular content and releasing a magnitude of platelet growth factors (PGFs), cytokines, and molecules capable of initiating tissue repair [9, 13]. The lesser-known angiogenesis cascade adds an additional layer of complexity to the wound healing process. It may not have been studied as extensively as the traditional wound healing cascade, but it plays an imperative role in wound healing because it involves recruitment of endothelial cells, differentiation, proliferation, and ultimately formation of new blood vessels from preexisting ones (angiogenesis) [14].

3. Outlining ABPs

Many biological treatments options are available to treat various clinical maladies (**Figure 2**). The preparation of ABPs can be categorized into cellular preparations (such as tSVF, cSVF, or culture expanded cell groups), acellular preparations, or combinations of these methods. Cell-based preparations can be classified into two categories: preparations derived from peripheral whole blood and preparations derived from stromal vascular fraction elements, including mesenchymal, pericytes, endothelial, peri- and paravascular stem cells, originating from bone marrow or adipose tissue. Preparations derived from blood are available in various compositions and characterizations, such as PRP, platelet-rich fibrin (PRF), platelet lysates (PL), or as a combined PRP and plasma protein preparation [15, 16].

Bone marrow aspirate (BMA) and BMC are frequently cited as autologous MSC and progenitor cell preparations [17, 18]. Adipose tissue-based preparations can be defined as autologous ATC, concentrated ATC, tissue stromal vascular fraction (t-SVF), and cellular stromal vascular fraction (c-SVF) [19, 20].

Acellular preparations consist of (concentrated) plasma proteins and protein fibers, containing a combination of insoluble and soluble molecules. Protein-based technologies

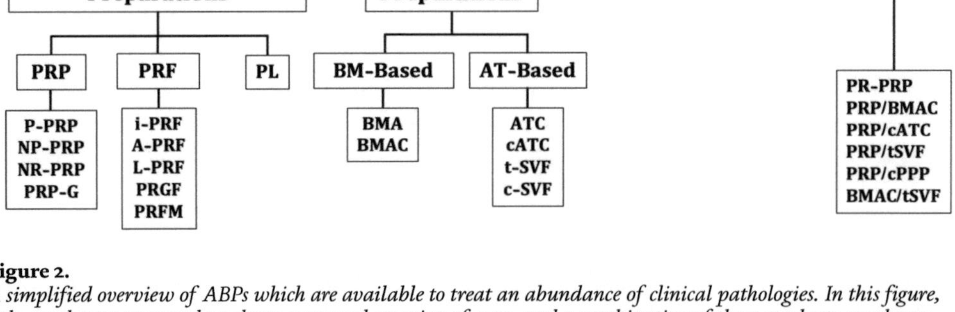

Figure 2.
A simplified overview of ABPs which are available to treat an abundance of clinical pathologies. In this figure, only autologous prepared products, prepared at point-of-care, and a combination of these products are shown. MSC: mesenchymal stem cell; PRP: platelet-rich plasma; PRF: platelet-rich fibrin; PL: platelet lysate; BM: bone marrow; AT: adipose tissue; P-PRP: pure PRP; NP-PRP: neutrophil-poor PRP; NR-PRP: neutrophil-rich PRP; PRP-G: PRP Gel; i-PRF: injectable platelet-rich fibrin; A-PRF: activated platelet-rich fibrin; L-PRF: leukocyte platelet-rich plasma; PRGF: platelets rich in growth factors; PRFM: platelet-rich fibrin matrix; BMA: bone marrow aspirate; BMAC: bone marrow aspirate concentrate; ATC: adipose tissue complex; cATC: compressed ATC; t-SVF: tissue stromal vascular fraction; c-SVF: cellular stromal vascular fraction; ACS: autologous conditioned serum; A2M: alpha-2-marcoglobulin; PPP-M: platelet-poor plasma matrix; PR-PPP: protein-rich platelet-poor plasma; PR-PRP: protein-rich platelet concentrate.

are a class of natural biomaterials that can be used either as standalone products (fibrin glue and sealant) or as scaffolds in combination with cellular-based products [21, 22].

3.1 Blood-derived biological preparations

Blood-derived platelet preparations are prepared from a unit of whole blood by centrifugation methods to facilitate gravitational cellular density separation [10]. The final prepared biomaterials are collectively termed autologous platelet concentrates.

The employment of autologous platelet concentrates has been of interest to clinicians and researchers for decades because of their potential to accelerate and support in numerous cellular activities that can lead to tissue repair, tissue regeneration, wound healing, and ultimately functional structural repair. However, contingent on the PRP device used, platelet preparations can contain varying platelet concentrations, as well as differences in bioformulations. It has been suggested the low-quality platelet concentrates, incorporating low platelet numbers and inconsistent other cellular content, are directly responsible for poor patient outcomes [23–27].

The differences in composition between PRP, plasma-based PRP preparations such as PRF, and blood plasma were described in a proteomic analysis [28]. A total of nearly 600 proteins were detected in human plasma, and an in-depth analysis revealed that PRP formulations contained significantly more proteins than both platelet poor plasma-based PRP products and whole blood plasma.

Although more positive than negative patient outcomes have been reported in the literature, no definitive and accepted standards have been realized for preparing PRP preparation methods and product classifications. A simplified categorization would be to divide platelet concentrates in PRP-buffy coat and plasma-based PRP technologies. The PRP technologies exploit higher patient whole blood volumes to prepare the final PRP products with higher platelet concentrations and preparation options in bioformulation.

Depending on the PRP device architecture, the flexibility to produce different bioformulations, and the employed centrifugation protocols, PRP device uses one spin or two spin centrifugation cycles [29]. Following the PRP manufacturer's instructions for use, and the practitioner's desired PRP bioformulation, PRP devices should be able to sequester a unit of freshly anticoagulated whole blood into a clear PPP fraction, a buffy coat stratum, and a red blood cell fraction, as illustrated in **Figure 3**. Indicatively, these PRP-based systems are capable of capturing platelets after processing that will increase the PRP platelet concentration between five to more than 12 times the baseline whole blood platelet concentration [30].

Alternatively, plasma-based devices utilize low patient blood volumes to a produce a low volume "PRP-like" product. These systems use mostly a single spin processing protocol designed to mainly isolate the PPP fraction from the whole blood, incorporating platelets that are present in this fraction. Their final platelet concentration ranges from 0.5 to 2.5 times the native platelet concentration [31].

As with PRP, plasma-based products can further be classified into leukocyte- and platelet-rich fibrin (L-PRF) and leukocyte-poor or pure platelet-rich fibrin (P-PRF) [32].

3.1.1 Buffy-coat-based PRP technology is rich in platelets

A variety of PRP bioformulations, terminologies, and product descriptions have been introduced to practitioners over the years [15, 31, 33]. As part of the healing and angiogenesis cascades, platelet biological components and mechanisms are crucial to tissue repair, regeneration, and wound healing [14]. In response to administered PRP

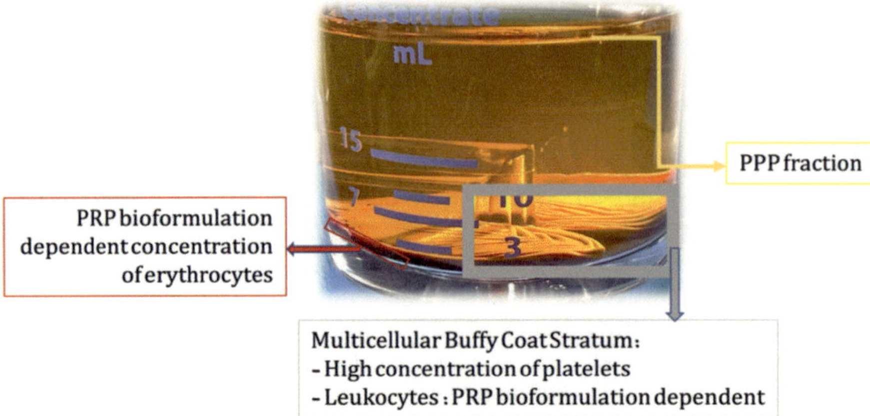

Figure 3.
An image of PRP preparation after the second centrifugation step. The concentrated platelets are present on the top of the buffy-coat stratum (device in picture is the PurePRP®SP, EmCyte Corporation®, Fort Myers FL, USA). PRP: platelet-rich plasma; PPP: platelet-poor plasma.

and the subsequent in situ tissue platelet activation, a number of regenerative and mitogenic components are released, which initiate cell differentiation, proliferation, and metabolic activity [34].

In the absence of consensus on standardization and classification of PRP devices and preparation methods to produce consistent effective PRP formulations, approximately 20 buffy coat PRP devices have been introduced to the market. These PRP devices can be categorized as pure PRP, leukocyte-poor PRP (LP-PRP), or leukocyte-rich PRP (LR-PRP) [35]. Considering the vast differences between the architecture of PRP devices, a great deal of variability has been reported on PRP platelet dosing and cellular characterization, which has led to poor and even negative patient outcomes [36].

As a best practice, different PRP formulations should be used at the same time in the same patient to treat multiple pathoanatomic conditions by using tissue-type-specific PRP formulations to optimize microenvironmental healing response and ultimately restore tissue structures that facilitate functional tissue repair [36], as portrayed in **Figure 4**. In particular, when treating chronic wounds, different PRP formulations should be utilized, based on the wound bed tissue appearances [5].

3.1.2 Plasma-based PRP technologies are poor in platelets

In plasma-based PRP procedures, a "PRP-like" suspension is prepared, excluding erythrocytes, and in most instances leukocytes [37]. In PRF plasma-based preparations, fibrin is the most important constituent of the final injectate [38]. This blood-derived plasma-based PRP product represents a plasma protein matrix which can contain processed platelets and eventual other cells that have cell stimulatory and immunological properties.

In more specific terms, this ABP consists of a fibrin-matrix compound containing platelets, with or without leukocytes, and other molecules [6, 39]. A notable aspect is that many plasma-based test-tube devices do not use anticoagulants when harvesting patient's blood prior to processing. It is anticipated that platelet activation will occur, leading to the release of clotting factors, including thrombin that will convert the PPP fibrinogen into a fibrin matrix after processing [40, 41], shown in **Figure 5**. It has

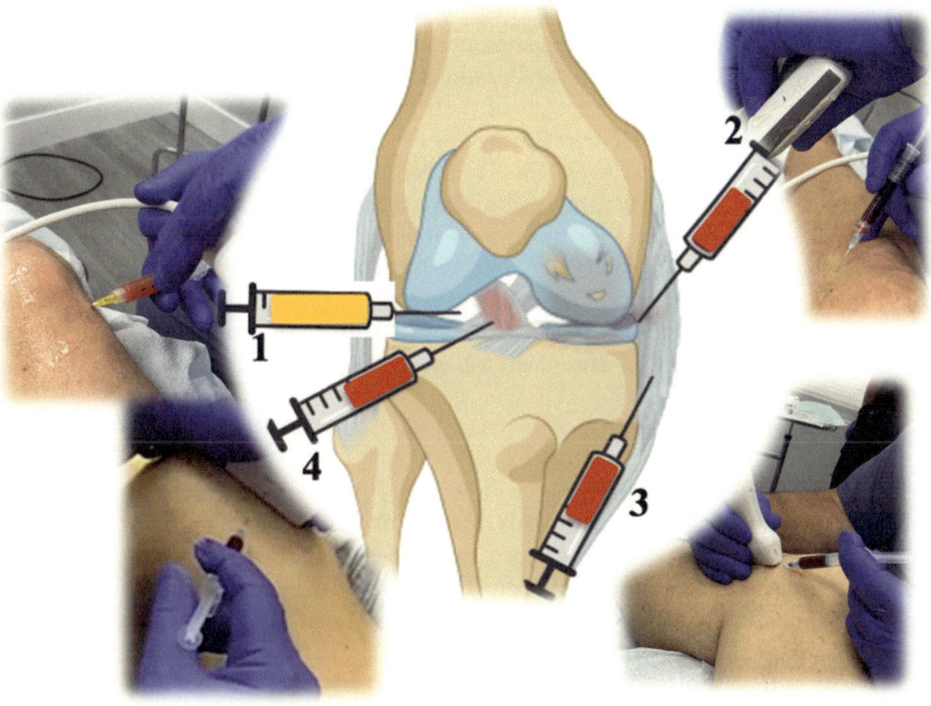

Figure 4.
A graphic illustration showing the administration of multiple different PRP formulations to treat various pathoanatomic tissue structures in the same patient, during the same session, to optimize total joint healing [36].

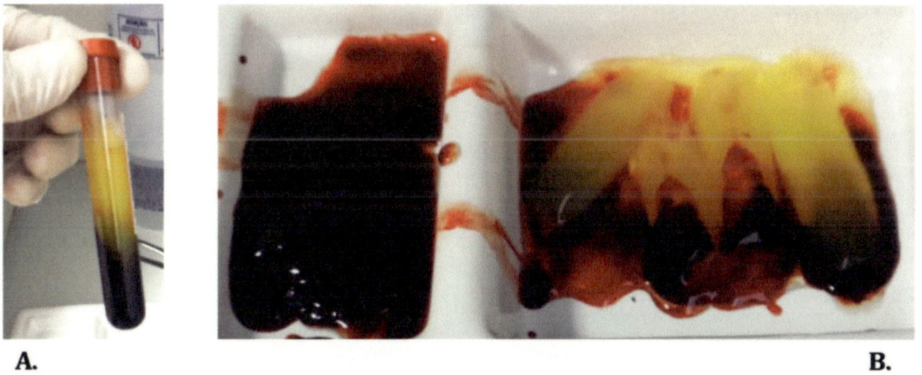

Figure 5.
Plasma-based test tube preparation (A). After a single centrifugation procedure, the whole blood (10 ml) is segmented and clotted. The clot is extracted from the test tube, and the erythrocyte fraction is separated from the clot, leaving a fibrin matrix for clinical application (B).

been demonstrated that fibrin polymerization, which is often induced by the addition of calcium chloride, results in a denser fibrin matrix when compared to non-activated PRP [42]. Thus, following therapeutic application, fibrinolysis of the cellular fibrin matrix will be initiated by plasminogen and plasmin, thereby liberating fibrin matrix components for a prolonged period of time compared to activated PRP clots which do not contain excessive amounts of plasma fibrin and other proteins [22].

In two major device comparison studies, Fadadu and Magalon evaluated many PRP devices, and they concluded that the platelet concentration was significantly lower in the low volume and single spin plasma-based PRP devices, when compared to buffy-coat PRP-based devices [31]. The results of these studies have been confirmed by others who have measured higher PGF concentrations following high preparation volume devices and double spin procedures [43]. Therefore, one might assume that the tissue repair, regeneration, and the wound healing capacities are less in plasma-based devices when compared to buffy-coat PRP systems. A striking observation is that some of the plasma-based platelet rich fibrin (PRF) devices have been presented with more than 20 different sub-formulations and preparation protocols by modifying the centrifugal force, the centrifuge speed, and the processing time [44]. **Table 1** summarizes the differences between buffy-coat-based PRP and plasma-based PRP technologies.

3.1.3 Platelet lysate preparations

Platelet lysates (PLs) are prepared following a PRP preparation procedure. As a result of freezing and thawing protocols, the membranes of PRP platelets are mechanically disrupted, allowing growth factors, cytokines, and other granular contents to be released. PLs are more than minimally manipulated ABPs, and they are a source of acellular, platelet-free, biologically active supernatants, which are rich in PGF and cytokines, as well as angiogenic factors. Additionally, as with PRP preparations, any

	Buffy coat-based PRP	**Plasma-based PRP**
Performance and technology features		
High volume preparation devices	++++	–
Double spin protocols	++++	+
Platelet capture rate %	++++	+
PRP volume range	++++	+
Platelet dosing strategies	++++	–
Flexibility in bioformulation	++++	–
Sustained release feature	++	++++
Cellular Features		
Platelet growth factor concentrations	++++	+
Immunomodulatory capacity	++++	+
Angiogenetic properties	++++	+
Nociceptive effects	++++	–
Collagen synthesis	++++	+
Fibroblast proliferation	++++	+
Leukocyte Control	+++	+
PRP to plasma protein ratio	+	++++

++++: *highly feasible;* ++: *feasible;* +: *potentially possible;* –: *not feasible.*

Table 1.
Differences illustrated between buffy coat-based PRP and plasma-based PRP technologies regarding general device performance characteristics and cellular features of both technologies.

concerns regarding immunogenicity can be dismissed as well [45]. The mechanisms of action of PL are poorly understood, but theoretically, there should be a similar mechanism of action between PL and PRP [46, 47]. Nonetheless, PGFs present in PLs have a short half-life, and they are reported to negatively affect endothelial cell proliferation as well as vascular tube formation in in vitro research [48].

The growth-promoting properties of PLs have been studied in multiple clinical indications, including wounds and soft tissue injuries, as early as the 1980s. A renewed interest in PLs has led to their use in specific musculoskeletal pathologies [49], in part due to their alleged anti-inflammatory properties [50]. Many advocates of PLs assert that their main advantage is that they can be stored in a freezer as well as that they are readily available for subsequent procedures or future applications [51].

Like PRP, there is neither consensus on the preparation of PL protocols nor is there a clear indication for its use, despite some reports citing PL applications in intra-articular procedures and tendinopathies, and in lumbar radiculopathies [50, 52].

4. MSC-based biological preparations

Adult MSCs are undifferentiated multipotent cells that are found in virtually all organs of the human body, and they are known for their self-renewal capacity. Easily accessible tissues to harvest MSCs include the red bone marrow and adipose tissue SVF [5]. In addition to their potential to promote immune modulation, angiogenic activity, anti-inflammatory activity, and anti-apoptotic activity, they also release numerous cytokines and growth factors that confer immunomodulatory, anti-apoptotic, and anti-inflammatory effects on many heterogeneous populations of cells [9]. Furthermore, MSCs have the ability to differentiate into various cells of mesodermal origin, including adipocytes, chondrocytes, myocytes, and osteoblasts, when exposed to specific signaling pathways [53].

Density centrifugation techniques are used to concentrate aspirated bone marrow and lipoaspirates to produce bone marrow aspirate concentrate (BMAC) and tSVF, respectively. Unfortunately, similar to PRP preparations, there is no consensus on classification, preparation standards including validation, and quality controls.

Adipose-derived MSCs (AD-MSCs) and BM-MSCs share many biological characteristics [54]. Several studies indicated that MSC transcriptome profiles from AD-MSCs and BM-MSCs showed the highest homology [55]. Although some differences in their immunophenotype, differentiation potential, proteome, and immunomodulatory activities have been reported [56]. Additionally, some clinicians have been reporting on using bone marrow aspirate (BMA) as an ABP, in particular in musculoskeletal pathologies [57].

4.1 Bone marrow aspirate: aspiration and direct injection

Cortical and trabecular bones, cartilage, and connective tissues comprise the bone. The bone marrow tissue, like the peripheral blood, is composed of soft spongy bone, fat-rich marrow, and sinusoidal arterial and venous blood vessels. Bone marrow is a life tissue as it is well recognized as an abundant and heterogeneous source of cells that reside in the trabecular part of long bones and are ultimately, continuously, released into the bloodstream [58].

Bone marrow aspirate (BMA) can be minimally invasive extracted from various anatomical sites using simple bone marrow harvesting needles or more sophisticated bone marrow aspiration systems. The posterior superior iliac spine (PSIS) and anterior superior iliac spine (ASIS) are frequently cited harvesting sites since these sites have the highest MSC concentration among other anatomical sites [59].

BMAs are ABPs with the intent to use an aspirate-collecting device only. In general, a single 10 ml syringe is used to extract bone marrow followed by direct administration of the harvested BMA to pathological treatment locations [57]. Using BMA only is intentionally done to avoid filtration techniques and BMA concentration processing steps, thus avoiding any methods to increase all native cell counts in the treatment specimen [60]. Only few articles have been published in the sports medicine and orthopedic literature regarding BMA applications [61]. Rarely, direct comparisons between BMA and BMAC have been executed and clinical benefits of BMA injections have not been clearly elucidated [60].

4.2 Bone marrow aspirate concentration: BM-MSC preparations

In contrast to BMA treatment vials, BMAC is prepared from a particular harvested volume of BMA, using gravitational density centrifugation processing steps, similar to PRP preparations [62].

BMAC contains concentrated bone marrow MSCs (BM-MSCs), hematopoietic stem cells (HSCs) as well as their multipotent progenitor cells (MPCs), platelets, leukocytes, and myeloid cells. Distinct differences between a BMA and a BMAC treatment specimen is that the latter has significantly more bone marrow cellular concentrations, and platelets when compared to BMA [60]. Importantly, the RBC content in BMAC is significantly lower due to the use of bone marrow tissue fragmentation as a result of centrifugation, decreasing the RBC concentration and thus avoiding all the negative effects related to the presence of native RBCs concentrations [63].

The cellular composition of BMAC is more complex and distinct when compared to PRP, as it contains BM-MSCs and HSCs, each with its own MPCs, which provide distinct reparative functions, other than concentrated PRP.

Prior to BMA harvesting, it is important to recognize that the bone marrow cavity is a well shielded cellular environment consisting of a particular structure and segmented in 4 main regions, niches, according to Lambertsen and Weis [64]. A bone marrow niche is a dynamic and complex environment, defined by its specific cellular content and molecular environment to regulate the function of stem cells and progenitors. Furthermore, the three-dimensional niches contain cells capable of intercellular communications and interactions with the extra cellular matrix (ECM). Cells present in bone marrow niches define stemness and regulate stem cell renewal and quiescence through cell signaling, proliferation, and differentiation [65]. In bone marrow niches, newly formed cells are retained until they mature and are then released into the peripheral circulation [66].

The vast majority of BM-MSCs are found within the endosteal and subendosteal regions of the bone marrow entity [67, 68]. Furthermore, BM-MSCs can be presented as pericytes in the perisinusoidal region [69]. As opposed to BM-MSCs, HSCs are located in the deeper bone marrow regions in the perivascular and perisinusoidal regions, and in the megakaryocyte niches. Most niche-specific processes are regulated by complex biochemical and mechanical signaling processes, followed by direct cell-to-cell interactions with platelet-derived chemokines, stem cell factors, and transforming growth factor [70].

BM-MSCs induce the production of cell-specific antigens, and their progenitors may differentiate into cells of the mesodermal lineage including osteoblasts, chondrocytes, tenocytes, endothelial cells, myocytes, fibroblasts, nerves, and adipocytes [71]. The differentiation of HSCs and progenitor cells into specialized blood cells plays a vital role in hemostasis, homeostatic mechanisms, and wound healing and angiogenesis in indirect ways [4]. Due to these reasons, BMAC has been regarded as an effective ABP to treat numerous clinical pathologies by altering local microenvironmental conditions through immunomodulatory activities, angiogenesis, and tissue repair.

4.3 Adipose tSVF based preparations

Adipose tissue preparations have been successfully used in minimally invasive reconstructive procedures and in guided injections into damaged, degenerative, or non-healing wounds. The rational to use tSVF is that it is a heterogeneous ABP, highly vascularized and stable connective tissue due to cell-to-cell or cell-to-matrix connections which are considered a pre-requisite for such stem cells to open the cellular send and receive signaling [72]. ATC, with its important bioactive scaffolding capabilities should therefore be recognized as a multifaceted microvascular organ, or better as an ATC, in the form of lipoaspirates, consisting of various cellular tissue components, including AD-MSCs [73], Furthermore, concentrated and compressed tSVF provides a physiological multicellular scaffold containing AD-MSCs along with other stromal vascular cells [19]. Minimally invasive access techniques are employed to harvest from several subcutaneous fat deposits, including the abdomen, perigluteal, thigh, and flank areas. During the procedure, a subcutaneous injection of a dilute local anesthetic solution (tumescent) is administered to numb the area of adipose harvesting and facilitate the creation of a tSVF suspension [74]. After a brief waiting period, a blunt-tipped atraumatic aspiration cannula is introduced through a small puncture or incision in the skin and attached to a syringe for manually controlled, low negative pressure, lipoaspiration [75]. A correctly performed lipoaspiration procedure preserves the neurovascular structures at the donor site with a minimal level of discomfort for the patient [76]. Furthermore, the cell yield and viability of AD-MSCs should not be affected by liposuction techniques [77, 78].

Harvested tSVF can be transferred to a syringe or adipose processing device and centrifugated. Centrifugation methods have proven to be an effective means to safely wash, rinse, eliminate the infranatant-extracellular fluid, separate free lipids, and residual oil, to prepare a clean, compressed tSVF specimen [79], as illustrated in **Figure 6**.

Following lipoaspirate centrifugation, isolation of tSVF-based preparations can be accessed, consisting of cellular and matrix components derived from adipose tissue and are used in advanced regenerative medicine procedures. The SVF is a complex mixture of various cell types including endothelial cells, immune cells, fibroblasts, and a significant population of AD-MSCs. These cells are embedded in a network of collagen fibers and other extracellular matrix components, which together contribute to the regenerative properties of the SVF.

Prior to regenerative applications, various SVF preparation protocols are obtainable to prepare either fully emulsified nanofat in small aggregates (tSVF) or cSVF [80]. cSVF preparation methods are based on enzymatic digestion techniques using collagenase [81]. tSVF preparations are created by mechanical emulsification, reducing the size of macrofat to either partially or fully emulsified aggregates, known as micronized fat or nanofat (**Figure** 7) [80]. Importantly, the fully emulsified, sized tSVF aggregates present an intact microenvironment, whereby the fully emulsified

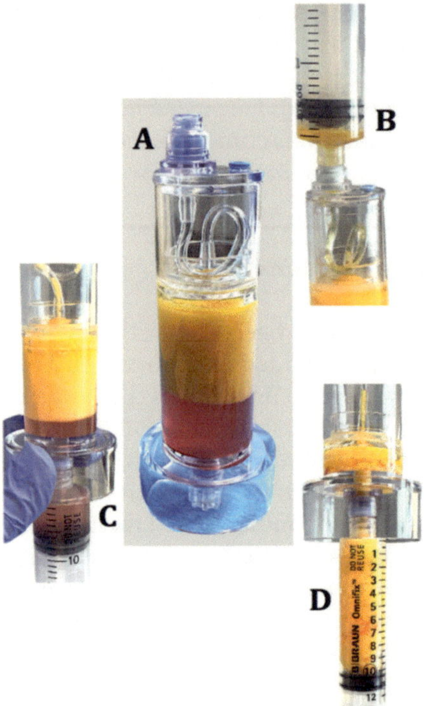

Figure 6.
An illustration following adipose tissue centrifugation to access tSVF (A). After centrifugation, first the residual oil (B) and then the infranatant solution (C) are removed, thereafter the tSVF is extracted (D). (Device shown in the picture is the Progenikine® Adipose Concentration System EmCyte Corporation®, Fort Myers FL, USA).

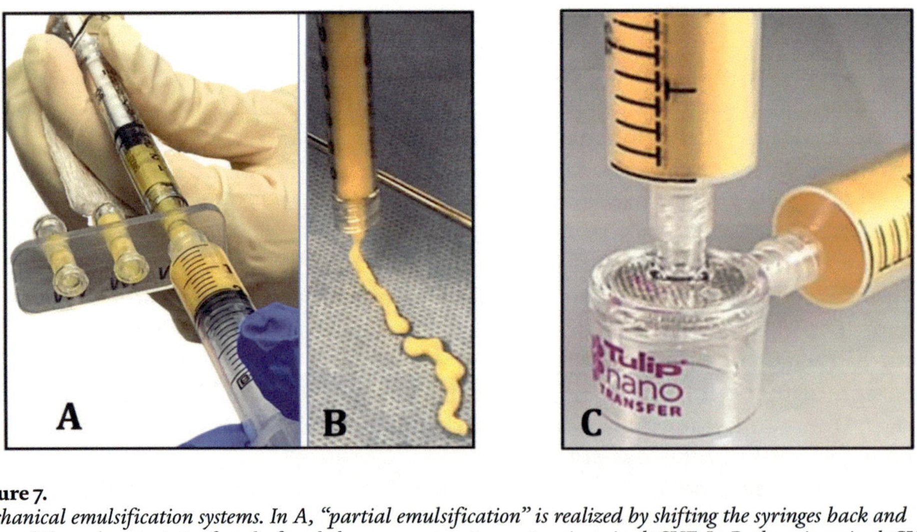

Figure 7.
Mechanical emulsification systems. In A, "partial emulsification" is realized by shifting the syringes back and forward through restraining female-female luer connectors to create micronized tSVF. In B, the micronized tSVF is ready for application. In C, adipose tissue is pushed through a 600/400micron screen, creating nanofat tSVF (devices shown are in A the Adicen™, a three phase micro-fragmentation accessory with 2.4, 1.4, and 1.2 mm emulsification sizes, EmCyte Corporation®, Fort Myers FL, USA. In C, the disposable Nanofat™ device is displayed, Tulip® Medical, San Diego CA, USA).

small nanofat aggregates essentially are devoid of adult adipocytes. Generally, nanofat tSVF preparations are considered the most potent valuable form of tSVF for regenerative and wound healing purposes.

4.3.1 Multicellular SVF components

The presence of SVF-based cells can be tested by enzymatic means and measured by advanced laboratory flow cytometry techniques. The typical, heterogenous cell distribution and the cellular ranges in SVF are shown in **Table 2** [82].

AD-MSCs are the most prominent stem cells in tSVF. They have the capability to differentiate into various cell types, including osteoblasts, adipocytes, chondrocytes tenocytes, and myocytes. Many researchers and clinicians believe that pericyte stem cells (PSC) are ubiquitous cells, representing the original "stem" cell originator [83] and are fully capable of all the functions of the MSCs. PSCs are located on the walls of capillaries, the perivascular/paravascular locations, and work intimately with the endothelial and intra-adventitial cells. Furthermore, PCS stabilize blood vessels and have the potential to differentiate into other cell types, contributing to tissue regeneration and repair. Endothelial cells can line blood vessels and play key roles in forming new blood vessels through angiogenesis. Immune cells, originating from hematopoietic cell linages (e.g., monocytes, lymphocytes, and various macrophage phenotypes) are involved in modulating the immune response. Lastly, fibroblasts are present in SVF and they are recognized for producing collagen and an extracellular matrix, providing structural support to tissues and they hold crucial roles in wound closure and the strength of the healed tissues [84].

Freshly prepared SVF can be directly administered to the patient without the need for cell expansion techniques or additional cell separation preparations. Unlike cSVF, emulsified tSVF is not solely a 100% cellular product, as it contains both cellular fragments and important native adipose structural ECM components) [80, 85, 86]. Following tSVF preparation, the product is ready for injection. An advantage of tSVF compared to cSVF is that it offers the ability to provide a bioactive cellular tissue

Stromal Cells:	15–30%	AD-MSC
		Pre-adipocytes
		Fibroblast
Stem cell and progenitors	< 0.1%	
Hematopoietic cell linages:		Platelets
		Erythrocyte
		Lymphocyte
		Neutrophil
		Monocyte – macrophage
Pericytes	3–5%	
Endothelial cells	10–20%	

Table 2.
Overview of identified multicellular components in SVF.

matrix that can be delivered to pathoanatomic treatment sites. In fact, following tSVF application, stromal supportive cells in their microenvironment are being transferred to recipient sites where these stromal elements start cell-cell communication and cell signaling [87].

4.3.2 The role of tSVF in wound healing, repair, and regenerative therapies

The application of tSVF in wound healing and regenerative therapies are based on its rich content of regenerative cells and factors. tSVF cells are capable of differentiation, cell-to-cell communication (paracrine, sending/receiving when attached, and may secrete ECM, and provide key elements in the response to damaged or degenerative cells [73]. tSVF aids in the promotion of angiogenesis as endothelial cells and growth factors promote the formation of new blood vessels, enhancing oxygen and nutrient supply to the wound or damaged tissue, thereby supporting healing [88]. Immune cells and anti-inflammatory cytokines present in tSVF support in modulating the body's immune response to reduce chronic inflammation while promoting a more conducive environment for tissue repair. Following tSVF preparation, the AD-MSCs can self-replicate and they are capable of differentiating into various cell types, secrete growth factors, help with creation of biologically active ECM, and may provide mesodermal, ectodermal, neuroectodermal cells that contribute and stimulate tissue regeneration [89]. This is particularly valuable in tissue repair and regeneration. Finally, fibroblasts contribute to the synthesis of collagen and other extracellular matrix components, essential for the structural integrity and function of repaired tissues [90].

5. Combined ABPs

PRP, BMAC, and tSVF are ABPs that contribute to immunomodulation, painkilling, wound healing, and functional tissue restoration with different intensities and distinctly different pathways.

Many studies have reported on the beneficial effects of PRP and MSC-based preparations for the treatment of acute cutaneous and chronic wounds, degenerative tissues, and burns [91, 92]. Some of the therapeutic effects of PRP are recognized by the release of the platelet granular content, following in-situ platelet activation [10]. Platelet have been found, among other activities, to stimulate fibroblast proliferation and differentiation and incite endothelial cellular pathways regarding angiogenesis and ECM secretion to regulate tissue inflammation [93]. In addition, following platelet activation, the PRP fibrin network provides an autologous cellular scaffold [6].

Individually, BM-MSCs and AD-MSCs have demonstrated their cellular differentiation potential and immunomodulatory effects. Not many studies have addressed the combination of both MSCs, but they are routinely being performed in regenerative medicine center. Wardner et al. concluded that the proliferation of peripheral blood mononuclear cells was more suppressed by AD-MSCs, however, combining them with BM-MSCs resulted in highly efficient immunomodulation, with significant responder cell suppression in a dose dependent manner, possibly reducing the inflammatory effects when BMAC is used as a stand-alone product [94].

The delivery of MSCs exert tissue repair effects primarily through the release of a wide range of soluble factors, growth factors, cytokines, and exosomes capable of proangiogenic and anti-inflammatory performances [95–97]. In contrast to PRP, both BM-MSCs and AD-MSCs can modify their cellular secretome according to the local microenvironment in which they have been injected or applied and maintain cell-signaling to neighboring cells for several days [98].

Based on the typical PRP, MSC, and plasma protein characteristics, it was suggested that potentially positive synergistically effects may occur if PRP is combined with BM and AD-MSC preparations. Additionally, PRP effects might be extended over a longer period of time when mixed with plasma protein concentrates and consolidated as one ABP [99].

5.1 Protein rich-platelet rich plasma (PR-PRP): concentrated platelet poor plasma mixed with PRP

PRP buffy-coat preparations are created by gravitational density separation that sequesters a unit of blood into three main fractions: a PPP fraction, a buffy coat stratum rich in platelets, and a RBC fraction. Normally, as part of the PRP preparation process, the PPP fraction is discarded after the platelet concentrate has been extracted from the PRP device.

One of the less well known, but equally important features of PPP is the presence of exosomes and other macrovesicles [100, 101]. They are considered to be important in cell-cell communication and cell signaling. Furthermore, some GF are not present in the platelet alpha granules, but instead, they reside in higher concentrations in the PPP fraction, outside of platelets. In particular insulin-like growth factor-1 (IGF-1) and hepatocyte growth factor (HGF).

In addition to their roles as angiogenesis activators, these plasma-based GFs are also known to promote keratinocyte migration and wound healing. Interestingly, Beitia et al. found a significant correlation between IGF-1 concentrations and cell proliferation [102]. Moreover, it has been shown that both IGF-1 and HGF can inhibit inflammation and fibrosis.

Technology advancements in ABPs have led to the development of more advanced biological processing methods and devices. By using new ultrafiltration technologies, it is possible to concentrate PPP, at point-of-care, in a fast and efficient manner producing a viable and viscous protein concentrate [103].

Microfiltration and ultrafiltration devices are made of high-performance medical grade polymers and offer an excellent biocompatibility and present a consistent performance eliminating plasma water. They have been used widely as blood-plasma contact devices in blood apheresis for decades [104]. Later, modified ultrafiltration techniques were successfully developed to alleviate systemic inflammatory responses caused by cytokines [105].

Currently, ultrafiltration techniques can incorporate PPP processing methods. The PPP fluid fraction is manually transported by syringes, exerting a positive transmembrane pressure, through the microporous membranes of the ultrafiltration device fibers. Once the PPP volume has frequently passed the ultrafiltration device, plasma water, cytokines, molecules, and plasma proteins with a molecular mass (weight), less than the pore size of the fibers, are all filtered out of the ultrafiltration device. This waste solution is collected in an effluent syringe, as demonstrated in **Figure 8**.

Reducing the PPP water component will result in a significant increase in the concentration of, functional, total proteins, like fibrinogen, albumen, and alpha-2-macroglobulin. Moreover, plasma levels of IGF-1 and HGF are also significantly higher after ultrafiltration when compared to their levels in the native PPP fraction before

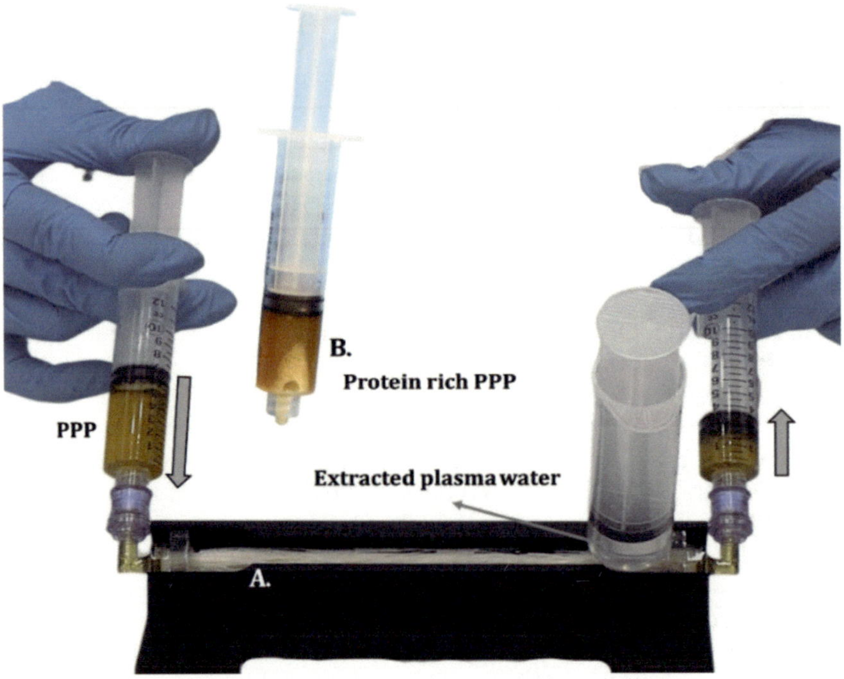

Figure 8.
The platelet-poor plasma (PPP) syringes are manually "pushed" through the ultrafiltration device (A). Plasma water, small proteins, and cytokines are eliminated through the filter membrane pores and captured in the effluent syringe. After a series of passes, the PPP volume is significantly reduced to a high viscous protein rich PPP volume, as shown in B. Note the clear visual difference between the unprocessed PPP and the final viscous protein rich PPP (the ultrafiltration device presented is the CORE™ Ultrafiltration System, developed by EmCyte Corporation®, Fort Myers FL, USA).

the filtration process [106]. Effectively, larger non-concentrated PPP volumes will be reduced to low volume protein rich PPP, up to 10-fold reductions can be achieved.

Recently, EmCyte Corporation® has introduced the concept of CORE™ protein rich platelet concentrate formulation. This consolidated ABP, combining a high concentration of PRP platelets with a high concentration of plasma proteins (**Figure 9**), has distinctive scaffolding features, protease inhibitor, and regenerative capabilities when compared with other similar ABPs on the market.

The creation and ultimate delivery of PR-PRP in tissue repair, regeneration, and wound healing procedures can be considered as a novel and powerful therapeutic.

Depending on the bioformulation of the prepared PRP, the PR-PRP scaffold retains and facilitates interactions between a variety of concentrated heterogeneous PRP components and molecules: activated and non-activated platelets, PGFs, dense platelet granular elements, plasma-based IGF and HGF, cytokines, plasma proteins, exosomes, and eventually leukocytes [107], as presented in **Figure 10**.

The use of PR-PRP preparations in non-surgical interventional procedures in musculoskeletal pathologies includes, among others, intra-articular injections in patients with OA, and patients with partial of full-thickness tendon tears. In OA, the PR-PRP specific protein alpha-2-macroglobulin (A2M), a macro protein molecule known to function as a broad-spectrum protease inhibitor, traps active joint proteases into the A2M typical molecular cage and subsequently eliminates them from the joint space [108]. In patients with partial or full thickness tendon and ligament tears,

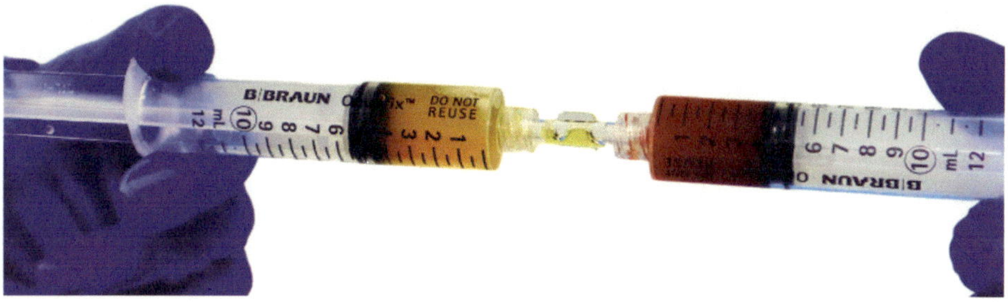

Figure 9.
PR-PRP preparation. A low volume of protein rich PPP (left syringe) is cautiously mixed with the same volume of highly concentrated PRP (right syringe) creating PR-PRP, at a ratio of 1:1. Before application, the consolidated volume is gently agitated to produce a uniform ABP treatment specimen. Abbreviations: PRP: platelet-rich plasma; PPP: platelet-poor plasma; PR-PRP: protein-rich platelet concentrate; ABP: autologous biological preparation.

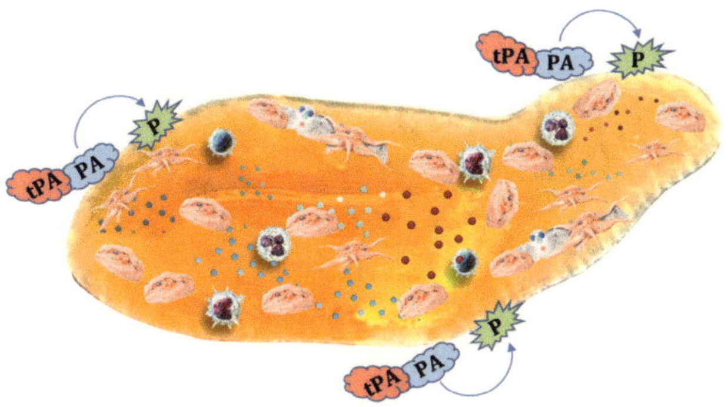

Figure 10.
A graphic illustration of a PR-PRP scaffold with the retained platelets, and leukocytes. Interactions between tissue plasminogen (tPA) and plasminogen (PA) binding to the scaffold with the subsequent production of plasmin (P) to accomplish fibrinolysis, leading to fibrinolysis with the release of the retained PR-PRP elements. Abbreviations: tPA: tissue plasminogen; PA: plasminogen; P: plasmin.

the PR-PRP proteins fibrinogen and albumen function as a biological active tissue scaffold, capable of filling tissue voids [109, 110]. Additionally, the scaffold facilitates a sustained platelet release of PGFs, cytokines, molecules, and eventual leukocytes, stimulating the local environment for a longer period to regulate inflammation, immunomodulation, and extend the tissue repair processes.

In chronic wound care management, autologously prepared PR-PRP grafts have been used as biological wound dressings [5, 111]. The wound healing process is meticulously controlled by various cytokines and growth factors that are secreted to the wound area [112], with platelets holding pivotal roles in wound healing by platelet plug formation, PGF release and the initiation of the angiogenesis cascade [14]. Platelets in PR-PRP matrix serve as vital scaffolds where platelets release PGF, cytokines, molecules, and other granular content that facilitate wound closure by acting as chemotactic cues to inflammatory cells and stimulate angiogenesis. In the protein matrix, the presence of thrombin facilitates platelet degranulation with the subsequent release of platelet content. Furthermore, concentrated plasma proteins such as thrombospondin, vitronectin, and fibronectin are important in cell adhesion and cell migration in the wound healing cascade [113]. Ultimately, these processes can result in wound re-epithelialization and wound contractions of connective tissue.

PR-PRP can either be injected in wound tissue structures, or it can be prepared and activated in a petri-dish and applied as a biological wound dressing to open chronic wounds, as demonstrated in **Figure 11** [114].

PR-PRP spray applications can be effectively used during surgical interventions, referred to as biosurgery, to support in post-operative wound healing (**Figure 12**). Specifically, the combination of PRP characteristics with protein rich fibrin scaffolding in a variety of biosurgical procedures, are effective in reducing dehiscent wounds, lowering infection rates, reducing scarring, as well as reducing seromata formation, thus improving overall patient outcomes [2, 3, 115–118].

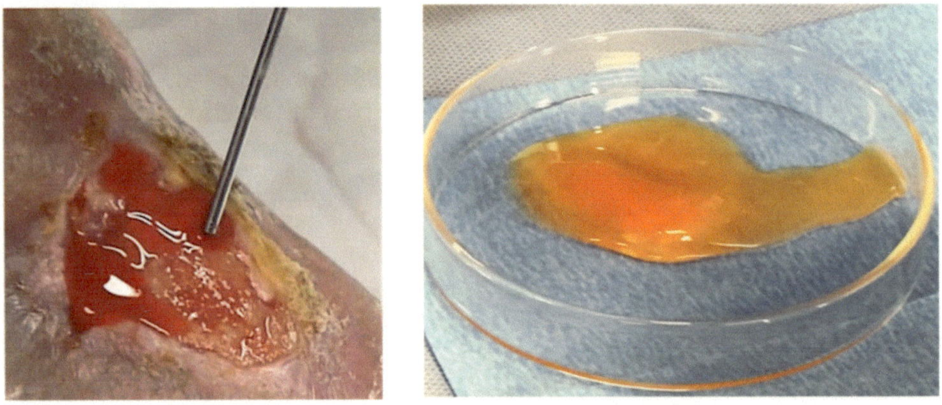

A **B**

Figure 11.
Different PR-PRP application modalities can be prepared to treat, open, chronic wounds. In A, a leukocyte-rich PR-PRP is administered as a topical and liquid ABP to a chronic leg ulcer. In B, a leukocyte-poor PR-PRP is prepared in a petri-dish as a solid biological graft which can be applied to chronic wounds as an autologous biological wound dressing.

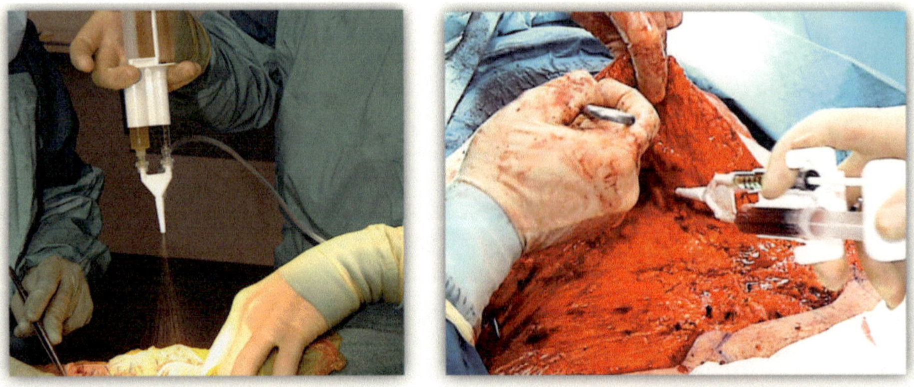

A. PRPC containing LP-PRP **B. PRPC containing LR-PRP**

Figure 12.
An illustration of PR-PRP applications in orthopedic (A) (total knee replacement) and plastic reconstructive (B) (lower body lift) biosurgical procedures. A dual syringe spray applicator is used to deliver the combined PR-PRP preparation and mix it with thrombin to support in post-surgical wound healing. Both, leukocyte-rich and leukocyte-poor PRP formulations can be combined with the protein concentrate. Abbreviations: PR-PRP: protein rich platelet concentrate; LP-PRP: leukocyte-poor platelet-rich plasma; LR-PRP: leukocyte-rich platelet-rich plasma.

After the PR-PRP scaffold has been delivered to tissue sites, the protein scaffold will start to breakdown due to the interaction of tissue plasminogen (tPA) with the inactive enzyme plasminogen (PA). Subsequently, PA will bind to the PR-PRP and will release the catalytically active nonspecific protease plasmin [119]. The proteolytic plasmin initiates plasma hydrolysis of cross-linked fibrin polymers within the scaffold [120]. In response, the PR-PRP scaffold will undergo a fibrinolytic breakdown (fibrinolysis), thereby releasing the cells that have been retained in the PR-PRP scaffold. A sustained release of concentrated cells and molecules in the PR-PRP scaffold over a longer period will transpire until the entire scaffold has been dissolved following fibrinolysis.

Future studies have to elucidate that this biologically created, sustained release-based, microenvironment holds an important role in tissue regeneration, immunomodulation, and ultimately functional tissue repair.

5.2 PRP and BMAC combined

Several studies have been indicating positive effects of combining PRP and BMAC as one consolidated ABP [121–124], although cellular and cytokine characterization revealed overlapping data [125]. While interleukin-1 receptor antagonist (IL-1RA), a potent natural anti-inflammatory cytokine, was significantly increased in BMAC when compared to PRP [126]. Combining PRP and BMAC may create a more biologically active graft, projected to optimize tissue repair, regeneration, and wound healing treatment outcomes as concentrated MSCs and HSCs are added to the PRP cellular components, including significantly more anti-inflammatory activity due to higher concentrations of IL-1RA (**Figure 13**). An analysis concluded that PRP stimulates BM-MSC proliferation and preserves MSC multipotency, as the interactions between PRP and MSCs did not affect multilineage cell differentiation [99]. Additionally, PRP had a positive effect on MSC senescent activities. In an in vivo ACL study, the combined stimulatory effects of PRP and MSCs demonstrated improved MSC proliferation, cellular growth, and ligament integrity [127].

According to a review, citing 57 articles, studies using PRP showed a reduction in the time necessary to double the number of BM-MSCs [99]. A further study showed

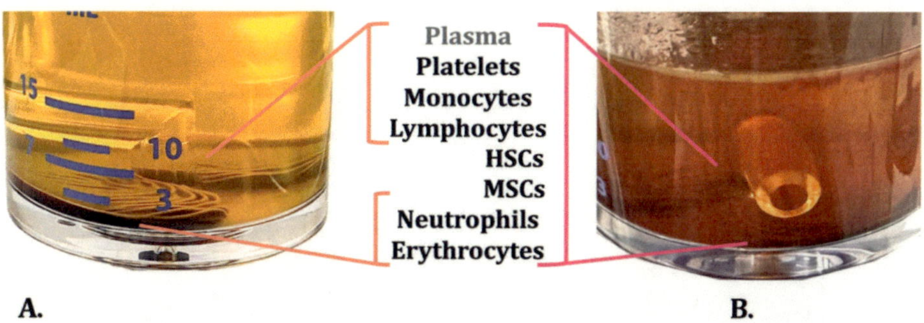

Figure 13.
A graphical comparison between leukocyte-rich PRP (LR-PRP) (A) and BMAC (B) cell distributions. When consolidating LR-PRP with BMAC, this ABP is characterized by high concentrations of platelets, BM-MSCs, and BM-HSCs. Noteworthy, the plasma color of the BMAC preparation is more orange than the yellow appearance of the LR-PRP preparation. This typical colorization aspect of a BMAC preparation is related to the higher shear forces employed when extracting bone marrow to liberate the BM-MSCs from their specific niches. Abbreviations: PRP: platelet-rich plasma; HSCs: hematopoietic stem cells; BM-MSCs: bone marrow mesenchymal stem cells; BMAC: bone marrow aspirate concentrate.

that MSCs cultured with PRP instead of fetal bovine serum altered the secretion of cytokines by T lymphocytes, B cells, and natural killer cells, demonstrating significant anti-inflammatory activities. In an animal study, the combination of PRP and BM-MSCs demonstrated an increase in the maturation of trabecular bone along with an increase in collagen type II expression and differentiation to chondrogenesis [128].

Improved VAS and functional scores were observed following combined PRP-BMAC injections in patients with partial rotator cuff tears, when compared to control patients [124]. It was thought that the PRP-BMAC consolidated biologic was responsible for the associated pain killing effects by downregulating various inflammatory mediators [127, 129].

PRP-BMAC complexes have revealed that PGFs and other platelet cytokines are influential in the BMAC reparative initiated processes as they stimulate multiple paracrine BM-MSC trophic effects, including endogenous tissue repair, while decreasing cell apoptosis expressing and releasing higher concentrations of therapeutic affecters [124, 125]. Additionally, a decrease in cell apoptosis and inflammation has been reported. Besides, combining PRP and concentrated BM-MSCs with a demineralized bone matrix (DBM) guaranteed the consistent release of high PGFs over time in an in-vitro model [130]. It was postulated that the clinical application of a PRP-BMAC graft in a bone matrix will allow for better healing in compromised tendons [98]. In another study, the response of BM-MSCs was measured in healthy human tendons, DBM, and a fibrin scaffold. MSC stromal cell adhesion, proliferation and differentiation assays indicated differences in cellular activity among the three different scaffolds. However, when PRP was added to the BM-MSCs, enhanced cellular function was observed in all three scaffolds, indicating significant synergistic effects by the combined PRP-BMAC biological preparation [131].

5.3 PRP and tSVF combined

The effectiveness of PRP and SVF modalities as biological treatment options for a variety of pathological conditions has been studied in numerous clinical trials.

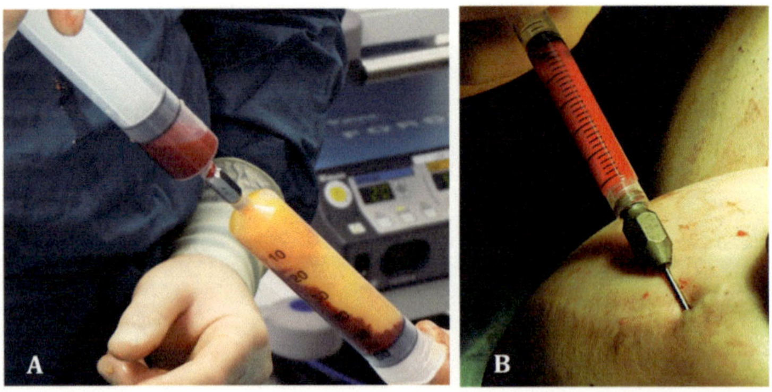

Figure 14.
In A, LR-PRP is mixed with processed tSVF to create a compounded ABP. In A, the less dense adipose tissue is mixed with the denser PRP, insinuating that proper agitation is required to create homogenously mixed graft prior to application [132]. Ideally, multiples smaller application syringes (B) are prepared after mixing both the PRP and compressed tSVF volumes to ensure proper distribution of the PRP-cATC graft, targeting for significant synergistic therapeutic effects. Abbreviations: LR-PRP: leukocyte-rich platelet rich plasma; cATC: compressed adipose tissue complex.

Recently, compounding PRP and tSVF as a combined ABP (**Figure 14**) have been used by practitioners in mainly esthetic and plastic reconstructive surgical procedures, and to treat patients with non-healing chronic wounds. The rationale behind this combination is to increase the survival rate of fat grafts, to decrease inflammation, and ultimately improve long term fat grafting outcomes [133, 134].

PRP combined with AD-MSCs was shown to significantly stimulate tissue vascularization in wounds as compared to PRP or AD-MSCs alone [135]. Similar findings were reported by others [136, 137]. According to their findings, PRP stimulates the angiogenic potential of AD-MSCs by activating the MSC secretome directly, which results in a stimulation of the VEGF and SDF-1 synthesis, thereby improving blood vessel formation and endothelial cell migration. Others observed a synergistic effect between tSVF and the PRP induced fibrin matrix, with regard to the secretion of high VEGF concentrations [138]. Another important finding was that PRP promoted the proliferation of AD-MSCs via various pathways [139]. Furthermore, van Dongen et al. concluded that the combination of PRP growth factors and the mechanically dissociated, emulsified ATC (tSVF) are proficient in parenchymal cell proliferation, and immunomodulation [140].

Intriguingly, PRP combined with AD-MSCs increased mitochondrial respiration and oxygen consumption, resulting in an increase in ATP production. The addition of PRP to AD-MSCs increased the AD-MSC metabolism and fat graft vascularization, ultimately resulting in improved fat graft survival and stimulation of the recipient tissue site [134]. Importantly, when PRP was mixed with adipose grafts, a reduction in inflammatory reactions, as well as a reduction in fat necrosis percentage was observed [141–143]. Synergistic cellular and GF specific effects, after mixing PRP with an adipose tissue graft, are presented in **Table 3**.

It is important to note that after mixing lipoaspirate formulations with PRP, a PRP-tSVF-fibrin scaffold will develop as a combined product. This scaffold serves as a cellular matrix and retains adipocytes, AD-MSCs, PGFs, cytokines, and other proteins for an extended period of time, serving as a sustained, extended-release medication [148]. In addition, it has been shown that the PRP-tSVF-fibrin scaffold inhibits apoptosis of adipocytes [149].

Despite some initial positive reports in chronic wound healing models [147], additional clinical research is needed to develop more synergistic formulations of

	Vascularization	Proliferation Osteoblasts	Proliferation Fibroblasts	ECM Synthesis	Chemotaxis
PDGF	*	++	++	++	+/−
TGF	*	+/−	+/−	++	+
VEGF	++	*	—	+	—
CTGF	++	+/−	++	+	—
IGF	—	++	+	++	++
Fibrin	++	—	—	++	—

**: indirect effect; +: increased; ++: highly increased; −: no effect [136, 144–147].*
Abbreviations: ECM: extra-cellular matrix; PDGF: platelet-derived growth factor; TGF: transforming growth factor; VEGF: vascular endothelial growth factor; CTCG: connective tissue growth factor; IGF: insulin-like growth factor.

Table 3.
The synergistical and contributing dynamics of specific PRP growth factors and plasma-fibrin fraction to adipose tissue grafting cellular processes.

ABPs and application strategies for the treatment of degenerative conditions, poorly healing chronic wounds, as well as to support in patient outcomes following biosurgical procedures.

6. Conclusions

ABPs, prepared with modern and dedicated devices and ultimately precisely delivered, are powerful high yielded cellular biological products.

The employment of properly prepared stand-alone or combined biologics is a valuable and safe therapy for clinicians to repair and regenerate tissues, aiming for functional restoration. Furthermore, they can be used as supportive armamentarium in wound healing treatments and biosurgical procedures to improve patient outcomes and decrease complications, as evidenced by an extensive body of clinical literature.

Lastly, we believe that more clinical and translational studies, as well as educational activities, are required in order for ABPs to be widely accepted as mainstream therapeutics.

Conflict of interest

Other authors declare no conflict of interest.

Author details

Peter A. Everts[1,2,3*], Luga Podesta[4,5] and Robert W. Alexander[6,7]

1 Gulf Coast Biologics, A Non-Profit Organization, Fort Myers, FL, USA

2 Max-Planck University (UniMAX), OrthoRegen International Course, Indaiatuba, São Paulo, Brazil

3 Medical School, Max-Planck University Center (UniMAX), Indaiatuba, São Paulo, Brazil

4 Bluetail Medical Group and Podesta Orthopedic Sports Medicine, Naples, FL, USA

5 Orlando College of Osteopathic Medicine, Orlando, FL, USA

6 Regenevita Biocellular Aesthetic and Reconstructive Surgery, Cranio-Maxillofacial Surgery, Regenerative and Wound Healing, Hamilton, MT, USA

7 School of Medicine and Dentistry, Department of Surgery and Maxillofacial Surgery, University of Washington, Seattle, WA, USA

*Address all correspondence to: peter@gulfcoastbiologics.com

References

[1] Wright DE, Wagers AJ, Gulati AP, Johnson FL, Weissman IL. Physiological migration of hematopoietic stem and progenitor cells. Science. 2001;**294**(5548):1933-1936

[2] Everts PAM, Devilee RJJ, Oosterbos CJM, Mahoney CB, Schattenkerk ME, Knape JTA, et al. Autologous platelet gel and fibrin sealant enhance the efficacy of total knee arthroplasty: Improved range of motion, decreased length of stay and a reduced incidence of arthrofibrosis. Knee Surgery, Sports Traumatology, Arthroscopy [Internet]. 2007;**15**(7):888-894. DOI: 10.1007/s00167-007-0296-x

[3] Poodt IGM, Van Dijk MM, Klein S, Hoogbergen MM. Complications of lower body lift surgery in postbariatric patients. Plastic and Reconstructive Surgery - Global Open [Internet]. 2016;**4**(9):e1030. Available from: https://journals.lww.com/01720096-201609000-00001

[4] Calvi LM, Link DC. The hematopoietic stem cell niche in homeostasis and disease. Blood [Internet]. 2015;**126**(22):2443-2451. Available from: https://ashpublications.org/blood/article/126/22/2443/34611/The-hematopoietic-stem-cell-niche-in-homeostasis

[5] Everts PA. Autologous platelet-rich plasma and mesenchymal stem cells for the treatment of chronic wounds. In: Hakan Dogan K, editor. Wound Healing - Current Perspectives [Internet]. London, UK: IntechOpen; 2019. Available from: https://www.intechopen.com/books/wound-healing-current-perspectives/autologous-platelet-rich-plasma-and-mesenchymal-stem-cells-for-the-treatment-of-chronic-wounds

[6] Lana JF, Purita J, Everts PA, De Mendonça Neto PAT, De Moraes Ferreira Jorge D, Mosaner T, et al. Platelet-rich plasma power-mix gel (ppm)—An orthobiologic optimization protocol rich in growth factors and fibrin. Gels [Internet]. 2023;**9**(7):553. Available from: https://www.mdpi.com/2310-2861/9/7/553

[7] Yamaguchi S, Silva S. PRP and BMAC for musculoskeletal conditions via biomaterial carriers. IJMS [Internet]. 2019;**20**(21):5328. Available from: https://www.mdpi.com/1422-0067/20/21/5328

[8] Everts PA, Flanagan G, Podesta L. Autologous Orthobiologics. In: Mostoufi SA, George TK, Tria AJ Jr, editors. Clinical Guide to Musculoskeletal Medicine: A Multidisciplinary Approach [Internet]. Cham: Springer International Publishing; 2022. pp. 651-679. DOI: 10.1007/978-3-030-92042-5_62

[9] Everts PA, Panero AJ. Basic science of autologous orthobiologics. Physical Medicine and Rehabilitation Clinics of North America [Internet]. 2023;**34**(1):25-47. Available from: https://linkinghub.elsevier.com/retrieve/pii/S1047965122000730

[10] Everts P, Onishi K, Jayaram P, Lana JF, Mautner and K. Plateletrich plasma: New performance understandings and therapeutic considerations in 2020. International Journal of Molecular Sciences. 2020;**21**:7794. DOI: 10.3390/ijms21207794

[11] Hasiba-Pappas SK, Tuca AC, Luze H, Nischwitz SP, Zrim R, Geißler JCJ, et al. Platelet-rich plasma in plastic surgery: A systematic review. Transfusion Medicine and Hemotherapy [Internet]. 2022;**49**(3):129-142. Available from: https://www.karger.com/Article/FullText/524353

[12] Andia I, Maffulli N. A contemporary view of platelet-rich plasma therapies: Moving toward refined clinical protocols and precise indications. Regenerative Medicine [Internet]. 2018;**13**(6):717-728. DOI: 10.2217/rme-2018-0042

[13] Zheng C, Zhu Q, Liu X, Huang X, He C, Jiang L, et al. Effect of platelet-rich plasma (PRP) concentration on proliferation, neurotrophic function and migration of Schwann cells *in vitro*: Effect of platelet-rich plasma on Schwann cells. Journal of Tissue Engineering and Regenerative Medicine [Internet]. 2016;**10**(5):428-436. DOI: 10.1002/term.1756

[14] Everts PA, Lana JF, Onishi K, Buford D, Peng J, Mahmood A, et al. Angiogenesis and tissue repair depend on platelet dosing and bioformulation strategies following orthobiological platelet-rich plasma procedures: A narrative. Review. Biomedicines. 2023;**11**:1922. DOI: 10.3390/biomedicines11071922

[15] Lana JFSD, Purita J, Paulus C, Huber SC, Rodrigues BL, Rodrigues AA, et al. Contributions for classification of platelet rich plasma – Proposal of a new classification: MARSPILL. Regenerative Medicine [Internet]. 2017;**12**(5):565-574. DOI: 10.2217/rme-2017-0042

[16] Acebes-Huerta A, Arias-Fernández T, Bernardo Á, Muñoz-Turrillas MC, Fernández-Fuertes J, Seghatchian J, et al. Platelet-derived bio-products: Classification update, applications, concerns and new perspectives. Transfusion and Apheresis Science [Internet]. 2020;**59**(1):102716. Available from: https://linkinghub.elsevier.com/retrieve/pii/S1473050219302897

[17] Arthur A, Gronthos S. Clinical application of bone marrow mesenchymal stem/stromal cells to repair skeletal tissue. IJMS [Internet]. 2020;**21**(24):9759. Available from: https://www.mdpi.com/1422-0067/21/24/9759

[18] PintoreA, Notarfrancesco D, Zar A, Oliviero A, Migliorini F, Oliva F, et al. Intra-articular injection of bone marrow aspirate conncentrate (BMAC) or adiposederived stemcells (ADSCs) for knee osteoarthritis: A prospective comparative clinical trial. Journal of Orthopaedic Surgery and Research. 2023;**18**:350. DOI: 10.1186/s13018-023-03841-2

[19] Alexander RW. Understanding mechanical emulsification (Nanofat) versus enzymatic isolation of tissue stromal vascular fraction (tSVF) cells from adipose tissue: Potential uses in biocellular regenerative medicine. Journal of Prolotherapy. 2016;**8**:e947-e960

[20] Zuk PA. The adipose-derived stem cell: Looking Back and looking ahead. MBoC. 2010;**21**(11):1783-1787. DOI: 10.1091/mbc.e09-07-0589

[21] Hadjipanayi E, Kuhn PH, Moog P, Bauer AT, Kuekrek H, Mirzoyan L, et al. The fibrin matrix regulates angiogenic responses within the hemostatic microenvironment through biochemical control. PLoS One [Internet]. 2015;**10**(8):e0135618. DOI: 10.1371/journal.pone.0135618

[22] Pavlovic V, Ciric M, Jovanovic V, Stojanovic P. Platelet rich plasma: A short overview of certain bioactive components. Open Medicine [Internet]. 2016;**11**(1):242-247. DOI: 10.1515/med-2016-0048

[23] Rodeo SA, Delos D, Williams RJ, Adler RS, Pearle A, Warren RF. The effect of platelet-rich fibrin matrix on rotator cuff tendon healing:

A prospective, randomized clinical study. The American Journal of Sports Medicine [Internet]. 2012;**40**(6):1234-1241. DOI: 10.1177/0363546512442924

[24] Linnanmäki L, Kanto K, Karjalainen T, Leppänen OV, Lehtinen J. Platelet-rich plasma or autologous blood do not reduce pain or improve function in patients with lateral epicondylitis: A randomized controlled trial. Clinical Orthopaedics and Related Research [Internet]. 2020;**478**(8):1892-1900. DOI: 10.1097/CORR.0000000000001185

[25] Longo UG, Castricini R, De Benedetto M, Panfoli N, Pirani P, Zini R, et al. Paper # 117: Platelet-rich fibrin matrix augmentation for arthroscopic rotator cuff repair: A randomized controlled trial. Arthroscopy: The Journal of Arthroscopic & Related Surgery [Internet]. 2011;**27**(10):e145-e146. Available from: https://linkinghub.elsevier.com/retrieve/pii/S0749806311008279

[26] Bennell KL, Paterson KL, Metcalf BR, Duong V, Eyles J, Kasza J, et al. Effect of intra-articular platelet-rich plasma vs placebo injection on pain and medial tibial cartilage volume in patients with knee osteoarthritis: The RESTORE randomized clinical trial. JAMA [Internet]. 2021;**326**(20):2021. Available from: https://jamanetwork.com/journals/jama/fullarticle/2786501

[27] Atiyeh B, Oneisi A, Ghieh F. Platelet-rich plasma facial rejuvenation: Myth or reality? Aesthetic Plastic Surgery. 2021;**45**(6):2928-2938. DOI: 10.1007/s00266-021-02300-9

[28] Miroshnychenko O, Chalkley RJ, Leib RD, Everts PA, Dragoo JL. Proteomic analysis of platelet-rich and platelet-poor plasma. Regenerative Therapy [Internet]. 2020;**15**:226-235. Available from: https://linkinghub.elsevier.com/retrieve/pii/S2352320420300730

[29] Ozer K, Kankaya Y, Colak O, Kocer U. The impact of duration and force of centrifugation on platelet content and mass in the preparation of platelet-rich plasma. Aesthetic Plastic Surgery [Internet]. 2019;**43**(4):1078-1084. DOI: 10.1007/s00266-019-01375-9

[30] Magalon J, Brandin T, Francois P, Degioanni C, De Maria L, Grimaud F, et al. Technical and biological review of authorized medical devices for platelets-rich plasma preparation in the field of regenerative medicine. Platelets [Internet]. 2021;**32**(2):200-208. DOI: 10.1080/09537104.2020.1832653

[31] Fadadu PP, Mazzola AJ, Hunter CW, Davis TT. Review of concentration yields in commercially available platelet-rich plasma (PRP) systems: A call for PRP standardization. Regional Anesthesia and Pain Medicine [Internet]. 2019;**44**(6):652-659. DOI: 10.1136/rapm-2018-100356

[32] Pietruszka P, Chruścicka I, Duś-Ilnicka I, Paradowska-Stolarz A. PRP and PRF—Subgroups and divisions when used in dentistry. JPM [Internet]. 2021;**11**(10):944. Available from: https://www.mdpi.com/2075-4426/11/10/944

[33] Chahla J, Cinque ME, Piuzzi NS, Mannava S, Geeslin AG, Murray IR, et al. A call for standardization in platelet-rich plasma preparation protocols and composition reporting: A systematic review of the clinical orthopaedic literature. The Journal of Bone and Joint Surgery [Internet]. 2017;**99**(20):1769-1779. Available from: http://Insights.ovid.com/crossref?an=00004623-201710180-00009

[34] Parrish WR. Physiology of blood components in wound healing: An

appreciation of cellular co-operativity in platelet rich plasma action. JESO [Internet]. 2017;**4**(2):1-14. Available from: https://symbiosisonlinepublishing.com/exercise-sports-orthopedics/exercise-sports-orthopedics56.php

[35] Giannotti L, Di Chiara SB, Spedicato F, Nitti P, Damiano F, Demitri C, et al. Progress in regenerative medicine: Exploring autologous platelet concentrates and their clinical applications. Genes [Internet]. 2023;**14**(9):1669. Available from: https://www.mdpi.com/2073-4425/14/9/1669

[36] Everts PA, Mazzola T, Mautner K, Randelli PS, Podesta L. Modifying orthobiological PRP therapies are imperative for the advancement of treatment outcomes in musculoskeletal pathologies. Biomedicine [Internet]. 2022;**10**(11):2933. Available from: https://www.mdpi.com/2227-9059/10/11/2933

[37] Piao L, Park H, Jo CH. Theoretical prediction and validation of cell recovery rates in preparing platelet-rich plasma through a centrifugation. PLoS One [Internet]. 2017;**12**(11):e0187509. DOI: 10.1371/journal.pone.0187509

[38] Saluja H, Dehane V, Mahindra U. Platelet-rich fibrin: A second generation platelet concentrate and a new friend of oral and maxillofacial surgeons. Annals of Maxillofacial Surgery [Internet]. 2011;**1**(1):53. DOI: 10.4103/2231-0746.83158

[39] Zumstein AM, Berger S, Schober M, Boileau P, Nyffeler WR, Horn M, et al. Leukocyte-and platelet-rich fibrin (L-PRF) for long-term delivery of growth factor in rotator cuff repair: Review, preliminary results and future directions. Current Pharmaceutical Biotechnology. 2012;**13**(7):1196-1206

[40] Dohan DM, Choukroun J, Diss A, Dohan SL, Dohan AJ, Mouhyi J, et al. Platelet-rich fibrin (PRF): A second-generation platelet concentrate. Part I: Technological concepts and evolution. Oral Surgery, Oral Medicine, Oral Pathology, Oral Radiology, and Endodontology. 2006;**101**(3):e37-e44

[41] Dohan DM, Choukroun J, Diss A, Dohan SL, Dohan AJ, Mouhyi J, et al. Platelet-rich fibrin (PRF): A second-generation platelet concentrate. Part II: Platelet-related biologic features. Oral Surgery, Oral Medicine, Oral Pathology, Oral Radiology, and Endodontology. 2006;**101**(3):e45-e50

[42] Matveeva VG, Senokosova EA, Sevostianova VV, Khanova MY, Glushkova TV, Akentieva TN, et al. Advantages of fibrin polymerization method without the use of exogenous thrombin for vascular tissue engineering applications. Biomedicine [Internet]. 2022;**10**(4):789. Available from: https://www.mdpi.com/2227-9059/10/4/789

[43] Oh JH, Kim W, Park KU, Roh YH. Comparison of the cellular composition and cytokine-release kinetics of various platelet-rich plasma preparations. The American Journal of Sports Medicine [Internet]. 2015;**43**(12):3062-3070. DOI: 10.1177/0363546515608481

[44] Miron RJ, Chai J, Fujioka-Kobayashi M, Sculean A, Zhang Y. Evaluation of 24 protocols for the production of platelet-rich fibrin. BMC Oral Health [Internet]. 2020;**20**(1):310. DOI: 10.1186/s12903-020-01299-w

[45] Da Fonseca L, Santos GS, Huber SC, Setti TM, Setti T, Lana JF. Human platelet lysate – A potent (and overlooked) orthobiologic. Journal of Clinical Orthopaedics and Trauma. [Internet]. 2021;**21**:101534. Available from: https://linkinghub.elsevier.com/retrieve/pii/S0976566221004185

[46] Jayaram P, Chia Yeh P, Epstein M, Patel SJ. 7 - autologous Orthobiologics. In: Williams CJ, WalterL S, Pitts J, editors. Atlas of Interventional Orthopedics Procedures [Internet]. London, UK: Elsevier; 2022. pp. 70-88. Available from: https://www.sciencedirect.com/science/article/pii/B9780323755146000078

[47] Molloy T, Wang Y, Murrell GAC. The roles of growth factors in tendon and ligament healing. Sports Medicine [Internet]. 2003;**33**(5):381-394. DOI: 10.2165/00007256-200333050-00004

[48] Chiara Barsotti M, Losi P, Briganti E, Sanguinetti E, Magera A, Al Kayal T, et al. Effect of platelet lysate on human cells involved in different phases of wound healing. PLoS One. 2013;**8**(12):e84753

[49] Dellera E, Bonferoni MC, Sandri G, Rossi S, Ferrari F, Del Fante C, et al. Development of chitosan oleate ionic micelles loaded with silver sulfadiazine to be associated with platelet lysate for application in wound healing. European Journal of Pharmaceutics and Biopharmaceutics[Internet]. 2014;**88**(3):643-650. Available from: https://www.sciencedirect.com/science/article/pii/S0939641114002410

[50] Centeno C, Markle J, Dodson E, Stemper I, Hyzy M, Williams C, et al. The use of lumbar epidural injection of platelet lysate for treatment of radicular pain. Journal of Experimental Orthopaedics.[Internet]. 2017;**4**(1):38. Available from: https://jeo-esska.springeropen.com/articles/10.1186/s40634-017-0113-5

[51] Bieback K. Platelet lysate as replacement for fetal bovine serum in mesenchymal stromal cell cultures. Transfusion Medicine and Hemotherapy [Internet]. 2013;**40**(5):326-335. DOI: 10.1159/000354061

[52] Al-Ajlouni J, Awidi A, Samara O, Al-Najar M, Tarwanah E, Saleh M, et al. Safety and efficacy of autologous intra-articular platelet lysates in early and intermediate knee osteoarthrosis in humans: A prospective open-label study. Clinical Journal of Sport Medicine [Internet]. 2015;**25**(6):524-528. Available from: https://journals.lww.com/cjsportsmed/fulltext/2015/11000/safety_and_efficacy_of_autologous_intra_articular.10.aspx

[53] Mohamed-Ahmed S, Fristad I, Lie SA, Suliman S, Mustafa K, Vindenes H, et al. Adipose-derived and bone marrow mesenchymal stem cells: A donor-matched comparison. Stem Cell Research & Therapy [Internet]. 2018;**9**(1):168. DOI: 10.1186/s13287-018-0914-1

[54] Izadpanah R, Trygg C, Patel B, Kriedt C, Dufour J, Gimble JM, et al. Biologic properties of mesenchymal stem cells derived from bone marrow and adipose tissue. Journal of Cellular Biochemistry. 2006;**99**(5):1285-1297. DOI: 10.1002/jcb.20904

[55] Heo JS, Choi Y, Kim HS, Kim HO. Comparison of molecular profiles of human mesenchymal stem cells derived from bone marrow, umbilical cord blood, placenta and adipose tissue. International Journal of Molecular Medicine. 2016;**37**(1):115-125. DOI: 10.3892/ijmm.2015.2413

[56] Dmitrieva RI, Minullina IR, Bilibina AA, Tarasova OV, Anisimov SV, Zaritskey AY. Bone marrow- and subcutaneous adipose tissue-derived mesenchymal stem cells: Differences and similarities. Cell Cycle [Internet]. 2012;**11**(2):377-383. DOI: 10.4161/cc.11.2.18858

[57] Scarpone M, Kuebler D, Chambers A, De Filippo CM,

Amatuzio M, Ichim TE, et al. Isolation of clinically relevant concentrations of bone marrow mesenchymal stem cells without centrifugation. Journal of Translational Medicine [Internet]. 2019;**17**(1):10. DOI: 10.1186/s12967-018-1750-x

[58] Hernigou J, Alves A, Homma Y, Guissou I, Hernigou P. Anatomy of the ilium for bone marrow aspiration: Map of sectors and implication for safe trocar placement. International Orthopaedics (SICOT) [Internet]. 2014;**38**(12):2585-2590. Available from: http://link.springer.com/10.1007/s00264-014-2353-7

[59] Cavallo C, Boffa A, de Girolamo L, Merli G, Kon E, Cattini L, et al. Bone marrow aspirate concentrate quality is affected by age and harvest site. Knee Surgery, Sports Traumatology, Arthroscopy [Internet]. 2023;**31**(6):2140-2151. DOI: 10.1007/s00167-022-07153-6

[60] Everts PA, Ferrell J, Mahoney CB, Ii GF, de Roman MI, Paul R, et al. A comparative quantification in cellularity of bone marrow aspirated with two new harvesting devices, and the non-equivalent difference between a centrifugated bone marrow concentrate and a bone marrow aspirate as biological injectates, using a bi-lateral patient model. Journal of Stem Cell Research & Therapeutics. 2020;**10**:1-10

[61] Tsitsilianos N, Shirazi Z, Lu J, Singh JR. Bone marrow aspirate injection for osteoarthritis of the hip; A pilot study. Interventional Pain Medicine [Internet]. 2022;**1**(4):100163. Available from: https://linkinghub.elsevier.com/retrieve/pii/S2772594422001613

[62] Centeno CJ. Bone marrow concentrate (BMC) therapy in musculoskeletal disorders: Evidence-based policy position statement of American society of interventional pain physicians (ASIPP). Pain Physician [Internet]. 2020;**23**(2):E85-E131. Available from: https://painphysicianjournal.com/current/pdf?article=NzAyNQ%3D%3D&journal=125

[63] Everts PA, Malanga GA, Paul RV, Rothenberg JB, Stephens N, Mautner KR. Assessing clinical implications and perspectives of the pathophysiological effects of erythrocytes and plasma free hemoglobin in autologous biologics for use in musculoskeletal regenerative medicine therapies. A review. Regenerative Therapy [Internet]. 2019;**11**:56-64. Available from: https://linkinghub.elsevier.com/retrieve/pii/S2352320419300033

[64] Lambertsen RH, Weiss L. Studies on the organization and regeneration of bone marrow: Origin, growth, and differentiation of endocloned hematopoietic colonies. American Journal of Anatomy [Internet]. 1983;**166**(4):369-392. DOI: 10.1002/aja.1001660402

[65] Spradling A, Drummond-Barbosa D, Kai T. Stem cells find their niche. Nature [Internet]. 2001;**414**(6859):98-104. Available from: http://www.nature.com/articles/35102160

[66] Li L, Xie T. Stem cell niche: Structure and function. Annual Review of Cell and Developmental Biology. 2005;**21**:605-631

[67] Yusop N, Battersby P, Alraies A, Sloan AJ, Moseley R, Waddington RJ. Isolation and characterisation of mesenchymal stem cells from rat bone marrow and the endosteal niche: A comparative study. Stem Cells International [Internet]. 2018;**2018**:1-14. Available from: https://www.hindawi.com/journals/sci/2018/6869128/

[68] Siclari VA, Zhu J, Akiyama K, Liu F, Zhang X, Chandra A, et al. Mesenchymal

progenitors residing close to the bone surface are functionally distinct from those in the central bone marrow. Bone [Internet]. 2013;**53**(2):575-586. Available from: https://linkinghub.elsevier.com/retrieve/pii/S8756328212014317

[69] Mangialardi G, Cordaro A, Madeddu P. The bone marrow pericyte: An orchestrator of vascular niche. Regenerative Medicine. [Internet]. 2016;**11**(8):883-895. DOI: 10.2217/rme-2016-0121

[70] Lana JFSD, da Fonseca LF, da Macedo RR, Mosaner T, Murrell W, Kumar A, et al. Platelet-rich plasma *vs* bone marrow aspirate concentrate: An overview of mechanisms of action and orthobiologic synergistic effects. WJSC [Internet]. 2021;**13**(2):155-167. Available from: https://www.wjgnet.com/1948-0210/full/v13/i2/155.htm

[71] Everts P, Flanagan G II, Rothenberg J, Mautner K. The rationale of autologously prepared bone marrow aspirate concentrate for use in regenerative medicine applications. In: Regenerative Medicine [Internet]. London, UK: IntechOpen; 2020. Available from: https://www.intechopen.com/online-first/the-rationale-of-autologously-prepared-bone-marrow-aspirate-concentrate-for-use-in-regenerative-medi

[72] Van Boxtel J, Vonk LA, Stevens HP, Van Dongen JA. Mechanically derived tissue stromal vascular fraction acts anti-inflammatory on TNF alpha-stimulated chondrocytes in vitro. Bioengineering [Internet]. 2022;**9**(8):345. Available from: https://www.mdpi.com/2306-5354/9/8/345

[73] Alexander R. Overview of cellular stromal vascular fraction (cSVF) & biocellular uses of stem/stromal cells & matrix (tSVF+ HD-PRP) in regenerative medicine, aesthetic medicine and plastic surgery. Journal of Stem Cells Research, Development & Therapy. 2019;**2**:304-312

[74] Klein JA. The tumescent technique: Anesthesia and modified liposuction technique. Dermatologic Clinics. 1990;**8**(3):425-437. Available from: https://www.sciencedirect.com/science/article/pii/S0733863518304741

[75] Simonacci F, Bertozzi N, Grieco MP, Raposio E. From liposuction to adipose-derived stem cells: Indications and technique. Acta Bio Medica Atenei Parmensis [Internet]. 2019;**90**(2):197-208. DOI: 10.23750/abm.v90i2.6619

[76] Illouz Y. Body contouring by lipolysis: A 5-year experience with over 3000 cases. Plastic and Reconstructive Surgery [Internet]. 1983;**72**(5):591-597. DOI: 10.1097/00006534-198311000-00001

[77] Kurita M, Matsumoto D, Shigeura T, Sato K, Gonda K, Harii K, et al. Influences of centrifugation on cells and tissues in liposuction aspirates: Optimized centrifugation for lipotransfer and cell isolation. Plastic and Reconstructive Surgery [Internet]. 2008;**121**(3):1033-1041. Available from: http://journals.lww.com/00006534-200803000-00041

[78] Gentile P, Calabrese C, De Angelis B, Pizzicannella J, Kothari A, Garcovich S. Impact of the different preparation methods to obtain human adipose-derived stromal vascular fraction cells (AD-SVFs) and human adipose-derived mesenchymal stem cells (AD-MSCs): Enzymatic digestion versus mechanical centrifugation. IJMS [Internet]. 2019;**20**(21):5471. Available from: https://www.mdpi.com/1422-0067/20/21/5471

[79] Argentati C, Morena F, Bazzucchi M, Armentano I, Emiliani C, Martino S.

Adipose stem cell translational applications: From bench-to-bedside. IJMS [Internet]. 2018;**19**(11):3475. Available from: http://www.mdpi.com/1422-0067/19/11/3475

[80] Alexander RW. Adipose tissue complex (ATC): Cellular and biocellular uses of stem/stromal cells and matrix in cosmetic plastic, reconstructive surgery and regenerative medicine. In: Duscher D, Shiffman MA, editors. Regenerative Medicine and Plastic Surgery: Skin and Soft Tissue, Bone, Cartilage, Muscle, Tendon and Nerves [Internet]. Cham: Springer International Publishing; 2019. pp. 45-69. DOI: 10.1007/978-3-030-19962-3_5

[81] Oberbauer E, Steffenhagen C, Wurzer C, Gabriel C, Redl H, Wolbank S. Enzymatic and non-enzymatic isolation systems for adipose tissue-derived cells: Current state of the art. Cell Regeneration [Internet]. 2015;**4**:7. Available from: https://linkinghub.elsevier.com/retrieve/pii/S2045976917300093

[82] Williams SK, Wang TF, Castrillo R, Jarrell BE. Liposuction-derived human fat used for vascular graft sodding contains endothelial cells and not mesothelial cells as the major cell type. Journal of Vascular Surgery [Internet]. 1994;**19**(5):916-923. Available from: https://linkinghub.elsevier.com/retrieve/pii/S0741521494700192

[83] Wong SP, Rowley JE, Redpath AN, Tilman JD, Fellous TG, Johnson JR. Pericytes, mesenchymal stem cells and their contributions to tissue repair. Pharmacology & Therapeutics. 2015;**151**:107-120

[84] Guo J, Nguyen A, Banyard DA, Fadavi D, Toranto JD, Wirth GA, et al. Stromal vascular fraction: A regenerative reality? Part 2: Mechanisms of regenerative action. Journal of Plastic, Reconstructive & Aesthetic Surgery [Internet]. 2016;**69**(2):180-188. Available from: https://linkinghub.elsevier.com/retrieve/pii/S1748681515004982

[85] Tonnard P, Verpaele A, Peeters G, Hamdi M, Cornelissen M, Declercq H. Nanofat grafting: Basic research and clinical applications. Plastic and Reconstructive Surgery [Internet]. 2013;**132**(4):1017-1026. Available from: http://journals.lww.com/00006534-201310000-00053

[86] Bianchi F, Maioli M, Leonardi E, Olivi E, Pasquinelli G, Valente S, et al. A new nonenzymatic method and device to obtain a fat tissue derivative highly enriched in pericyte-like elements by mild mechanical forces from human lipoaspirates. Cell Transplantation [Internet]. 2013;**22**(11):2063-2077. DOI: 10.3727/096368912X657855

[87] Jiang W, Cai J, Guan J, Liao Y, Lu F, Ma J, et al. Characterized the adipogenic capacity of adipose-derived stem cell, extracellular matrix, and microenvironment with fat components grafting. Frontiers in Cell and Development Biology [Internet]. 2021;**9**:723057. DOI: 10.3389/fcell.2021.723057/full

[88] Tate-Oliver K, Alexander RW. Combination of autologous adipose-derived tissue stromal vascular fraction plus high density platelet-rich plasma or bone marrow concentrates in Achilles tendon tears. Journal of Prolotherapy. 2013;**5**:e895-e912

[89] Tapp H, Hanley EN, Patt JC, Gruber HE. Adipose-derived stem cells: Characterization and current application in orthopaedic tissue repair. Experimental Biology and Medicine (Maywood, N.J.) [Internet]. 2009;**234**(1):1-9. DOI: 10.3181/0805-MR-170

[90] Blaber SP, Webster RA, Hill CJ, Breen EJ, Kuah D, Vesey G, et al. Analysis of in vitro secretion profiles from adipose-derived cell populations. Journal of Translational Medicine [Internet]. 2012;**10**(1):172. DOI: 10.1186/1479-5876-10-172

[91] Everts PA, Warbout M, de Veth D, Cirkel M, Spruijt NE, Buth J. Use of epidermal skin grafts in chronic wounds: A case series: Epidermal skin grafts in chronic wounds. International Wound Journal [Internet]. 2017;**14**(6):1213-1218. DOI: 10.1111/iwj.12787

[92] Gentile P, Garcovich S. Systematic review—The potential implications of different platelet-rich plasma (PRP) concentrations in regenerative medicine for tissue repair. IJMS [Internet]. 2020;**21**(16):5702. Available from: https://www.mdpi.com/1422-0067/21/16/5702

[93] Oklu R, Walker TG, Wicky S, Hesketh R. Angiogenesis and current antiangiogenic strategies for the treatment of cancer. Journal of Vascular and Interventional Radiology. 2010;**21**(12):1791-1805

[94] Waldner M, Zhang W, James IB, Allbright K, Havis E, Bliley JM, et al. Characteristics and immunomodulating functions of adipose-derived and bone marrow-derived mesenchymal stem cells across defined human leukocyte antigen barriers. Frontiers in Immunology [Internet]. 2018;**9**:1642. DOI: 10.3389/fimmu.2018.01642/full

[95] Wang X, Thomsen P. Mesenchymal stem cell-derived small extracellular vesicles and bone regeneration. Basic & Clinical Pharmacology & Toxicology. 2021;**128**(1):18-36

[96] Sánchez M, Anitua E, Delgado D, Sanchez P, Prado R, Orive G, et al. Platelet-rich plasma, a source of autologous growth factors and biomimetic scaffold for peripheral nerve regeneration. Expert Opinion on Biological Therapy [Internet]. 2017;**17**(2):197-212. DOI: 10.1080/14712598.2017.1259409

[97] Bohren Y, Timbolschi DI, Muller A, Barrot M, Yalcin I, Salvat E. Platelet-rich plasma and cytokines in neuropathic pain: A narrative review and a clinical perspective. European Journal of Pain [Internet]. 2022;**26**(1):43-60. DOI: 10.1002/ejp.1846

[98] Thomi G, Joerger-Messerli M, Haesler V, Muri L, Surbek D, Schoeberlein A. Intranasally administered exosomes from umbilical cord stem cells have preventive neuroprotective effects and contribute to functional recovery after perinatal brain injury. Cells. 2019;**8**(8):855

[99] Rubio-Azpeitia E, Andia I. Partnership between platelet-rich plasma and mesenchymal stem cells: in vitro experience. Biological Effects. Muscles Ligaments Tendons Journal. 2014;**8**;4(1):52-62

[100] Delgado D, Garate A, Sánchez P, Bilbao AM, Garcia Del Cano G, Salles J, et al. Biological and structural effects after intraosseous infiltrations of age-dependent platelet-rich plasma: An in vivo study. Journal of Orthopaedic Research. 2020;**38**(9):1931-1941

[101] Harrison P, Martin CE. Platelet α-granules. Blood Reviews [Internet]. 1993;**7**(1):52-62. Available from: https://www.sciencedirect.com/science/article/pii/0268960X9390024X

[102] Sánchez-González DJ, Méndez-Bolaina E, Trejo-Bahena NI. Platelet-rich plasma peptides: Key for regeneration. International Journal of Peptides

[Internet]. 2012;**2012**:1-10. Available from: https://www.hindawi.com/archive/2012/532519/

[103] Everts PA, Lana JF, Alexander RW, Dallo I, Kon E, Ambach MA, et al. Profound properties of protein-rich, platelet-rich plasma matrices as novel, multi-purpose biological platforms in tissue repair, regeneration, and wound healing. IJMS [Internet]. 2024;**25**(14):7914. Available from: https://www.mdpi.com/1422-0067/25/14/7914

[104] Senthilkumar S, Rajesh S, Mohan D, Soundararajan P. Preparation, characterization, and performance evaluation of poly(ether-imide) incorporated cellulose acetate ultrafiltration membrane for Hemodialysis. Separation Science and Technology [Internet]. 2013;**48**(1):66-75. DOI: 10.1080/01496395.2012.674603

[105] Suzuki H, Oshima N, Watari T. Effect of modified ultrafiltration on cytokines and hemoconcentration in dogs undergoing cardiopulmonary bypass. The Journal of Veterinary Medical Science. 2020;**82**(11):1589-1593. Available from: https://www.jstage.jst.go.jp/article/jvms/82/11/82_20-0143/_article

[106] Mercader Ruiz J, Beitia M, Delgado D, Sánchez P, Guadilla J, Pérez De Arrilucea C, et al. Method based on ultrafiltration to obtain a plasma rich in platelet and plasma growth factors. JCM [Internet]. 2023;**12**(18):5941. Available from: https://www.mdpi.com/2077-0383/12/18/5941

[107] Muir SM, Reisbig N, Baria M, Kaeding C, Bertone AL. The concentration of plasma provides additional bioactive proteins in platelet and autologous protein solutions. The American Journal of Sports Medicine [Internet]. 2019;**47**(8):1955-1963. DOI: 10.1177/0363546519849671

[108] Vandooren J, Itoh Y. Alpha-2-macroglobulin in inflammation, immunity and infections. Frontiers in Immunology [Internet]. 2021;**12**:803244. Available from: https://www.frontiersin.org/articles/10.3389/fimmu.2021.803244/full

[109] Yan Z, Yin H, Nerlich M, Pfeifer CG, Docheva D. Boosting tendon repair: Interplay of cells, growth factors and scaffold-free and gel-based carriers. Journal of Experimental Orthopaedics [Internet]. 2018;**5**(1):1. DOI: 10.1186/s40634-017-0117-1

[110] Lomas AJ, Ryan CNM, Sorushanova A, Shologu N, Sideri AI, Tsioli V, et al. The past, present and future in scaffold-based tendon treatments. Advanced Drug Delivery Reviews [Internet]. 2015;**84**:257-277. Available from: https://linkinghub.elsevier.com/retrieve/pii/S0169409X14002956

[111] Li S, Xing F, Yan T, Zhang S, Chen F. The efficiency and safety of platelet-rich plasma dressing in the treatment of chronic wounds: A systematic review and meta-analysis of randomized controlled trials. JPM [Internet]. 2023;**13**(3):430. Available from: https://www.mdpi.com/2075-4426/13/3/430

[112] Anitua E, Andia I, Ardanza B, Nurden P, Nurden A. Autologous platelets as a source of proteins for healing and tissue regeneration. Thrombosis and Haemostasis [Internet]. 2004;**91**(01):4-15. DOI: 10.1160/TH03-07-0440

[113] Bilgen F, Ural A, Bekerecioglu M. Platelet-rich fibrin: An effective chronic wound healing accelerator. Journal of Tissue Viability [Internet].

2021;**30**(4):616-620. Available from: https://linkinghub.elsevier.com/retrieve/pii/S0965206X21000656

[114] Pinto NR, Ubilla M, Zamora Y, Del Rio V, Dohan Ehrenfest DM, Quirynen M. Leucocyte- and platelet-rich fibrin (L-PRF) as a regenerative medicine strategy for the treatment of refractory leg ulcers: A prospective cohort study. Platelets [Internet]. 2018;**29**(5):468-475. DOI: 10.1080/09537104.2017.1327654

[115] Calisir A, Ece I, Yormaz S, Colak B, Kirazli H, Sahin M. The effects of platelet-rich plasma to decrease the risk of Seroma formation after mastectomy and axillary dissection. Journal of Surgical Research [Internet]. 2020;**256**:156-162. Available from: https://linkinghub.elsevier.com/retrieve/pii/S0022480420304303

[116] Chen TM, Tsai JC, Burnouf T. A novel technique combining platelet gel, skin graft, and fibrin glue for healing recalcitrant lower extremity ulcers. Dermatologic Surgery. 2010;**36**(4):453-460

[117] Nourizadeh N, Sedaghat Sharifi N, Bakhshaee M, Ghiasi S, Rasoulian B, Hamidi AD. PRP-fibrin glue for pain reduction and rapid healing in tonsillectomy. Iranian Journal of Otorhinolaryngology [Internet]. 2022;**34**(6):289. DOI: 10.22038/ijorl.2022.40429.2532

[118] Micovic S, Everts P, Calija B, Strugarevic E, Grubor N, Boricic M, et al. Novel autologous, high concentrated fibrin as advanced hemostatic agent for coronary surgery. Transfusion and Apheresis Science [Internet]. 2021;**60**(4):103171. Available from: https://linkinghub.elsevier.com/retrieve/pii/S1473050221001373

[119] Hassan MM, Sharmin S, Kim HJ, Hong ST. Identification and characterization of plasmin-independent thrombolytic enzymes. Circulation Research [Internet]. 2021;**128**(3):386-400. DOI: 10.1161/CIRCRESAHA.120.317245

[120] Weisel JW, Litvinov RI. Fibrin formation, structure and properties. In: Parry DAD, Squire JM, editors. Fibrous Proteins: Structures and Mechanisms [Internet], Subcellular Biochemistry. Vol. 82. Cham: Springer International Publishing; 2017. pp. 405-456. DOI: 10.1007/978-3-319-49674-0_13

[121] Lian Z, Yin X, Li H, Jia L, He X, Yan Y, et al. Synergistic effect of bone marrow-derived mesenchymal stem cells and platelet-rich plasma in Streptozotocin-induced diabetic rats. Annals of Dermatology [Internet]. 2014;**26**(1):1. DOI: 10.5021/ad.2014.26.1.1

[122] Sassoli C, Vallone L, Tani A, Chellini F, Nosi D, Zecchi-Orlandini S. Combined use of bone marrow-derived mesenchymal stromal cells (BM-MSCs) and platelet rich plasma (PRP) stimulates proliferation and differentiation of myoblasts in vitro: New therapeutic perspectives for skeletal muscle repair/regeneration. Cell and Tissue Research [Internet]. 2018;**372**(3):549-570. DOI: 10.1007/s00441-018-2792-3

[123] Muiños-López E, Delgado D, Sánchez P, Paiva B, Anitua E, Fiz N, et al. Modulation of synovial fluid-derived mesenchymal stem cells by intra-articular and intraosseous platelet rich plasma administration. Stem Cells International [Internet]. 2016;**2016**:1-10. Available from: https://www.hindawi.com/journals/sci/2016/1247950/

[124] Kim SJ, Kim EK, Kim SJ, Song DH. Effects of bone marrow aspirate concentrate and platelet-rich plasma on patients with partial tear

of the rotator cuff tendon. Journal of Orthopaedic Surgery and Research [Internet]. 2018;**13**(1):1. DOI: 10.1186/s13018-017-0693-x

[125] Cassano JM, Kennedy JG, Ross KA, Fraser EJ, Goodale MB, Fortier LA. Bone marrow concentrate and platelet-rich plasma differ in cell distribution and interleukin 1 receptor antagonist protein concentration. Knee Surgery, Sports Traumatology, Arthroscopy [Internet]. 2018;**26**(1):333-342. DOI: 10.1007/s00167-016-3981-9

[126] Ziegler CG, Van Sloun R, Gonzalez S, Whitney KE, DePhillipo NN, Kennedy MI, et al. Characterization of growth factors, cytokines, and chemokines in bone marrow concentrate and platelet-rich plasma: A prospective analysis. The American Journal of Sports Medicine [Internet]. 2019;**47**(9):2174-2187. DOI: 10.1177/0363546519832003

[127] Dhillon MS, Karna SK, Dhatt SS, Behera P, Bhatia A. Can platelet rich plasma stimulate human ACL growth in culture? A preliminary experience. Muscles Ligaments Tendons Journal. 2015;**5**(3)156-161

[128] Bai M, Yin H, Han C, Du Z, Meng G, Jiang D. Bone marrow-derived mesenchymal stem cell composited with platelet rich plasma improved repair of annulus fibrosus rupture. International Journal of Clinical and Experimental Medicine. 2017;**10**(6):8989-8998

[129] Desando G, Bartolotti I, Vannini F, Cavallo C, Castagnini F, Buda R, et al. Repair potential of matrix-induced bone marrow aspirate concentrate and matrix-induced autologous chondrocyte implantation for talar osteochondral repair: Patterns of some catabolic, inflammatory, and pain mediators. Cartilage. 2017;**8**(1):50-60

[130] Brewer JM, McCarthy MB, Pauzenburger L, Cote MP, Mazzocca AD. Combining platelet rich plasma and concentrated bone marrow with a demineralized bone matrix scaffold enhances growth factor release over time. Muscle Ligaments and Tendons J [Internet]. 2021;**11**(03):484. Available from: http://www.mltj.online/combining-platelet-rich-plasma-and-concentrated-bone-marrow-with-a-demineralized-bone-matrix-scaffold-enhances-growth-factor-release-over-time/

[131] Hoberman AR, Cirino C, McCarthy MB, Cote MP, Pauzenberger L, Beitzel K, et al. Bone marrow-derived mesenchymal stromal cells enhanced by platelet-rich plasma maintain adhesion to scaffolds in arthroscopic simulation. Arthroscopy: The Journal of Arthroscopic & Related Surgery. 2018;**34**(3):872-881

[132] Martin JF, Shaw T, Heggie J, Penington DG. Measurement of the density of human platelets and its relationship to volume. British Journal of Haematology [Internet]. 2008;**54**(3):337-352. DOI: 10.1111/j.1365-2141.1983.00337.x

[133] Li F, Guo W, Li K, Yu M, Tang W, Wang H, et al. Improved fat graft survival by different volume fractions of platelet-rich plasma and adipose-derived stem cells. Aesthetic Surgery Journal [Internet]. 2015;**35**(3):319-333. Available from: http://academic.oup.com/asj/article/35/3/319/200513/Improved-Fat-Graft-Survival-by-Different-Volume

[134] Smith OJ, Jell G, Mosahebi A. The use of fat grafting and platelet-rich plasma for wound healing: A review of the current evidence. International Wound Journal [Internet]. 2019;**16**(1):275-285. DOI: 10.1111/iwj.13029

[135] Hersant B, Sid-Ahmed M, Braud L, Jourdan M, Baba-Amer Y, Meningaud JP, et al. Platelet-rich plasma improves the wound healing potential of mesenchymal stem cells through paracrine and metabolism alterations. Stem Cells International [Internet]. 2019;**2019**:1-14. Available from: https://www.hindawi.com/journals/sci/2019/1234263/

[136] Blanton MW, Hadad I, Johnstone BH, Mund JA, Rogers PI, Eppley BL, et al. Adipose stromal cells and platelet-rich plasma therapies synergistically increase revascularization during wound healing. Plastic and Reconstructive Surgery [Internet]. 2009;**123**(Supplement):56S-64S. Available from: http://journals.lww.com/00006534-200902001-00009

[137] Chen CF, Liao HT. Platelet-rich plasma enhances adipose-derived stem cell-mediated angiogenesis in a mouse ischemic hindlimb model. WJSC [Internet]. 2018;**10**(12):212-227. Available from: https://www.wjgnet.com/1948-0210/full/v10/i12/212.htm

[138] Siegel KR, Clevenger TN, Clegg DO, Proctor DA, Proctor CS. Adipose stem cells incorporated in fibrin clot modulate expression of growth factors. Arthroscopy: The Journal of Arthroscopic & Related Surgery [Internet]. 2018;**34**(2):581-591. Available from: https://linkinghub.elsevier.com/retrieve/pii/S0749806317310629

[139] Lai F, Kakudo N, Morimoto N, Taketani S, Hara T, Ogawa T, et al. Platelet-rich plasma enhances the proliferation of human adipose stem cells through multiple signaling pathways. Stem Cell Research & Therapy [Internet]. 2018;**9**(1):107. DOI: 10.1186/s13287-018-0851-z

[140] Van Dongen JA, Tuin AJ, Spiekman M, Jansma J, Van Der Lei B, Harmsen MC. Comparison of intraoperative procedures for isolation of clinical grade stromal vascular fraction for regenerative purposes: A systematic review: Intraoperative procedures for stromal vascular fraction isolation. Journal of Tissue Engineering and Regenerative Medicine [Internet]. 2018;**12**(1):e261-e274. DOI: 10.1002/term.2407

[141] Rodríguez-Flores J, Palomar-Gallego MA, Enguita-Valls AB, Rodríguez-Peralto JL, Torres J. Influence of platelet-rich plasma on the histologic characteristics of the autologous fat graft to the upper lip of rabbits. Aesthetic Plastic Surgery. 2011;**35**:480-486

[142] Chignon-Sicard B, Kouidhi M, Yao X, Delerue-Audegond A, Villageois P, Peraldi P, et al. Platelet-rich plasma respectively reduces and promotes adipogenic and myofibroblastic differentiation of human adipose-derived stromal cells via the TGFβ signalling pathway. Scientific Reports [Internet]. 2017;**7**(1):2954. Available from: https://www.nature.com/articles/s41598-017-03113-0

[143] Wu M, Karvar M, Liu Q, Orgill DP, Panayi AC. Comparison of conventional and platelet-rich plasma-assisted fat grafting: A systematic review and meta-analysis. Journal of Plastic, Reconstructive & Aesthetic Surgery [Internet]. 2021;**74**(11):2821-2830. Available from: https://linkinghub.elsevier.com/retrieve/pii/S1748681521002989

[144] Kakudo N, Minakata T, Mitsui T, Kushida S, Notodihardjo FZ, Kusumoto K. Proliferation-promoting effect of platelet-rich plasma on human adipose-derived stem cells and human dermal fibroblasts. Plastic and Reconstructive Surgery. 2008;**122**(5):1352-1360. Available from: http://journals.lww.com/00006534-200811000-00007

[145] Chun SY, Lim JO, Lee EH, Han MH, Ha YS, Lee JN, et al. Preparation and characterization of human adipose tissue-derived extracellular matrix, growth factors, and stem cells: A concise review. Tissue Engineering and Regenerative Medicine [Internet]. 2019;**16**(4):385-393. DOI: 10.1007/s13770-019-00199-7

[146] De Lima BR, Stellet Lourenço E, De Azevedo Dos Santos JV, Rodrigues Santiago Rocha N, Mourão CF, Alves GG. The effects of platelet-rich fibrin in the behavior of mineralizing cells related to bone tissue regeneration—A scoping review of In vitro evidence. JFB [Internet]. 2023;**14**(10):503. Available from: https://www.mdpi.com/2079-4983/14/10/503

[147] D'Esposito V, Passaretti F, Perruolo G, Ambrosio MR, Valentino R, Oriente F, et al. Platelet-rich plasma increases growth and motility of adipose tissue-derived mesenchymal stem cells and controls adipocyte secretory function. Journal of Cellular Biochemistry [Internet]. 2015;**116**(10):2408-2418. DOI: 10.1002/jcb.25235

[148] Kang YH, Jeon SH, Park JY, Chung JH, Choung YH, Choung HW, et al. Platelet-rich fibrin is a bioscaffold and reservoir of growth factors for tissue regeneration. Tissue Engineering Part A [Internet]. 2011;**17**(3-4):349-359. DOI: 10.1089/ten.tea.2010.0327

[149] Aoyagi Y, Kuroda M, Asada S, Tanaka S, Konno S, Tanio M, et al. Fibrin glue is a candidate scaffold for long-term therapeutic protein expression in spontaneously differentiated adipocytes in vitro. Experimental Cell Research [Internet]. 2012;**318**(1):8-15. Available from: https://www.sciencedirect.com/science/article/pii/S0014482711004010

Chapter 2

New Formulations of Platelet-Rich Plasma: The Relevance of Extraplatelet Molecules

Jon Mercader Ruiz, Maider Beitia, Diego Delgado, Pello Sánchez, Ane Miren Bilbao, Nicolas Fiz, Beatriz Aizpurua, Juan Azofra and Mikel Sánchez

Abstract

Platelet-rich plasma (PRP) is a biological product with regenerative capacity. It is used in different fields of medicine such as traumatology, dentistry and dermatology, among others. Classically, PRP has been obtained by centrifugation, which generates a plasma enriched in platelets and their components compared to basal levels. However, this process does not enrich all the biomolecules present outside the platelets. Recently, different collection systems have been developed based on different processes such as filtration, sedimentation, ultrasound, microfluidics or water absorption. These systems often provide a more efficient collection in terms of enrichment or speed of collection. Importantly, some of them also favor the enrichment of extraplatelet components. This is potentially an advantage over other systems, given that extraplatelet factors such as IGF-1 or HGF have been reported to play a key role in contributing to the regenerative capacity of PRP.

Keywords: platelet-rich plasma, biomolecules, growth factors, cytokines, platelets

1. Introduction

In recent years, regenerative medicine has spread widely in both research and clinical use. One of the reasons is that both the goal and the treatments framed in this field can be cross-cutting and common to many medical specialties. This main objective is to restore and recover the function of damaged tissues by promoting cellular repair and regeneration processes [1]. Thus, therapies such as blood-derived or cell-based products have emerged to generate these biological processes through which different pathologies can be solved. While cell therapies are still in its infancy and have to overcome several challenges [2], blood derivatives such as platelet-rich plasma (PRP) have been applied for more than 15 years becoming a well-established treatment for certain conditions [3].

IntechOpen

However, despite the progress made in the field of PRP, there are still many questions surrounding this treatment, which hinder the achievement of optimal clinical results. Factors that affect the efficacy of PRP can arise from different sources such as the patient, the pathology, the product applied or the application protocol [4]. Indeed, the medico-scientific community has already recognized the importance of collecting and analyzing data of this nature, and that conditions the clinical outcomes of PRP treatment [5].

Much of this data focuses on aspects related to the analysis of PRP composition, such as the presence of leukocytes or platelet concentration. In fact, the platelet has been the main element to which the efficacy of PRP is attributed so far. Because of this, the goal of many PRP systems is to achieve great platelet recovery in order to achieve a high platelet concentration [6–8]. Although this may be reasonable because of the importance of platelet content in tissue repair, high platelet concentrations do not guarantee optimal cell behavior [9]. Furthermore, it is necessary to emphasize that the effect of PRP does not depend only on platelets but also on other extraplatelet elements present in the plasma [10]. The synergistic action of all the components of PRP is one of the main factors responsible for the efficacy of this treatment [11]. However, increasing the levels of plasma molecules requires the development of techniques and systems that allow not only platelet but also molecular enrichment, which is not possible with conventional centrifugation.

Therefore, the intention of this chapter is to describe the main effector components of PRP, including and highlighting the extraplatelet components. In addition, a review of current systems for obtaining PRP is also made, focusing mainly on those that propose alternative methods to centrifugation and those that aim to obtain high levels of non-platelet molecules.

2. Platelet-rich plasma

Platelet-rich plasma or PRP is a hemoderivative product classified as a biological therapy [12]. It is used in regenerative medicine due to its reparative capacity of injured tissues. Its restorative capacity lies in its enrichment in platelets and the biomolecules stored in them, such as growth factors or interleukins among others. Although this capacity has traditionally been thought to be driven by platelets and their factors, in recent years, it has been reported the essential role of the extraplatelet factors in these regenerative processes.

2.1 Platelets

Platelets are anucleate subcellular fragments derived from megakaryocytes. Megakaryocytes are large (30 μm diameter) polynucleated cells that are generated in the bone marrow and migrate to the endothelial barrier and pulmonary vasculature, where, through fragmentation, give rise to platelets [13]. These small discoid cell fragments called platelets are 2–5 μm in diameter and have a lifespan of 7–10 days [14]. They are found in the bloodstream and when blood vessels are disrupted by an injury, they adhere to the affected area by the binding of the von Willebrand factor (vWF) from the platelets to the exposed collagen of the affected vessel. In this manner, platelets aggregate with each other and plug the vessel injury, also being the first barrier of defense against external agents. Thus, platelets play an essential role in the generation of the blood clot in a wound. However, beyond that function, platelets are involved in the maintenance of hemostasis, immune system regulation and tissue repair. Notably, these functions are carried out by the molecular content of platelets.

2.2 Molecular content of the platelets

The molecular content of platelets is mainly stored in α-, δ- and λ-granules, although the most abundant are the former. The α-granules contain membrane-bound proteins (integrin and other receptors) as well as soluble bioactive proteins, such as growth factors and cytokines [15]. In turn, δ-granules, also called dense bodies, store proteins that trigger the clot formation, like bioactive amines such as serotonin and histamine, adenosine, polyphosphates and cations like calcium, among others [16]. Finally, λ-granules, also known as lysosomal type organelles, preserve the enzymes responsible for the degradation of proteins, lipids and carbohydrates to ensure the removal of affected tissue residues and infectious agents [17]. In addition, it is important to mention the presence of microvesicles, and exosomes in particular. These vesicles contain, on the one hand, the components synthesized by the megakaryocyte. Additionally, new molecular content is acquired from the medium and, in turn, released in a controlled manner as the platelet travels through the bloodstream [17–20].

When platelets are activated, these granules are released into the extraplatelet medium, providing the medium with bioactive compounds. Among these, it is included the platelet-derived growth factor (PDGF) [21]. This factor has the capacity to stimulate the chemotaxis of immune system cells, stimulate the proliferation and differentiation of mesenchymal cells, osteoblasts and fibroblasts, among others, and regulate the secretion and synthesis of collagenases and collagen, respectively. Transforming growth factor-β (TGF-β) overall promotes the proliferation and

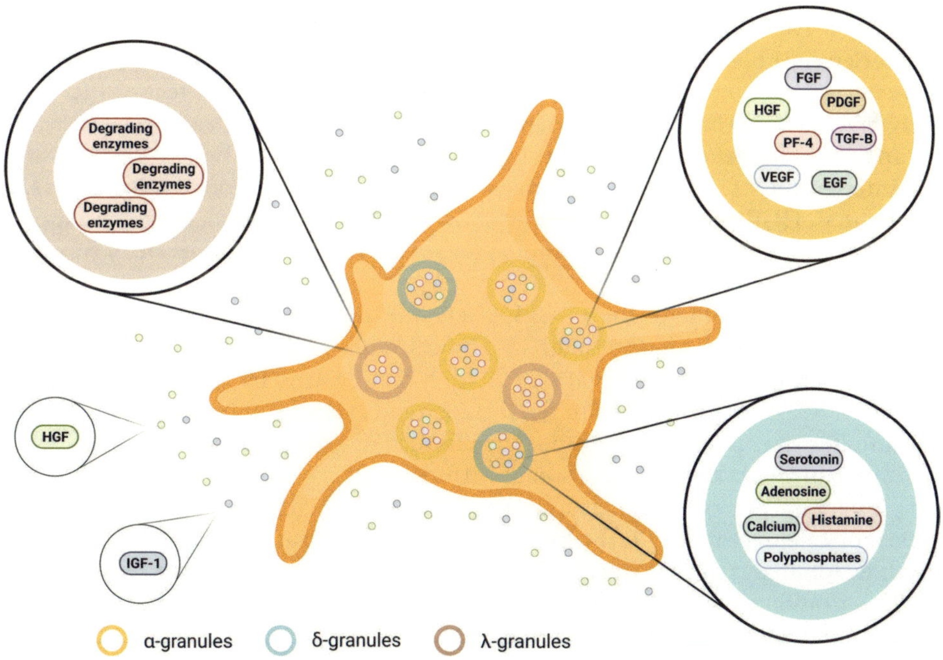

Figure 1.
Schematic representation of the platelet content. α-granules (yellow) contain mainly growth factors (PDGF, TGF-β, VEGF, among others), while δ-granules (blue) contain ADP, ATP, Ca^{2+}, neurotransmitters and hormones. Finally, λ-granules (purple) include degrading enzymes. In the extraplatelet medium other exclusive growth factors such as HGF or IGF-1 are present.

differentiation of mesenchymal stem cells, fibroblasts and keratinocytes among others, and inhibits immune system cell proliferation, stimulates collagen production, inhibits metalloproteinase activity and promotes angiogenesis. However, its effects can vary on the basis of the interacting cells and molecules [21–23]. Vascular endothelial growth factor (VEGF) promotes angiogenesis and endothelial cell proliferation and migration [24, 25]. Epidermal growth factor (EGF) acts by stimulating the proliferation of keratinocytes, endothelial cells and fibroblasts [26]. Fibroblast growth factor (FGF) promotes the proliferation and migration of fibroblasts, as well as mesenchymal cells, chondrocytes and osteoblasts [27]. Platelet factor-4 (PF-4) acts by regulating the immune system, recruiting leukocytes to the injured area [28].

The bioactive molecular content of platelets is, thus, composed of a vast number of biomolecules that overall regulate coagulation and hemostasis, tissue repair and regeneration and inflammation among others (**Figure 1**).

2.3 Extraplatelet biomolecules

Beyond the molecular content of the platelets, there are also extraplatelet growth factors and cytokines that exert essential functions in the restoration and reparation of the damaged tissues.

The hepatocyte growth factor (HGF) is present both inside and outside platelets. This factor takes an important part in the modulation of inflammatory processes. In a study by Zhang et al., they analyzed whether HGF had an anti-inflammatory function in tendons. To do this, they performed *in vitro* tests on tenocytes and *in vivo* tests on mouse's Achilles tendon. In both cases, they added, in addition to PRP, recombinant HGF protein and measured cyclooxygenase-1 (COX-1) and 2 (COX-2) and interleukin 1 beta (IL-1β) in the *in vitro* model and prostaglandin E2 (PGE2) in the *in vivo* model. The conclusion was that the anti-inflammatory effect of PRP is largely mediated by HGF in a dose-dependent manner [29, 30]. In another study, they used an *in vitro* model of chondrocytes where they found that when PRP is activated, HGF, interleukin-4 (IL4) and tumor necrosis factor alpha (TNFα), among others, are concentrated. HGF and TNFα have been shown to inhibit the nuclear factor kappa (NF-κB) pathway, thus playing an important role in the anti-inflammatory function of PRP [31].

IGF-1, in turn, is a factor found exclusively outside platelets. In fact, according to some studies, it has been found that IGF-1 levels in both PRP and platelet-poor plasma (PPP) were similar, indicating that this factor is synthesized by other cell types. Concretely, IGF-1 is synthesized in the liver, smooth muscle, chondrocytes and placenta and it is transported throughout the plasma [32–35]. Its main functions include its ability to promote the proliferation of different cell types. A study conducted in an *in vitro* model of skin fibroblasts concluded that the higher the concentration of the extraplatelet factor IGF-1, the higher the proliferation at 96 h. IGF-1 was the only growth factor analyzed that was statistically significant when it came to proliferation [10]. This proliferative capacity has been found in different cell types such as chondrocytes, tenocytes, neurons and retinal cells [36–39].

In addition to proliferation, it has also been shown to play a role in the regulation of inflammation and specifically neuroinflammation, through the interaction with the growth hormone (GH) [40–42]. Moreover, IGF-1 secreted by chondrocytes has been shown to promote increased proteoglycan and collagen II synthesis and reduce matrix metalloproteinase-13 (MMP-13) synthesis [43]. As such, it helps to reduce the harmful effects of osteoarthritis. In addition, IGF-1 lowers the production of reactive oxygen species (ROS), producing an anti-apoptotic effect in a rat model [44]. All thisimplies that IGF-1 plays an important role in regenerative processes. In fact, in a study by Ortolani et al., PRP and a solution containing PDGF and IGF-1 were added to a rabbit animal model. In the study, they observed greater tissue regeneration when cultured with PDGF and IGF-1 than when cultured with PRP or the negative control (methyl cellulose gel) [45].

3. PRP obtaining systems

At present, there is a wide range of methods to obtain PRP that can be classified as standard and novel. In accordance with this, there are a plenty of commercially available kits to obtain these products, which differ from each other according to certain variables such as platelet, leukocyte and erythrocyte content. On the one hand, it is important to mention that although PRP may contain different concentrations of platelets, an increase in platelets is not directly related to better effectiveness. This could be explained by the possible antagonistic effect that an excess of certain growth factors may cause [46]. Different studies have shown that the optimal platelet concentration could be between 1.5 and 6 times compared to baseline levels in many treatments, with 1.5–3 being the most favorable concentration in most pathologies [9, 47–50]. Regarding leukocytes, there is controversy as to whether their presence could have a beneficial or detrimental effect on the effectiveness of PRP. While some studies say that leukocytes may have an advantage in the antimicrobial response and, therefore, favor the release of more growth factors and proteinases [17, 51], others claim that leukocytes may increase the inflammatory response, as they induce the release of pro-inflammatory cytokines [52–54]. In addition, they may increase ROS levels by the action of the neutrophils and affect the wound-healing process [55]. Regarding the presence of erythrocytes, the vast majority of studies state that it can lead to hemolysis and erythrocytosis, generating products that promote inflammation, cellular stress and even cell death [50, 56]. **Table 1** lists the systems described below and their properties.

3.1 Standard systems for PRP obtaining

Most of the systems currently used commercially to obtain PRP are based on the centrifugation of blood and subsequent separation of the fractions obtained. The product varies depending on the speed and time parameters applied in the centrifugation, as well as the number of centrifugations carried out in the process (**Figure 2**). Furthermore, it is important to highlight the collection of the sample, since depending on the fraction or fractions collected, the composition of the PRP may vary. These collection steps have been modified to obtain different commercial PRP formulations. In fact, the final formulation may vary in its content in various aspects such as the number of platelets and the presence or absence of white and red blood cells [72, 73]. Furthermore, depending on the processing of the sample after centrifugation, it is possible to obtain, in addition to liquid formulations, gel formulations for wound application [74].

Although centrifugation is the standard method for obtaining PRP, in recent years different methods have been investigated to obtain it more efficiently. These systems, in addition to minimizing user intervention, allow obtaining larger or smaller

Commercial name or developers	System	Processing time	Platelet fold	Extraplatelet molecule concentration	Cytokine enrichment	Ref.
Jacofsky et al.	Filtration	7 min	4.3 ± 0.6	No	No	[57]
Schmolz et al.	Sedimentation and filtration	60 min	—	No	No	[58]
Wu et al.	Ultrasounds	10 min	2.11 ± 0.1	No	No	[59]
Gifford et al.	Sedimentation	180 min	5.45	No	No	[60]
Laxmi et al.	Microfluidics	0.4 mL min^{-1}	3–8	No	No	[61]
Dickson et al.	Microdevice filtering system	30 min	Variable	No	No	[62]
Kim et al.	Lab-on-a-disc filter system unit	10–15 min	>4	No	No	[63]
nStride®	Absorption by polyacrylamide gel	30–45 min	2.7 ± 0.6	Yes	Yes	[64, 65]
Orthokine®	Monocyte activation by $CrSO_4$ spheres	24 h	—	—	Yes	[66]
Qrem®	Anabolic and anti-inflammatory cytokine solution	36 min	—	No	Yes	[67]
ART PRP Plus®	Filtration	15–20 min	—	Yes	No	[68]
Mercader Ruiz et al.	Evaporation	20 min	2	Yes	—	[69]
Mercader Ruiz et al.	Filtration	90 min	2	Yes	—	[70]
Mercader Ruiz et al.	Absorption	20 min	2	Yes	—	[71]

Table 1.
Comparison of the different systems analyzed for the production of PRP for the concentration of platelet and plasma molecules. Different parameters such as type of PRP obtaining system, platelet enrichment fold, time of processing, modulation of extraplatelet factors and concentration of cytokines are evaluated.

volumes of PRP depending on the desired application. The systems developed make use of filtration, sedimentation, ultrasound and even microfluidic systems for the separation and elimination of erythrocytes and leukocytes and platelet concentration.

3.2 Novel systems for PRP obtaining

3.2.1 Platelet-derived factor enrichment

Concerning to novel methods for the obtaining of PRP formulations, Jacofsky et al. developed a disposable system to achieve platelet enrichment by filtration. To do this, 60 mL of blood was drawn into a syringe. The contents of the syringe, after mixing them with an aqueous solution, were then passed through a blood filter where the platelets were trapped and all other blood components were removed. To recover

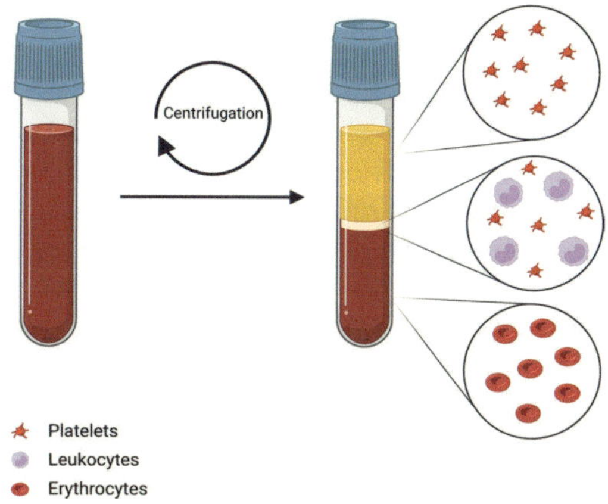

Figure 2.
Schematic representation of the centrifugation method to obtain the PRP. The blood collecting tube is centrifuged at a specific speed and time at certain cycles. After that, blood is fragmented into different layers. The lower one corresponds to the erythrocyte layer; the small white layer, or buffy coat, contains mostly erythrocytes and platelets; the upper layer corresponds to plasma and contains a gradient of platelets with higher concentration as it approaches the leukocyte layer.

the platelets, 7 mL aqueous solution was added, allowing their release and subsequent recovery. This PRP was compared to another one achieved by standard centrifugation where the same volume of PRP was obtained. Although the two products showed similar platelet levels, the collection time was significantly reduced in the new system, from 14 to 7 min [57].

Another system developed by Schmolz describes a PRP obtained by sedimentation and filtration. In short, they collected 8 mL of blood in a syringe with anticoagulant and a sedimentation accelerator. Thus, using a device developed by the group, after 1 h of incubation they achieve a separation of the different components of the blood, which allows the collection of the plasma fraction. This plasma was passed through a filter that traps platelets and removes all traces of the sedimentation accelerator by means of a washing buffer. They then added an aqueous solution to dissolve the platelets and collect the enriched fraction. Subsequent analyses were performed in comparison to baseline levels of unenriched plasma. The results of the study showed a significant increase in TGFβ and PDGF in the new product, compared to baseline levels [58].

In another system, PRP was obtained by ultrasound technology. They collected blood in a 10 mL syringe and applied ultrasounds using two piezoelectric ceramics to generate pressure nodes, causing the red blood cells to settle and, thus, fractionate the blood. In this manner, they obtained 4 mL PRP in 10 minutes. They compared this product with a PRP obtained using a commercial product that requires double centrifugation. Although the results showed a higher platelet fold increase in the new PRP than in the standard double centrifugation, the levels of the platelet growth factor PDGF were not increased [59].

Gifford et al. proposed a system for obtaining PRP by sedimentation and subsequent passage through a microfluidic device. A total of 250 mL of blood was drawn in a bag for blood collection and allowed to settle at a 10° inclination with the aid of two plates exerting pressure on the bag, so that the blood was segmented into fractions of erythrocytes, leukocytes and plasma. Sedimentation took 2.5 h, after which the plasma fraction was recovered. It was then passed through a microfluidic system where platelets were concentrated. As a comparison control, PRP obtained by a standard centrifugation system was used. Measurement of platelet counts revealed that, although both systems enriched the platelets, the standard PRP performed better. However, the new method had a lower percentage of platelets activated by the collection process than the centrifugation-based one [60].

An alternative method, also based on a microfluidic device, was developed by Laxmi et al. This polydimethylsiloxane (PDMS) device enables the Fåhraeus effect, which is based on the fact that when blood is applied at a certain flow rate in a small diameter channel, red blood cells are deformed causing them to move through the center of the channel [75]. Platelets, on the other hand, move through the periphery, where the plasma collection outlets of the channel are located. In this way, a plasma enriched in platelets, but devoid of red blood cells, is obtained. The results showed a platelet enrichment of 8.7% compared to baseline levels [61].

Dickson et al. proposed a microdevice that uses a filter to enrich platelets. To obtain PRP, they apply a constant blood flow through a device containing two filters. In the first one, the red blood cells are retained and only the plasma with platelets passes through to the second filter. In the second filter, only the plasma water passes through, but not the platelets, which are continuously transferred to a collector. The remaining plasma without platelets rejoins the whole blood to continue filtering continuously. It was found that by varying the size of the device and the flow rate applied, a high throughput could be achieved, obtaining up to 50 mL of plasma in as little as half an hour [62].

Something similar was proposed by Kim et al., using a device with two filters to first remove leukocytes and erythrocytes and then part of the plasma, concentrating the PRP. In this case, they used a lab-on-a-disc with a CD format device where they made use of tangential flow filtration. Using this system, a fold of four was obtained compared to baseline levels [63].

3.2.2 Platelet- and extraplatelet-derived factors and cytokine enrichment

To our knowledge, none of these systems have been commercialized and remain in the research phase. All of them focus solely on the enrichment of platelet components, but none take into account bioactive molecules outside platelets, such as IGF-1 and HGF. It is also important to note that pro- and anti-inflammatory cytokines are concentrated during the production of PRP. These play a key role in different biological processes, especially in the inflammatory response. However, there are commercially available novel devices that regulate the concentration of these cytokines in the final formulation.

On the one hand, Zimmer Biomed marketed a protein-based solution called nStride® where PRP enriched in anabolic growth factors and anti-inflammatory cytokines is obtained. To do this, PRP is generated by centrifugation and then passed through a polyacrylamide gel that absorbs part of the water. In addition to platelets, this system concentrates both red and white blood cells [64, 65].

The Orthokine® kit, on the other hand, obtains a serum with an increase in anti-inflammatory cytokines, such as IL-4, IL-10 and IL-1RA. To do this, they incubate a syringe of blood with $CrSO_4$ spheres for 24 hours at 37°C. This causes the monocytes to become activated and the cytokines are released into the blood [76]. Then, by centrifugation, a plasma fraction enriched in anti-inflammatory cytokines is obtained. As a result, it is possible to enrich 140-fold IL-1RA, which, being an IL-1β antagonist, eliminates IL-1β as well [66].

Qrem® cytokine kit is an automatic device that requires no user intervention. It has two chambers, one for the separation of blood components and the other for the activation of both platelets and white blood cells, for the subsequent production of a serum enriched in growth factors and cytokines [67].

These commercial kits focus primarily on cytokine modulation. However, they do not focus on enriching extraplatelet factors. In fact, tissue repair is favored by the physiological balance of growth factors and cytokines, which contain anabolic and catabolic functions in supraphysiologic concentrations, directly into the site of injury optimizing the healing environment. Preserving a natural ratio of these biomolecules may allow the maintenance of the body's homeostatic environment, which theoretically would provide an abundance of healing factors without disrupting *in vivo* cellular functions [55, 77, 78].

Concerning the above mention molecular balance, Celling Biosciences launched a device called ART PRP Plus® that is based on filtration. The device is filled with blood, centrifuged and the plasma obtained is passed through fibers with a pore size of 25 kDa several times to remove some of the water and keep all the molecules above this size. This results in PRP enriched not only in platelets but also in the growth factors VEGF, PDGF, TGFβ, alpha-2-macroglobulin (A2M), IL-1RA and fibrinogen. However, this system does not concentrate on the extraplatelet factor IGF-1, as it is smaller than the pore size of the fibers [34, 68].

Recently, new systems have been developed that focus on obtaining PRP by removing water to concentrate all components equally. For this purpose, three water removal systems have been used. The first common step in all three methods is to perform a centrifugation to obtain a PRP with blood-like levels of platelets. One system consists of evaporating the water from the plasma using a rotary evaporator, after applying a certain temperature and pressure. The second method uses centrifuge filtration units to remove some of the water content from the plasma. The last method is based on the use of acrylamide hydrogels to absorb approximately half of the plasma water. Although all three systems are able to enrich platelets and total plasma proteins in a similar way, they do not all succeed in concentrating growth factors equally. The evaporation method fails to concentrate HGF, while the other two systems do. Platelet activation is also higher in the evaporation system, which may be a drawback. In terms of the ability of the final PRP to promote the proliferation of dermal fibroblasts, the absorption system showed greater proliferative capacity, although in all three cases, it was better than that of a standard PRP [69–71].

4. PRP classification

Taking into account all these systems and the fact that the presence or absence and even the level of enrichment of different cellular components can affect the efficacy of the PRP product, the comparison between different products is difficult. This would explain the controversy in the literature on the properties of PRP. Because of this various classification systems have attempted to classify and code PRP products for consistency in both application and research.

Thus, Dohan Ehrenfest et al. proposed four categories of platelet concentrates depending on their leucocyte and fibrin content [79, 80]. Years later, Mishra et al. [81] and DeLong et al. [82] also gave importance to the activation of PRP in addition to the number of platelets. In the following classifications, there was also mentioned the presence of erythrocytes [83], the recovery efficiency or centrifugation and application methods addressed [84, 85], trying to classify as much as possible the different PRP products.

4.1 Universal classification system

After these classification systems, Kon et al. proposed a way of PRP coding by which all basic as well as clinical research groups, could make comparisons between results [86]. This system proposed the assignment of a six-digit code grouped in pairs to each PRP that indicates parameters of several variables with the aim of unifying the way PRP is classified for comparison. The code provides the number of basal and enriched platelets, the presence or absence of leukocytes and erythrocytes, and whether platelet activation has been carried out and, if so, which method has been used.

In addition, it is accompanied by informative tables that include data on the preparation and application of PRP, depending on whether the study is *in vitro*, *in vivo* or clinical. Finally, the nature of this system allows the code to evolve and expand to take into account future factors such as the extraplatelet molecules discussed in this chapter. Thus, this system extends and adapts the parameters for the Studies Evaluating Biologics in Orthopedics (MIBO) system to the PRP [87].

5. Conclusions

In conclusion, contrary to what has been considered in the past, platelet factors are not the only ones that play an important role in PRP but also extraplatelet factors are of importance, as demonstrated in multiple studies conducted in recent years. These molecules could enhance PRP effects such as cellular modulation, which would have an impact on its therapeutic potential. Thus, the development of novel systems that allow the enrichment of these factors is encouraged for their potential to improve the biological therapies.

Conflict of interest

The authors declare no conflict of interest.

Author details

Jon Mercader Ruiz[1†], Maider Beitia[1†], Diego Delgado[1], Pello Sánchez[1,2], Ane Miren Bilbao[2], Nicolas Fiz[2], Beatriz Aizpurua[2], Juan Azofra[2] and Mikel Sánchez[1,2*]

1 Advanced Biological Therapy Unit, Hospital Vithas Vitoria, Vitoria-Gasteiz, Spain

2 Arthroscopic Surgery Unit, Hospital Vithas Vitoria, Vitoria-Gasteiz, Spain

*Address all correspondence to: mikel.sanchez@ucatrauma.com

† These authors contributed equally to this work.

References

[1] Salgado AJ, Oliveira JM, Martins A, Teixeira FG, Silva NA, Neves NM, et al. Tissue engineering and regenerative medicine: Past, present, and future. International Review of Neurobiology. 2013;**108**:1-33. DOI: 10.1016/B978-0-12-410499-0.00001-0

[2] Vizoso FJ, Costa LA, Eiro N. New era of mesenchymal stem cell-based medicine: Basis, challenges and prospects. Revista Clínica Española. 2023;**223**:619-628. DOI: 10.1016/j.rceng.2023.11.002

[3] Cole BJ, Gilat R, DiFiori J, Rodeo SA, Bedi A. The 2020 NBA orthobiologics consensus statement. Orthopaedic Journal of Sports Medicine. 2021;**9**:23259671211002296. DOI: 10.1177/23259671211002296

[4] Sánchez M, Jorquera C, de Dicastillo LL, Fiz N, Knörr J, Beitia M, et al. Real-world evidence to assess the effectiveness of platelet-rich plasma in the treatment of knee degenerative pathology: A prospective observational study. Therapeutic Advances in Musculoskeletal Disease. 2022;**14**:1759720X221100304. DOI: 10.1177/1759720X221100304

[5] Hurley ET, Sherman SL, Stokes DJ, Rodeo SA, Shapiro SA, Mautner K, et al. Experts achieve consensus on a majority of statements regarding platelet-rich plasma treatments for treatment of musculoskeletal pathology. Arthroscopy: The Journal of Arthroscopic and Related Surgery: Official Publication of the Arthroscopy Association of North America and the International Arthroscopy Association. 2023:S0749-8063(23)00673-4;**40**:470-477.e1. DOI: 10.1016/j.arthro.2023.08.020

[6] Muthu S, Krishnan A, Ramanathan KR. Standardization and validation of a conventional high yield platelet-rich plasma preparation protocol. Annals of Medicine and Surgery. 2022;**82**:104593. DOI: 10.1016/j.amsu.2022.104593

[7] Perez AGM, Lana JFSD, Rodrigues AA, Luzo ACM, Belangero WD, Santana MHA. Relevant aspects of centrifugation step in the preparation of platelet-rich plasma. ISRN Hematology. 2014;**2014**:176060. DOI: 10.1155/2014/176060

[8] Rossi R, Garg AK, Kurtzman GM. Novel protocols for the production of autologous blood concentrates with High platelet volume. Compendium of Continuing Education in Dentistry (Jamesburg, N.J.: 1995). 2022;**43**:140-145; quiz 146

[9] Giusti I, D'Ascenzo S, Mancò A, Di Stefano G, Di Francesco M, Rughetti A, et al. Platelet concentration in platelet-rich plasma affects tenocyte behavior in vitro. BioMed Research International. 2014;**2014**:630870. DOI: 10.1155/2014/630870

[10] Beitia M, Delgado D, Mercader J, Sánchez P, López de Dicastillo L, Sánchez M. Action of platelet-rich plasma on in vitro cellular bioactivity: More than platelets. International Journal of Molecular Sciences. 2023;**24**:5367. DOI: 10.3390/ijms24065367

[11] van der Bijl I, Vlig M, Middelkoop E, de Korte D. Allogeneic platelet-rich plasma (PRP) is superior to platelets or plasma alone in stimulating fibroblast proliferation and migration, angiogenesis, and chemotaxis as relevant processes for wound healing. Transfusion (Paris). 2019;**59**:3492-3500. DOI: 10.1111/trf.15535

[12] Alves R, Grimalt R. A review of platelet-rich plasma: History, biology, mechanism of action, and classification. Skin Appendage Disorders. 2018;**4**:18-24. DOI: 10.1159/000477353

[13] Patel SR, Hartwig JH, Italiano JE. The biogenesis of platelets from megakaryocyte proplatelets. The Journal of Clinical Investigation. 2005;**115**:3348-3354. DOI: 10.1172/JCI26891

[14] Josefsson EC, Vainchenker W, James C. Regulation of platelet production and life span: Role of Bcl-xL and potential implications for human platelet diseases. International Journal of Molecular Sciences. 2020;**21**:7591. DOI: 10.3390/ijms21207591

[15] Blair P, Flaumenhaft R. Platelet α–granules: Basic biology and clinical correlates. Blood Reviews. 2009;**23**:177-189. DOI: 10.1016/j.blre.2009.04.001

[16] Sharda A, Flaumenhaft R. The life cycle of platelet granules. F1000Research. 2018;**7**:236. DOI: 10.12688/f1000research.13283.1

[17] Pavlovic V, Ciric M, Jovanovic V, Stojanovic P. Platelet rich plasma: A short overview of certain bioactive components. Open Medicine. 2016;**11**:242-247. DOI: 10.1515/med-2016-0048

[18] Boilard E, Nigrovic PA. Platelets. In: Kelley and Firestein's Textbook of Rheumatology. Amsterdam: Elsevier; 2017. pp. 264-273.e3. DOI: 10.1016/B978-0-323-31696-5.00016-4

[19] Boswell SG, Cole BJ, Sundman EA, Karas V, Fortier LA. Platelet-rich plasma: A milieu of bioactive factors. Arthroscopy: The Journal of Arthroscopic and Related Surgery: Official Publication of the Arthroscopy Association of North America and the International Arthroscopy Association. 2012;**28**:429-439. DOI: 10.1016/j.arthro.2011.10.018

[20] Maynard DM, Heijnen HFG, Horne MK, White JG, Gahl WA. Proteomic analysis of platelet alpha-granules using mass spectrometry. Journal of Thrombosis and Haemostasis. 2007;**5**:1945-1955. DOI: 10.1111/j.1538-7836.2007.02690.x

[21] Qian Y, Han Q, Chen W, Song J, Zhao X, Ouyang Y, et al. Platelet-rich plasma derived growth factors contribute to stem cell differentiation in musculoskeletal regeneration. Frontiers in Chemistry. 2017;**5**:89. DOI: 10.3389/fchem.2017.00089

[22] Yang EY, Moses HL. Transforming growth factor beta 1-induced changes in cell migration, proliferation, and angiogenesis in the chicken chorioallantoic membrane. The Journal of Cell Biology. 1990;**111**:731-741. DOI: 10.1083/jcb.111.2.731

[23] Morikawa M, Derynck R, Miyazono K. TGF-β and the TGF-β family: Context-dependent roles in cell and tissue physiology. Cold Spring Harbor Perspectives in Biology. 2016;**8**:a021873. DOI: 10.1101/cshperspect.a021873

[24] Ferrara N. Role of vascular endothelial growth factor in the regulation of angiogenesis. Kidney International. 1999;**56**:794-814. DOI: 10.1046/j.1523-1755.1999.00610.x

[25] Ballmer-Hofer K. Vascular endothelial growth factor, from basic research to clinical applications. International Journal of Molecular Sciences. 2018;**19**:3750. DOI: 10.3390/ijms19123750

[26] Kurten RC, Chowdhury P, Sanders RC, Pittman LM, Sessions LW,

Chambers TC, et al. Coordinating epidermal growth factor-induced motility promotes efficient wound closure. American Journal of Physiology-Cell Physiology. 2005;**288**:C109-C121. DOI: 10.1152/ajpcell.00024.2003

[27] Farooq M, Khan AW, Kim MS, Choi S. The role of fibroblast growth factor (FGF) signaling in tissue repair and regeneration. Cells. 2021;**10**:3242. DOI: 10.3390/cells10113242

[28] Field DJ, Aggrey-Amable AA, Blick SK, Ture SK, Johanson A, Cameron SJ, et al. Platelet factor 4 increases bone marrow B cell development and differentiation. Immunologic Research. 2017;**65**:1089-1094. DOI: 10.1007/s12026-017-8951-x

[29] Zhang J, Middleton KK, Fu FH, Im H-J, Wang JH-C. HGF mediates the anti-inflammatory effects of PRP on injured tendons. PLoS ONE. 2013;**8**:e67303. DOI: 10.1371/journal.pone.0067303

[30] Nakamura T. Structure and function of hepatocyte growth factor. Progress in Growth Factor Research. 1991;**3**:67-85. DOI: 10.1016/0955-2235(91)90014-U

[31] Bendinelli P, Matteucci E, Dogliotti G, Corsi MM, Banfi G, Maroni P, et al. Molecular basis of anti-inflammatory action of platelet-rich plasma on human chondrocytes: Mechanisms of NF-κB inhibition via HGF. Journal of Cellular Physiology. 2010;**225**:757-766. DOI: 10.1002/jcp.22274

[32] El-Sharkawy H, Kantarci A, Deady J, Hasturk H, Liu H, Alshahat M, et al. Platelet-rich plasma: Growth factors and pro- and anti-inflammatory properties. Journal of Periodontology. 2007;**78**:661-669. DOI: 10.1902/jop.2007.060302

[33] Wen Y-H, Lin W-Y, Lin C-J, Sun Y-C, Chang P-Y, Wang H-Y, et al. Sustained or higher levels of growth factors in platelet-rich plasma during 7-day storage. Clinica Chimica Acta: International Journal of Clinical Chemistry. 2018;**483**:89-93. DOI: 10.1016/j.cca.2018.04.027

[34] Laron Z. Insulin-like growth factor 1 (IGF-1): A growth hormone. Molecular Pathology. 2001;**54**:311-316

[35] Nilsson A, Isgaard J, Lindahl A, Dahlström A, Skottner A, Isaksson OG. Regulation by growth hormone of number of chondrocytes containing IGF-I in rat growth plate. Science. 1986;**233**:571-574. DOI: 10.1126/science.3523759

[36] de Figueiredo CS, Raony Í, Medina SV, de Mello SE, Dos Santos AA, Giestal-de-Araujo E. Insulin-like growth factor-1 stimulates retinal cell proliferation via activation of multiple signaling pathways. Current Research in Neurobiology. 2023;**4**:100068. DOI: 10.1016/j.crneur.2022.100068

[37] Zhang B, Hu L, Zhang J, Wu H, Li W, Gou L, et al. Insulin growth factor-1 enhances proliferation and inhibits apoptosis of neural progenitor cells by phosphorylation of Akt/mTOR/p70S6K molecules and triggering intrinsic apoptosis signaling pathway. Cell and Tissue Banking. 2022;**23**:459-472. DOI: 10.1007/s10561-021-09956-2

[38] Zhong J, Zhang J, Zhou Z, Pan D, Zhao D, Dong H, et al. Novel insights into the effect of deer IGF-1 on chondrocyte viability and IL-1β-induced inflammation response. Journal of Biochemical and Molecular Toxicology. 2023;**37**:e23227. DOI: 10.1002/jbt.23227

[39] Disser NP, Sugg KB, Talarek JR, Sarver DC, Rourke BJ, Mendias CL. Insulin-like growth factor 1 signaling in tenocytes is required for adult tendon growth. FASEB Journal: Official

Publication of the Federation of American Societies for Experimental Biology. 2019;**33**:12680-12695. DOI: 10.1096/fj.201901503R

[40] Labandeira-Garcia JL, Costa-Besada MA, Labandeira CM, Villar-Cheda B, Rodríguez-Perez AI. Insulin-like growth factor-1 and neuroinflammation. Frontiers in Aging Neuroscience. 2017;**9**:365

[41] Sukhanov S, Higashi Y, Shai S-Y, Vaughn C, Mohler J, Li Y, et al. IGF-1 reduces inflammatory responses, suppresses oxidative stress, and decreases atherosclerosis progression in ApoE-deficient mice. Arteriosclerosis, Thrombosis, and Vascular Biology. 2007;**27**:2684-2690. DOI: 10.1161/ATVBAHA.107.156257

[42] Heemskerk VH, Daemen MA, Buurman WA. Insulin-like growth factor-1 (IGF-1) and growth hormone (GH) in immunity and inflammation. Cytokine & Growth Factor Reviews. 1999;**10**:5-14. DOI: 10.1016/s1359-6101(98)00022-7

[43] Zhang M, Zhou Q, Liang Q-Q, Li C-G, Holz JD, Tang D, et al. IGF-1 regulation of type II collagen and MMP-13 expression in rat endplate chondrocytes via distinct signaling pathways. Osteoarthritis and Cartilage. 2009;**17**:100-106. DOI: 10.1016/j.joca.2008.05.007

[44] Hossain MA, Adithan A, Alam MJ, Kopalli SR, Kim B, Kang C-W, et al. IGF-1 facilitates cartilage reconstruction by regulating PI3K/AKT, MAPK, and NF-kB signaling in rabbit osteoarthritis. Journal of Inflammation Research. 2021;**14**:3555-3568. DOI: 10.2147/JIR.S316756

[45] Ortolani E, Guerriero M, Coli A, Giannuario AD, Minniti G, Polimeni A. Effect of PDGF, IGF-1 and PRP on the implant osseointegration. An histological and immunohistochemical study in rabbits. Annali di Stomatologia (Roma). 2014;**5**:66

[46] Verma R, Kandwal A, Negi G, Chandra H. Factors affecting the quantity and quality of platelet-rich plasma and platelet-derived growth factor-BB: An observational study. Journal of Bio-X Research. 2021;**4**:67. DOI: 10.1097/JBR.0000000000000091

[47] Sánchez M, Anitua E, Azofra J, Andía I, Padilla S, Mujika I. Comparison of surgically repaired Achilles tendon tears using platelet-rich fibrin matrices. The American Journal of Sports Medicine. 2007;**35**:245-251. DOI: 10.1177/0363546506294078

[48] Torricelli P, Fini M, Filardo G, Tschon M, Pischedda M, Pacorini A, et al. Regenerative medicine for the treatment of musculoskeletal overuse injuries in competition horses. International Orthopaedics. 2011;**35**:1569-1576. DOI: 10.1007/s00264-011-1237-3

[49] Hee HT, Majd ME, Holt RT, Myers L. Do autologous growth factors enhance transforaminal lumbar interbody fusion? European Spine Journal: Official Publication of the European Spine Society, the European Spinal Deformity Society, and the European Section of the Cervical Spine Research Society. 2003;**12**:400-407. DOI: 10.1007/s00586-003-0548-5

[50] Everts PA, Malanga GA, Paul RV, Rothenberg JB, Stephens N, Mautner KR. Assessing clinical implications and perspectives of the pathophysiological effects of erythrocytes and plasma free hemoglobin in autologous biologics for use in musculoskeletal regenerative medicine therapies. A review.

Regenerative Therapy. 2019;**11**:56-64. DOI: 10.1016/j.reth.2019.03.009

[51] Zimmermann R, Jakubietz R, Jakubietz M, Strasser E, Schlegel A, Wiltfang J, et al. Different preparation methods to obtain platelet components as a source of growth factors for local application. Transfusion (Paris). 2001;**41**:1217-1224. DOI: 10.1046/j.1537-2995.2001.41101217.x

[52] Wang S, Fan W, Jia J, Ma L, Yu J, Wang C. Is exclusion of leukocytes from platelet-rich plasma (PRP) a better choice for early intervertebral disc regeneration? Stem Cell Research & Therapy. 2018;**9**:199. DOI: 10.1186/s13287-018-0937-7

[53] Xu Z, Yin W, Zhang Y, Qi X, Chen Y, Xie X, et al. Comparative evaluation of leukocyte- and platelet-rich plasma and pure platelet-rich plasma for cartilage regeneration. Scientific Reports. 2017;**7**:43301. DOI: 10.1038/srep43301

[54] Liu T, Zhang L, Joo D, Sun S-C. NF-κB signaling in inflammation. Signal Transduction and Targeted Therapy. 2017;**2**:1-9. DOI: 10.1038/sigtrans.2017.23

[55] Anitua E, Andia I, Ardanza B, Nurden P, Nurden A. Autologous platelets as a source of proteins for healing and tissue regeneration. Thrombosis and Haemostasis. 2004;**91**:4-15. DOI: 10.1160/TH03-07-0440

[56] Braun HJ, Kim HJ, Chu CR, Dragoo JL. The effect of platelet-rich plasma formulations and blood products on human synoviocytes. The American Journal of Sports Medicine. 2014;**42**:1204-1210. DOI: 10.1177/0363546514525593

[57] Jacofsky D, Scott M, Smith R, Jennings L, Sowemimo-Coker S, Long M, et al. Method to Prepare Platelet Rich Concentrate From Blood Without a Centrifuge. Vol. 30. Poster presented in the 51st Annual Meeting of the Orthopaedic Research Society. Feb 2005. pp. 20-35

[58] Schmolz M, Stein GM, Hübner W-D. An innovative, centrifugation-free method to prepare human platelet mediator concentrates showing activities comparable to platelet-rich plasma. Wounds: A Compendium of Clinical Research and Practice. 2011;**23**:13

[59] Wu Y, Kanna MS, Liu C, Zhou Y, Chan CK. Generation of autologous platelet-rich plasma by the ultrasonic standing waves. IEEE Transactions on Biomedical Engineering. 2016;**63**:1642-1652. DOI: 10.1109/TBME.2015.2449832

[60] Gifford SC, Strachan BC, Xia H, Vörös E, Torabian K, Tomasino TA, et al. A portable system for processing donated whole blood into high quality components without centrifugation. PLoS ONE. 2018;**13**:e0190827. DOI: 10.1371/journal.pone.0190827

[61] Laxmi V, Tripathi S, Joshi SS, Agrawal A. Separation and enrichment of platelets from whole blood using a PDMS-based passive microdevice. Industrial and Engineering Chemistry Research. 2020;**59**:4792-4801. DOI: 10.1021/acs.iecr.0c00502

[62] Dickson MN, Amar L, Hill M, Schwartz J, Leonard EF. A scalable, micropore, platelet rich plasma separation device. Biomedical Microdevices. 2012;**14**:1095-1102. DOI: 10.1007/s10544-012-9675-2

[63] Kim C-J, Ki DY, Park J, Sunkara V, Kim T-H, Min Y, et al. Fully automated platelet isolation on a centrifugal microfluidic device for molecular diagnostics. Lab on a Chip. 2020;**20**:949-957. DOI: 10.1039/C9LC01140D

[64] Higgins JC, Woodell-May J, Hoeppner JC. Use of a Device for Obtaining Interleukin-1 Receptor Antagonist Rich Solutions. EP2567692A1; 2013

[65] Muir SM, Reisbig N, Baria M, Kaeding C, Bertone AL. The concentration of plasma provides additional bioactive proteins in platelet and autologous protein solutions. The American Journal of Sports Medicine. 2019;**47**:1955-1963. DOI: 10.1177/0363546519849671

[66] Meijer H, Reinecke J, Becker C, Tholen G, Wehling P. The production of anti-inflammatory cytokines in whole blood by physico-chemical induction. Inflammation Research: Official Journal of the European Histamine Research Society … [et al.]. 2003;**52**:404-407. DOI: 10.1007/s00011-003-1197-1

[67] Qrem Cytokine. 2023. Available from: https://qrem-regenerative.com/ [Accessed July 7, 2023]

[68] Kyle MR, Coull T. Fluid Concentrator, Autologous Concentrated Body Fluids, and Uses Thereof. WO2009002849A2; 2008

[69] Mercader Ruiz J, Beitia M, Delgado D, Sánchez P, Sánchez MB, Oraa J, et al. Method to obtain a plasma rich in platelet- and plasma-growth factors based on water evaporation. PLoS One. 21 Feb 2024;**19**(2):e0297001. DOI: 10.1371/journal.pone.0297001. PMID: 38381708; PMCID: PMC10880971

[70] Mercader Ruiz J, Beitia M, Delgado D, Sánchez P, Guadilla J, Pérez de Arrilucea C, et al. Method based on ultrafiltration to obtain a plasma rich in platelet and plasma growth factors. Journal of Clinical Medicine. 2023;**12**:5941. DOI: 10.3390/jcm12185941

[71] Mercader Ruiz J, Beitia M, Delgado D, Sánchez P, Arnaiz MJ, López de Dicastillo L, et al. New formulation of platelet-rich plasma enriched in platelet and extraplatelet biomolecules using hydrogels. International Journal of Molecular Sciences. 2023;**24**:13811. DOI: 10.3390/ijms241813811

[72] Collins T, Alexander D, Barkatali B. Platelet-rich plasma: A narrative review. EFORT Open Reviews. 2021;**6**:225-235. DOI: 10.1302/2058-5241.6.200017

[73] Magalon J, Brandin T, Francois P, Degioanni C, De Maria L, Grimaud F, et al. Technical and biological review of authorized medical devices for platelets-rich plasma preparation in the field of regenerative medicine. Platelets. 2021;**32**:200-208. DOI: 10.1080/09537104.2020.1832653

[74] Gude W, Hagan D, Abood F, Clausen P. Aurix gel is an effective intervention for chronic diabetic foot ulcers: A pragmatic randomized controlled trial. Advances in Skin & Wound Care. 2019;**32**:416-426. DOI: 10.1097/01.ASW.0000577140.19174.9e

[75] Fåhraeus R. The suspension stability of the blood. Physiological Reviews. 1929;**9**:241-274. DOI: 10.1152/physrev.1929.9.2.241

[76] Schutte RJ, Parisi-Amon A, Reichert WM. Cytokine profiling using monocytes/macrophages cultured on common biomaterials with a range of surface chemistries. Journal of Biomedical Materials Research. Part A. 2009;**88**:128-139. DOI: 10.1002/jbm.a.31863

[77] Creaney L, Hamilton B. Growth factor delivery methods in the management of sports injuries: The state of play. British Journal of Sports Medicine. 2008;**42**:314-320. DOI: 10.1136/bjsm.2007.040071

[78] Mishra A, Woodall J, Vieira A. Treatment of tendon and muscle using platelet-rich plasma. Clinics in Sports Medicine. 2009;**28**:113-125. DOI: 10.1016/j.csm.2008.08.007

[79] Dohan Ehrenfest DM, Rasmusson L, Albrektsson T. Classification of platelet concentrates: From pure platelet-rich plasma (P-PRP) to leucocyte- and platelet-rich fibrin (L-PRF). Trends in Biotechnology. 2009;**27**:158-167. DOI: 10.1016/j.tibtech.2008.11.009

[80] Marín, Fermín T, Calcei JG, Della Vedova F, Martinez Cano JP, Arias Calderon C, Imam MA, et al. Review of Dohan Eherenfest et al. (2009) on "Classification of platelet concentrates: From pure platelet-rich plasma (P-PRP) to leucocyte- and platelet-rich fibrin (L-PRF)". Journal of ISAKOS: Joint Disorders and Orthopaedic Sports Medicine. 2023;**9**:S2059-7754(23)00545-X. DOI: 10.1016/j.jisako.2023.07.010

[81] Mishra A, Harmon K, Woodall J, Vieira A. Sports medicine applications of platelet rich plasma. Current Pharmaceutical Biotechnology. 2012;**13**:1185-1195. DOI: 10.2174/138920112800624283

[82] DeLong JM, Russell RP, Mazzocca AD. Platelet-rich plasma: The PAW classification system. Arthroscopy: The Journal of Arthroscopic and Related Surgery. 2012;**28**:998-1009. DOI: 10.1016/j.arthro.2012.04.148

[83] Mautner K, Malanga GA, Smith J, Shiple B, Ibrahim V, Sampson S, et al. A call for a standard classification system for future biologic research: The rationale for new PRP nomenclature. PM & R : The Journal of Injury, Function, and Rehabilitation. 2015;**7**:S53-S59. DOI: 10.1016/j.pmrj.2015.02.005

[84] Magalon J, Chateau AL, Bertrand B, Louis ML, Silvestre A, Giraudo L, et al. DEPA classification: A proposal for standardising PRP use and a retrospective application of available devices. BMJ Open Sport & Exercise Medicine. 2016;**2**:e000060. DOI: 10.1136/bmjsem-2015-000060

[85] Lana JFSD, Purita J, Paulus C, Huber SC, Rodrigues BL, Rodrigues AA, et al. Contributions for classification of platelet rich plasma—Proposal of a new classification: MARSPILL. Regenerative Medicine. 2017;**12**:565-574. DOI: 10.2217/rme-2017-0042

[86] Kon E, Di Matteo B, Delgado D, Cole BJ, Dorotei A, Dragoo JL, et al. Platelet-rich plasma for the treatment of knee osteoarthritis: An expert opinion and proposal for a novel classification and coding system. Expert Opinion on Biological Therapy. 2020;**20**(12):1-14. DOI: 10.1080/14712598.2020.1798925

[87] Murray IR, Geeslin AG, Goudie EB, Petrigliano FA, LaPrade RF. Minimum information for studies evaluating biologics in orthopaedics (MIBO): Platelet-rich plasma and mesenchymal stem cells. The Journal of Bone and Joint Surgery. American Volume. 2017;**99**:809-819. DOI: 10.2106/JBJS.16.00793

Chapter 3

Regenerative Medicine in the Treatment of Traumatic Skin Wounds in Dogs and Cats Using Platelet-Rich Fibrin (PRF) Therapy

Carla S. Soares, Pedro P. Carvalho and Maria dos Anjos Pires

Abstract

Regenerative medicine has gained prominence in recent decades and originated from the growing need for medical intervention in degenerative diseases associated with age. This need is believed to be enhanced also by the increase in the average life expectancy of pets, aliased with the growing social integration of pets into human lives, and the development of specialized veterinary medical care. Platelet-rich products, such as platelet-rich fibrin (PRF), have received attention in clinical veterinary settings. PRF therapy has been proposed for the treatment of skin wounds of various etiologies. Traumatic skin wounds are a frequent occurrence in veterinary practice, constituting an opportunity for PRF therapy application, as an adjunct to medical and surgical treatments. The PRF biomaterial is a hemoderivative obtained after single whole-blood centrifugation. In the process, platelets and leukocytes are activated, resulting in a fibrin clot rich in growth factors and cytokines. Considering the young age of PRF regenerative therapy, it is imperative to promote well-characterized PRF biomaterials using standardized preparation methods in both clinical and research scenarios. This step is critical to promote the comparison and allow a critical analysis of platelet-based therapies, allowing its development and rational clinical use.

Keywords: platelet-rich fibrin, veterinary regenerative medicine, wound healing, growth factor, biological therapy, biomaterial

1. Introduction

1.1 Contextualization

The veterinary regenerative medicine is an emerging field and has gained prominence in recent decades. Regenerative medicine for veterinary patients will follow a translational model, encouraged by the investment and biotechnological advances achieved in humans [1, 2].

Regenerative medicine originated from the growing need for medical intervention in degenerative diseases associated with age, such as osteoarthritis. It is believed to

IntechOpen

be enhanced also by pets' life expectancy increase, aliased with the growing social integration of pets into human families, and the development of specialized veterinary medical care [1, 3].

Regenerative medicine is a clinical area whose main objective is to promote the regeneration of damaged tissues, restoring the human/animal healthy state or improving the condition and well-being, with the application of the individual's biological products [4–6].

Therapy with platelet-derived products (PDPs) and with adult stem cells derived from tissues such as fat or bone marrow is increasingly being used as valid and effective therapeutic options, often in combination with pharmacological therapies [1, 7].

PDPs are hemoderivatives, being obtained from whole blood separation, attained from simple blood harvesting. They have been explored mainly as autologous or allogeneic sources of growth factors, cytokines, and structural proteins, with immunological, healing, and regenerative potential for both tissue engineering approaches and regenerative therapies [1]. PDPs, also frequently addressed as platelet-based therapies, have been used primarily in the treatment of traumatic injury or degenerative processes, with the main objective of promoting the restoration of tissue homeostasis (assessed later, Section 6). This is based on inflammation triggering, involving biochemical and metabolic phenomena, and proliferation and differentiation of several cell populations, with strong emphasis on angiogenesis [6].

1.2 Summary of the most important PDPs: platelet-rich plasma (PRP) and PRF (platelet-rich fibrin)

The various PDPs used in human and veterinary medicine can be broadly classified into platelet-poor and platelet-rich products, distinguished mainly by the presence of platelets. Depending on the platelet and fibrin content, blood-derived biomaterials include platelet concentrate (recognized as PC, but sometimes referred to as platelet-rich plasma, PRP), platelet-poor plasma (also nominated as PPP), and platelet-rich fibrin (PRF), among others [1, 8]. Nowadays, the leukocyte quantification in the formulation is also considered as inherent to the categorization of the related PDP [9]. This feature is explained by the prominence of several cytokines associated with immunological features in the local of their action, when the formulation is applied *in situ*, which happens in clinical applications [10, 11].

The term PRP was first used in the 1970s by human hematologists. It refers to plasma with a platelet count higher than that of peripheral blood and was initially used to treat patients with thrombocytopenia. Ten years later, PRP was first used in maxillofacial surgery as platelet-rich fibrin (PRF). Furthermore, these blood-derived products have been used in various surgical areas, including cardiology, pediatric surgery, gynecology, urology, plastic surgery, and ophthalmology [6, 12].

PRP is produced by centrifugation of anticoagulated blood, *which means, whole blood with anticoagulant solution.* This process separates the blood fractions based on the density of its components. Typically, the formulation of PRP involves two sequential centrifugations. The first centrifugation separates erythrocytes from the plasma, and the second one concentrates the platelets and the leukocytes [1]. In addition, single centrifugation protocols are described [13]. Furthermore, PPP is a plasmatic solution containing low to vestigial platelets and other blood element concentration, rich in fibrinogen. PPP is obtained from the centrifugation of anticoagulated blood, as a subproduct of PRP manufacture [1, 14]. The presence of angiogenic factors and biomolecules in PPP has been associated with bone repair in human and canine studies.

On the other hand, the hemoderivative PRF has been relevant in recent years. Also entitled as leukocyte-PRF (L-PRF), it was developed by Choukroun, in France, in oral and maxillofacial surgical areas, to improve bone healing in implant dentistry [15]. The PRF is produced by a single centrifugation of whole blood deprived anti-coagulant, which allows the natural formation of a clot, with simultaneous platelet activation [9, 16]. PRF is a reliable PDP, mentioned as second-generation platelet concentrate, and its production is the only one that is consistently described among all hemoderivatives [17]. The manufacturing procedure for PRF production is minimalistic, safe, easy, and cost-effective and does not require advanced manufacturing skills, once that its preparation has low variables, being a highly reproducible methodology [1].

2. Inclusion of platelet-derived products (PDPs) in veterinary regenerative dermatology: a brief introduction

In the last decade, there has been a significant clinical and biotechnological investment in platelet-rich products [1, 18–20]. Both autologous PRP and PRF therapy is advocated in human dermatology, in different etiology wound treatment and, allogenic platelet therapy has also been proposed [21–24]. Regarding veterinary medicine, PRF and even PRP therapy has been advocated for wound regeneration, using autologous, allogenic, and xenogenic administration [3, 25–28].

PDPs, due to their characteristic of being 'ready to use' in clinical facilities, have become increasingly embraced by clinicians. Platelets are well-known for their role in hemostasis and thrombogenesis, as well as their crucial contribution to the initiation and development of the healing process. This complex process begins with the event of inflammation, stimulating the recruitment of leukocytes and progenitor cells, as well as the stimulation of angiogenesis. Products rich in platelets are eminently suitable for wound healing [1, 29, 30].

2.1 Traumatic skin wounds in dogs and cats: an occasional problem or a frequent complaint?

Bite wounds in companion animals are understudied compared to the incidence of bite wounds in humans. Isolated reports estimate that 10–15% of veterinary trauma cases in pets are bite wounds [31].

Traumatic skin lesions are a frequent occurrence in pets' veterinary practice and can have various causes. In dogs and cats, many of these lesions become colonized by bacteria either during the initial trauma or during the healing process.

The skin is the body's largest organ, and it is composed of various cell populations, including epithelial, mesenchymal, and cells with immunological functions such as resident Langerhans and dendritic cells, T lymphocytes, macrophages, and mast cells, and also stem cells [32]. Physical assault to the skin leads to loss of integrity and invasion by saprophytes and pathogens/microorganisms into sterile compartments within the organism; as a consequence, the infected tissue becomes necrotized, increasing the inflammatory response. Severe tissue trauma, with or without infection, can trigger a systemic inflammatory response syndrome (SIRS), which potentiates inflammation, with multiple exponential cascades of cytokines, coagulation, and fibrinolytics. In severe cases, the infection can lead to sepsis [33].

Normal and intact skin is intended to control the surface microbial populations and to prevent the underlying tissue from being colonized and invaded by potential pathogens. The presence and proliferation of bacteria in wounds has been identified as a major cause of overdue healing and infection in both acute and chronic wounds [34].

In 2018, a study was conducted on bacterial contamination in 45 skin wounds (36 dogs and 9 cats). The study found that *Staphylococcus* spp. was the most frequently isolated agent from contaminated wounds. The study also revealed that the most common cause of skin injury was animal bites (26.67%), followed by the dehiscence of surgical wounds (22.22%). Injuries of unknown origin accounted for 11.11% [35].

In a different study involving 79 dogs and 8 cats, the most common agents were from the genera *Staphylococcus* spp. and *Pseudomonas* spp. It is important to note that this is a subjective evaluation, and further research is needed to confirm these findings [36]. In this study, only gentamicin and amikacin demonstrated resistance rates below 50.0%. Infections can delay wound healing, increasing the animal and owner's stress and costs of treatment, requiring the use of antibiotics. In recurrent situations, antibiotics are often applied empirically, which can contribute to the emergence of antimicrobial resistance [26, 36]. Nevertheless, studies have found a high incidence of resistant bacterial strains in open wounds when compared, highlighting the need for alternatives to antibiotics [37].

In veterinary medicine, the contaminated wound healing occurs through secondary intention, or *per secundam*, where the wound repairs itself without surgical intervention or suturing. In this case, the clinician's role is to provide medical support, including systemic administration of antimicrobials if necessary. Moreover, the wound healing is achieved after granulation tissue formation, followed by contraction and epithelialization of the lesion [38, 39].

3. The PRF biomaterial as an emergent therapy

3.1 Definition and PRF biomaterial preparation

The veterinary clinical use of PRF is gaining attention. The PRF clots are prepared during a single whole blood centrifugation process, without biochemical blood handling, where platelets are activated by the endogenous coagulation cascade, through the action of autologous thrombin [40, 41]. Fibrinogen polymerizes into fibrin, resulting in a clot formation that is composed of three distinct zones (**Figure 1**): (1) the red zone at the bottom of the tube, which comprises erythrocytes; (2) a flexible fibrin matrix, which retains in its mesh platelets and leukocytes, corresponding to the volume of blood collected, located immediately above the interface with the red zone (also designated the phlogistic region); and (3) the acellular zone, corresponding to serum [1, 42]. Furthermore, the structure of the fibrin matrix can also be divided into three distinct zones based on histological and ultrastructural analysis: the proximal zone (immediately after the phlogistic region), the intermediate zone (middle region of the white fibrin matrix), and the distal zone (located in the upper part of the tube) [3, 41]. This is mainly due to its composition that PRF is described as a biodegradable material, which acts as a reservoir of growth factors and cytokines, fundamental to regeneration, also behaving as a biological scaffold for regenerative and tissue engineering strategies [43].

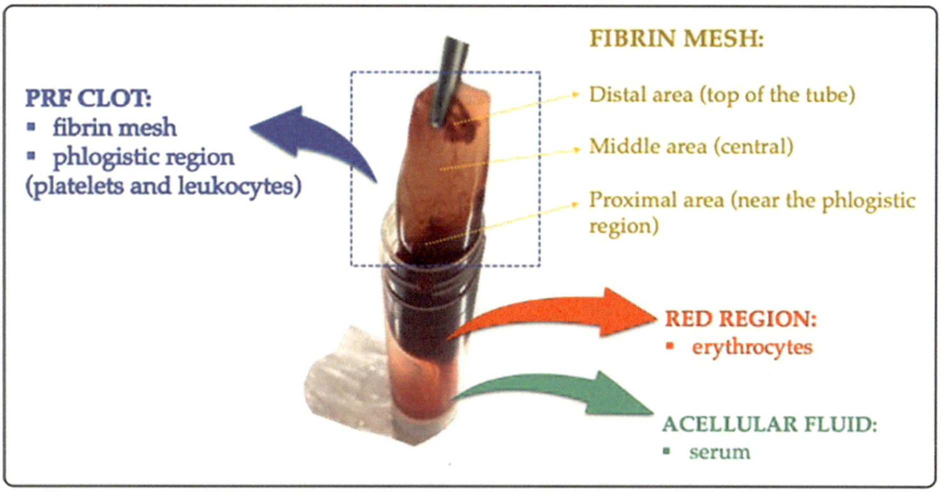

Figure 1.
After centrifugation of whole blood without anticoagulants, a platelet-rich fibrin (PRF) is obtained.

The platelet concentration within the PRFs is generally not stated in the scientific works, contrary to that stated for platelet-rich formulations, settled as having higher levels of platelets when compared with baseline whole blood [44].

This happens because it is technically difficult to calculate with precision the platelet within a solid material (the clot). Historically, Marx has defined PRP formulations should contain 1,000,000 platelets/mL in a 5 mL volume of plasma, due to the scientific evidence of bone and soft tissue healing enhancement [45]. PRF contains platelets which are concentrated in a specific region of the clot, as explained in the previous section. Especially because the single spin allows the recovery of all platelets within the fibrin clot that is formed during the process, with no loss of any plasmatic fraction as may occur in PRP produced using the double centrifugation method, it is assumed that all the platelets from the blood sample are concentrated and used in the clot. The protocol established by our group uses 5 mL of whole blood to produce one PRF clot, without the use of anticoagulant solutions. Thus, dilution does not occur. Considering that domestic dogs and cats have a median of 350×10^3 platelets/mL in baseline whole blood, a PRF clot produced from 5 mL whole blood contains 1.75×10^9 platelets/mL, overcoming platelet-rich formulation such as PRP [3].

Overall, in PRP methodology, the fraction is rich in platelets, with vestigial or low leukocytes according to the protocol, involving more manipulation and the addition of an anticoagulant solution. In the PRF method, the formulation is platelet and leukocyte concentrated with these elements being condensed in a natural fibrin matrix, also involving less manipulation and less platelet loss.

3.2 Structural and biochemical characteristics of PRF biomaterial

The regenerative properties of PRFs are due to the presence of growth factors that are released from the clot after its formation. This occurs actively and progressively over time as the PRF degrades and incorporates itself into the lesion [3, 25, 41, 46].

In tissue regeneration, cytokines, along with growth factors, play a crucial role due to their regulatory effects on inflammatory and their ability to promote cell

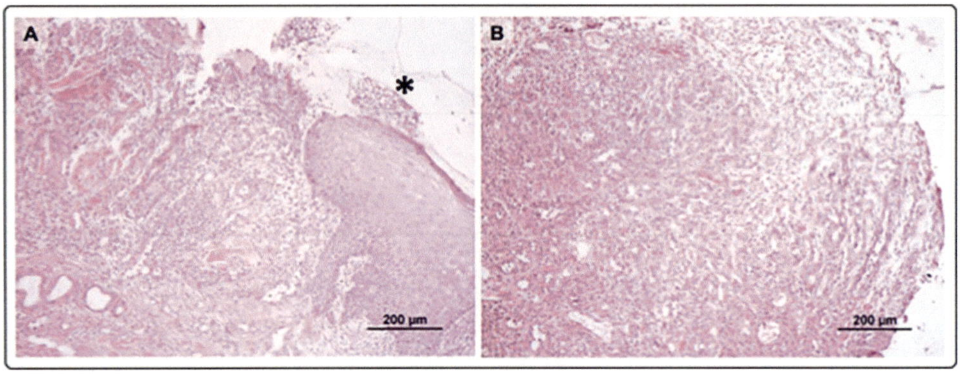

Figure 2.
Histological images of a wound after two autologous PRFs treatments in a dog with a road traffic accident wound. (A) The margin of the lesion is visible with epidermis and granulation tissue, without any bacterial contamination. Fibrin and a small amount of necrosis are observed on the surface (*). (B) Another area of the previous lesion, with granulation tissue under the surface fibrin matrix. Inflammatory cells in necrosis can be observed, but there is no bacterial contamination (H&E).

differentiation, proliferation, and regeneration. Recent scientific research indicates that leukocytes play a pivotal function, actively participating in wound healing by providing local immune protection (e.g., macrophages, whose main function is phagocytosis) and growth factor production in a manner analogous to thrombocytes and platelets [47].

Our research group conducted an in vitro study which confirmed that canine and feline PRFs, obtained using a standardized protocol, released PDGF-BB, TGF-β1, and VEGF-A by day 10. In addition, both PRFs initially release IL-8, a prominent driver of neutrophil recruitment and degranulation [3, 48]. The use of platelet-rich fibrin (PRF) on wounds results in the promotion of significant granulation tissue production, even in cases of extensive tissue loss, and induces normal epithelialization [26, 49, 50]. Macroscopically, the granulation tissue (**Figure 2**) is characterized by an intense red color and is friable to touch as a consequence of the content of numerous microvessels (formed by neovascularization), which are essential for the oxygenation of the area after a period of hypoxia in which anabolic and catabolic events occurred [25].

PRFs of human, equine, canine (**Figure 3**), and feline origin (**Figure 4**) share a similar structure [51–53]. In PRFs, the high density of platelets and leukocytes is in the proximal region of the clot, immediately above the typical red fraction (which is discarded). This region is estimated to contain around 97% of the platelets and at least 50% of the leukocytes of the clot, as compared to circulating whole blood. This is particularly true in the case of human PRFs [54]. Platelets are positioned in an organized pattern, with their presence decreasing along the axis of the PRF toward its most distal end. The fibrin mesh also exhibits a distinct organization along the PRF axis, with a reticular and dense pattern in the proximal area and an elongated arrangement in the distal area [3, 55].

4. Standardized PRF therapy in veterinary wound regeneration

Within the first hour after the preparation of the PRF clot, cytokines and growth factors such as PDGF-BB, VEGF-V, TGF-β1, and IL-8 are released by

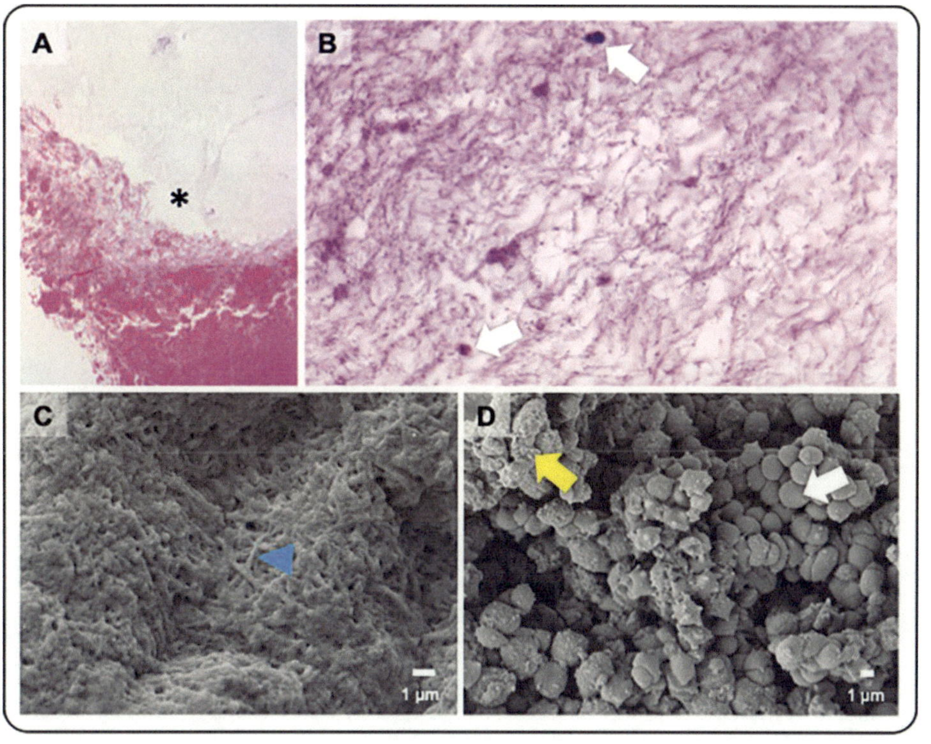

Figure 3.
Canine-origin PRF: This is a histological image of the intermediate region of the clot. The red fraction is observed, along with the central zone where leukocytes and platelets are concentrated and the initial part of the fibrin matrix (*). The image was taken using a 10x objective and stained with H&E. (B) The proximal region of the fibrin matrix is located immediately after the anterior or phlogistic region. This region contains small cellular elements such as platelets and rare leukocytes (white arrow). The background has a fibrillar appearance, which is due to fibrin (blue arrowhead) (100x objective, H&E). (C, D) the ultra-dimensional structure of the PRF is composed of fibrin fibrils (blue arrowhead) that retain leukocytes, erythrocytes, and platelets (scanning electron microscopy).

platelets and leukocytes retained in the PRF matrix. To maximize the collection of platelets and leukocytes present in the phlogistic region of the fibrin clot, it is essential to cut the PRF at the level of the red fraction [3]. The region rich in cellular elements that produce cytokines and growth factors must be placed in direct contact with the lesion, or in the deeper areas of the wound (when the injury has significant tissue loss). PRFs will be applied immediately after their polymerization, or in the first hours after their preparation, so that growth factors and cytokines are released directly at the site of the lesion, with direct application in situ, in a technique similar to that performed in epidermal grafts, in which the PRF is the material to be implanted.

When applied directly to the damaged skin tissue, PRF acts as a bioactive dressing and is therefore a methodology to be considered in companion animals, aiming the regeneration of skin injuries such as lacerations, ulcers, fistulas, burns, and abscesses being chronic or critical injuries [3, 26]. In addition, skin trauma that involves deep structures or infected soft tissues is also suitable for PRF therapy.

The group has optimized the technique for the preparation of canine and feline PRFs in order to obtain a standardized protocol for both species, using reduced volumes of peripheral blood (**Figure 5**) [26].

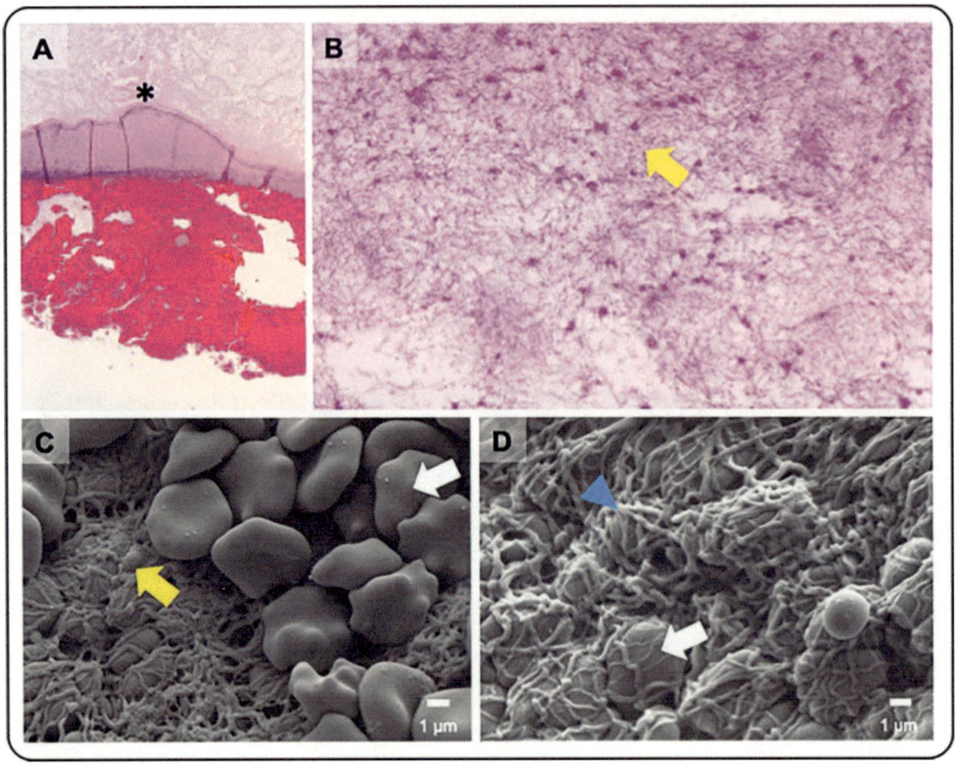

Figure 4.
Feline-origin PRF: The intermediate region of the clot is shown, highlighting the red fraction, the central zone of concentration of platelets and leukocytes, and the beginning of the fibrin clot (*) (10x, H&E). (B) The fibrin matrix is located immediately after the anterior region (proximal fibrin zone). It contains cellular elements such as platelets and occasional leukocytes, arranged under a background with a reticular appearance, which corresponds to fibrin fibrils (blue arrowhead) (100x, H&E). (C, D) scanning electron microscopy shows fibrin fibrils (blue arrowhead), leukocytes, and platelets.

Feline PRFs are typically slightly smaller than those of dogs and have a shiny appearance [3]. The risk of accidental contamination during preparation should be minimal because only one centrifugation is required to obtain PRFs, in a sterile, closed tube and the red fraction removing with sterility. Therefore, it can be easily carried out in surgical environment [3].

After the initial phase, PRF treatments are typically administered two times within the first week, being prolonged until the second week in more extended wounds, followed by single weekly treatments from the second/third week onward.

Skin wounds should ideally be mechanically debrided on the day of presentation to remove any necrotic tissue, if present. All skin lesions should be irrigated with sterile 0.9% saline or ringer and dried immediately prior to the grafting of the new PRF treatments to remove any inflammatory exudate or debris.

PRF treatment consisted of the application of freshly prepared PRFs to the recipient site. At the end of the PRF application, a closed dressing is applied using sterile petroleum jelly or paraffin-embedded gauzes, to maintain the clot at the recipient wound site. The number of PRFs applied to the recipient site depended on the size of the individual wound. The average PRF application was one PRF per 2.5 cm^2 of the wound surface. Contact between the platelet and leukocyte rich area of the clot and

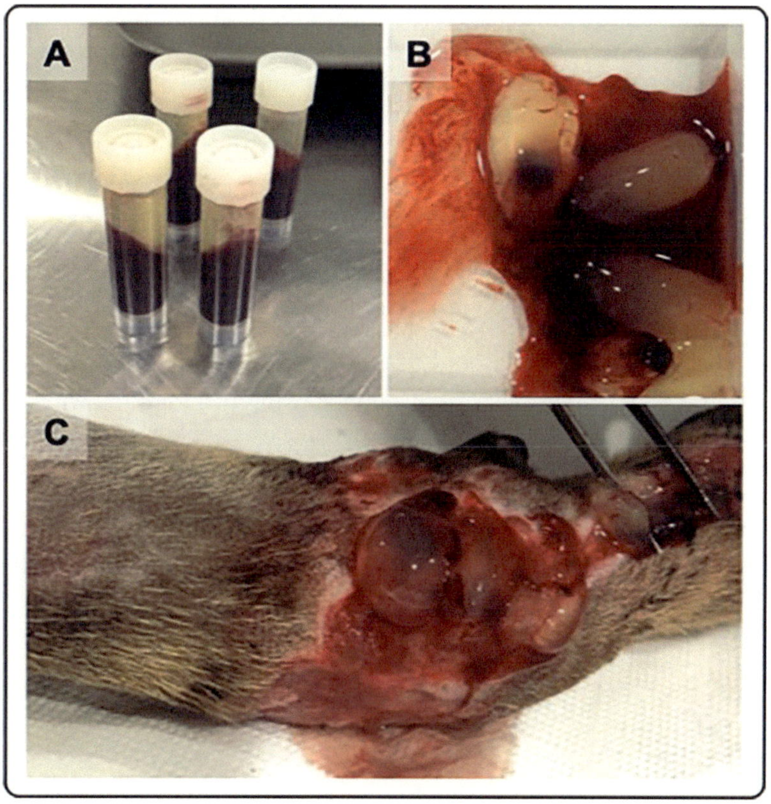

Figure 5.
Preparation and application of PRFs. (A) Appearance of the tubes immediately after centrifuging the blood. (B) White component of the blood clot, which constitutes the PRF, ready to be applied. (C) PRFs applied to the wound bed.

the lesion's bed is essential to guarantee the grafting of the biomaterial. PRF clots are naturally gelatinous and tend to slide over the wound, which facilitates the healing process. It is important to apply and immobilize the PRFs conveniently in the wound bed, as explained previously.

The treatment is finalized only when significant wound contraction is observed, preceded by the formation of granulation with exophytic characteristics (noticeable proliferation of granulation tissue that extends beyond the wound boundaries), with the formation of epithelial tissue being observed. Continuity of the dressing procedure is carried out only by applying a dressing with fatty material and compresses, until the wound has completely healed [56, 57].

Wounds treated using PRF biomaterials do not receive topical antiseptics, antibiotics, or topical drugs to promote wound healing during the treatment. PRF therapy has been claimed to have effective topical antimicrobial activity, and this has been confirmed by our group (under submission) [58–60]. The absence of wound infection during PRF therapy may reveal an important intrinsic antimicrobial property of the clots, especially considering that no local antiseptic or antibiotic was used during the treatments of the wounds addressed in the research of our group.

The search for biodegradable and biological solutions to reduce the ecological footprint must also consider healthcare for human and veterinary patients, following the One Health approach. To develop a method that is easy to perform in a clinical-veterinary environment, we obtain PRFs using polypropylene tubes. This plastic is recommended for medical use due to its shock-resistant, durable, economical, recyclable, thermo-resistant, and sterilizable properties, making it ideal for our purposes [3, 61]. Thus, PRF therapy is defined as an ecologically sustainable technique. It can be used on infected and contaminated wounds without the need for topical antiseptics or antimicrobials. This helps to reduce waste accumulation in the environment. The polypropylene tubes used in the therapy can be reused if they are properly sanitized and sterilized [26]. Alternatively, glass tubes may be used, respecting the same dimensions to provide the adequate concentration of platelets and leukocytes.

Larger wounds require a higher number of PRFs. The number of clinic visits for wound treatment and bandage change is reduced using PRF therapy when compared to the bandage changes/wound treatment necessary on conventional medical wound bandaging/treatments, that are required for 2–3 days until wound closure is achieved [39]. This represents less visits to the clinic, less wound manipulation, and indirect decrease in the associated cost (such as travel and hospital waste generated). Dogs and cats treated with PRF therapy in our clinical trials tolerated the repeated wound manipulation of PRF grafting and subsequent dressings extremely well without the use of topical anesthesia. In fact, the analgesic effect associated with PRF therapy has been confirmed by recent reports [26, 62, 63].

In addition, the PRF therapy technique can be highlighted as an environmentally sustainable technique as the polypropylene tubes used to produce the standardized PRFs could be reused, thereby reducing waste and supporting ecological practices in clinical research.

5. PRF as a natural homeostasis-mimetic patch for regenerative dermatology

Clinical performance of PRFs can be compared to natural and physiological in situ thrombus formation, which occurs whenever there is tissue damage (see **Figure 6**) [55]. Effectively, PRF acts as a biological filling material accompanied by the release, by the platelets and leukocytes concentrated in it, of bioactive structural proteins, in quantities greater than physiological ones, which promote angiogenesis and remodeling of the surrounding tissue [3].

Tissue regeneration can be characterized by four phases. When tissue damage occurs, such as a skin wound, two phases begin almost simultaneously: hemostasis and inflammation, which lasts for 1–3 days [64]. During these stages, platelets migrate to the site of injury where they become activated, a process known as platelet degranulation, in which chemotactic proteins are released and a clot forms. Other factors, such as the presence of bacteria or necrotic tissue, can promote degranulation [65]. This leads to the build-up of the fibrin matrix, which is essential for tissue healing as it acts as a scaffold for cells that arrive at the site by chemotaxis, such as immune cells, fibrocytes, keratinocytes, and even stem cells [40, 66, 67].

The inflammatory phase occurs simultaneously, and neutrophils are the initial leukocytes to be recruited to the site. Following the involvement of neutrophils, macrophages migrate to the site and undergo polarization, a process that alters their phenotype [68, 69].

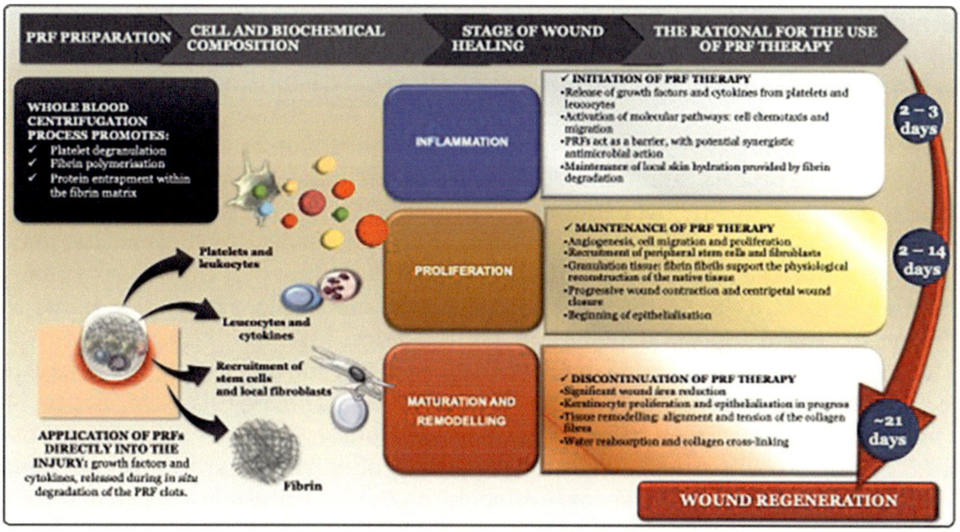

Figure 6.
Characterization of the physiological events that occur during tissue regeneration using PRF therapy, describing the physiological events that occur during the clinical application of PRF biomaterials.

Subsequently, these cells differentiate into M1 or M2 macrophage populations. The former exhibit pro-inflammatory action upon exposure to endotoxins such as lipopolysaccharides (LPS) or interferon gamma (IFN-gamma), inducing a humoral immune response and expressing tumor necrosis factor-alpha (TNF-alpha) and cytokines IL-1, IL-6, IL-12, and IL-23 (36, 52). M2 macrophages display anti-inflammatory properties, with a goal of controlling and resolving inflammation, with a high expression of IL-10 and low expression of IL-12, subdivided into M2a, M2b, M2c, and M2d. M2a polarization is stimulated by IL-4, IL-13, and infections associated with helminth parasites or fungi and is associated with the humoral Th2 response. M2b macrophages are activated by toll-Like receptors (TLR) and their binding proteins or by IL-1, which subsequently moderates the immune response. M2c polarization is stimulated by IL-10 and TGF-beta (peptide secreted by PRF), contributing to tissue remodeling and extracellular matrix synthesis, while M2d macrophages are stimulated by IL-6 and adenosine [70, 71].

Inflammation is a response to tissue damage, such as wounds, and triggers a series of events, beginning with hemostasis. The loss of cellular integrity activates immunological factors, including Danger/Damage Associated Molecular Patterns (DAMPs). DAMPs trigger stress signals in the body, leading to innate immune responses. These responses begin with the chemotaxis of neutrophils and other leukocytes to respond to and resolve the injury. The inflammatory response aims to eliminate the antigen that caused it and restore tissue homeostasis, minimizing damage. Platelet-rich formulations are utilized in regenerative medicine to enhance the regeneration of damaged tissues. They contain proteins from intraplatelet granules, such as platelet-derived growth factor (PDGF), transforming growth factor 1 beta (TGF-1 beta), and epidermal growth factor (EGF). These proteins trigger paracrine interactions and signaling pathways at the site of injury [72].

The proliferation phase of cell growth commences 2–3 days after the trauma. This is marked by the formation of granulation tissue, which is composed of fibroblasts and angioblasts. Additionally, there is a decrease in the population of inflammatory cells at the site [64]. Granulation tissue forms as a result of the migration of various cell types, stimulated by the release of PDGF and TGF-1 beta from the inflammatory cells and platelets previously present in the area. Fibroblasts, cells responsible for matrix synthesis, myofibroblasts, responsible for contraction of the lesion throughout the regenerative process, and endothelial cells, which induce the process of neoangiogenesis, are stimulated by the peptides VEGF and FGF (fibroblast growth factor) and form granulation tissue [64, 73]. The process of re-epithelialization occurs later and is characterized by the migration and proliferation of keratinocytes from the periphery of the lesion toward the centre of the wound. At the same time, granulation tissue develops to fill and approximate the edges of the defect [31].

The final stage is remodeling, which can take longer, starting around 3 weeks after the initial damage and lasting for more than a year [64]. During this stage, all previously initiated processes are halted, and many previously active cells undergo apoptosis. The stage is hallmarked by intense deposition of extracellular matrix composed of fibronectin, glycosaminoglycans, proteoglycans, and hyaluronic acid, with type III collagen being the most predominant and gradually replaced by type I collagen [73].

In vitro studies have predominantly been conducted in humans [54, 67] and horses [74] to evaluate the release kinetics of various proteins and growth factors contained in PRF. These studies have shown an active pattern up to 20 days after the production of this biomaterial. Recent in vitro studies in canine and feline species have also demonstrated a progressive release of these compounds over time, up to a maximum of 10 days [3]. However, in a real biological context, PRFs applied directly to the lesion are degraded on site within 3–5 days and are rarely macroscopically visible between dressing changes.

6. Advantages and disadvantages of PRF therapy

Autologous hemoderivatives are frequently used in both human and veterinary regenerative interventions, addressing biosafety requirements. This method helps to prevent the recipient from being at the risk of secondary infection. It is a widely documented approach [75, 76].

Nonetheless, considering that the use of allogenic blood products is currently widespread and properly regulated (e.g., blood transfusions are essentially allogeneic), the same principle can be extended to the use of PRFs in skin regenerative interventions. No adverse side effects of allogenic (in canine species) or even xenogenic use of PRFs were found in several studies, including the ones performed by our group [26, 75]. Allogenic PRF therapy was assessed within canine species, and in the xenogenic approach, canine-origin PRFs were applied compromised in cats (**Figure** 7) [26].

Cats produce reduced volumes of blood, limiting autologous production of PRF, which is in itself contraindicated in the presence of concomitant hematological, immunological, and/or metabolic disorders [77, 78]. Xenogenic use should be seen as one of the advantages conferred on PRF therapy as an innovative regenerative interventionist methodology. When considering this methodology, it is important to strictly comply with requirements aimed at ensuring the biosafety of the recipient. This includes screening for infectious diseases and considering the principles and guidelines applied to veterinary blood transfusions, as well as the geographic

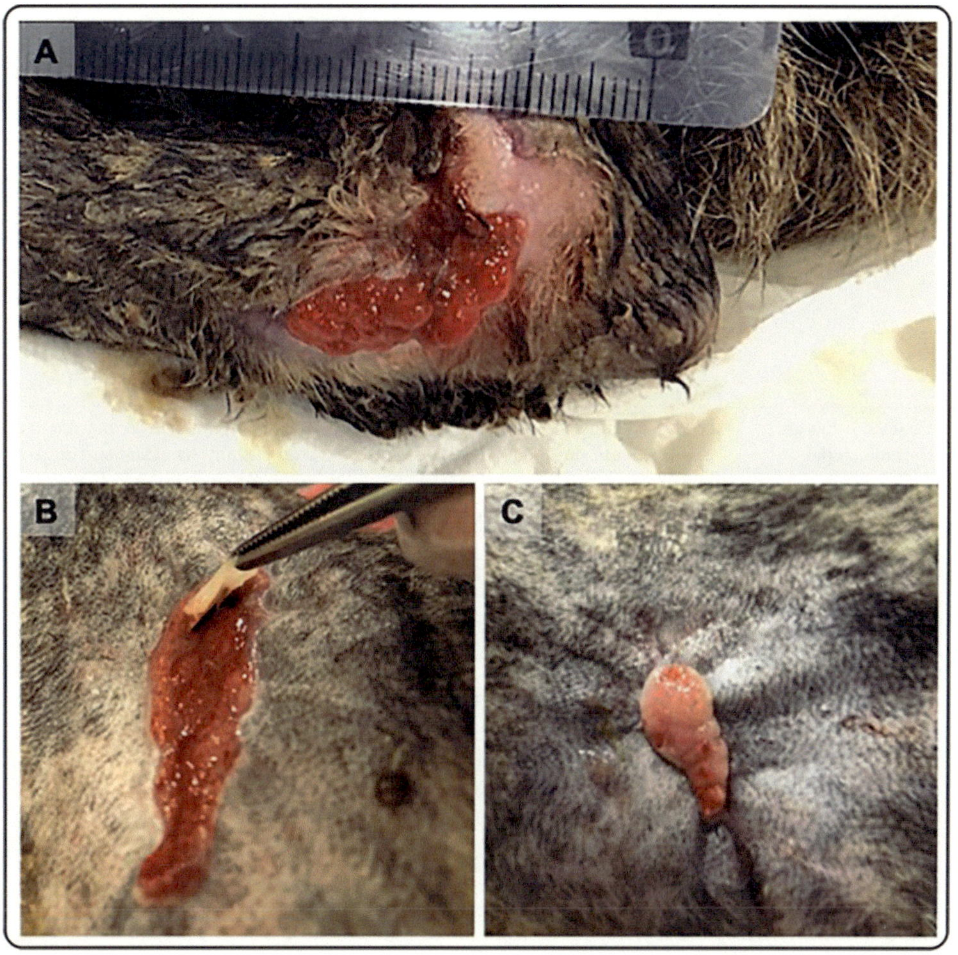

Figure 7.
This study documents the phases of healing evolution in different lesions treated with PRF therapy using various approaches. (A) Laceration in a cat that received xenogenic PRFs from a donor dog; evidence of exophytic granulation tissue after treatments with PRFs, displaying an intense red color. (B) PRFs incorporated into the wound, in a dog referred for autologous PRF therapy, after three treatments with PRFs. (C) The presence of exophytic granulation tissue with the formation of epithelium and contraction of the lesion, dog treated with an autologous approach, after four treatments.

prevalence of blood-transmitted diseases. It is also important to consider emerging pathologies that are intrinsically associated with current climate changes [1, 79, 80].

To date, blood typing for PDPs which are intended to be applied topically (for example, treatment of skin wounds) is considered unnecessary to date, considering the few clinical studies that exist to date [1, 22, 26–28, 81, 82].

PRF therapy for wound management has been described as an ecological technique, as it avoids the use of topical antiseptics. This is directly associated with antimicrobial, anti-inflammatory, and analgesic properties attributed to the PRF biomaterial, both in in vitro and in vivo studies [26, 59, 60, 83]. Our research indicates that the direct application of PRFs to the wound bed reduces the requirement for additional antimicrobial or chemical agents and may even obviate the need for some soft tissue surgery (**Table 1**) [26].

Domain	Advantages	Disadvantages
Technique	Easy to prepare: • Reduced peripheral blood volume • Equipment accessible in the clinic (centrifuge) • Economical technique, without the use of other reagents • Fast and easily reproducible technique (low operator dependence) Used autologously in most cases Allogenic and xenogenic uses are equally possible	Consider a single centrifuge for processing PRFs The aseptic technique must be used systematically throughout the preparation process
Characteristics of the biomaterial	• Biological, biocompatible, and biomimetic of physiological tissue regeneration • Moldable/easily adaptable to the defect	• Fibrin polymerization may not occur after 60 minutes after centrifugation (rare; e.g., hematological, hepatic pathology, etc.)
Clinical use	• Allows temporal release of growth factors and cytokines directly at the site • Possible actions: o Antibiotic/antiseptic o Anti-inflammatory/analgesic • The interval between dressings using the PRFs biomaterial is longer (in the initial phase of treatment) compared to conventional dressings	• PRF therapy does not apply to extensive skin lesions (on the surface)
Biological risks	• The risk of contamination during processing is low	• If allogenic and xenogenic: screened donors are mandatory: o Consider the possibility of a subclinical period of infectious disease o Consider the geographic area and associated blood-borne diseases o Use indoor living donors, with no travel history
Environmental Issues	• Biological and biodegradable • Ecologically sustainable technique: o Avoid the use of topical antiseptics and antimicrobials, contributing to reducing the accumulation of hospital waste o Polypropylene tubes are reusable (after decontamination and sterilization, it is possible by autoclaving)	

Table 1.
Summary of the advantages and disadvantages of PRF therapy in skin wounds.

The interval between dressings using the PRF biomaterial is lengthier than in other wound medical treatments, even in the initial phase of treatment, in which large (or deep) wounds appear quite exudative, contaminated, or even infected [39, 75].

Our experience with PRF therapy in wound treatment indicates advantages over other methodologies such as bandages with chemical hydrogels, healing ointments, or commercial wound materials. This results in the need for fewer dressings and less systemic antibiotic therapy for majority of cases [26].

The benefits of PRF therapy outweigh the drawbacks, which are primarily viewed as risks and critical points. The primary limitation of this therapy is linked to extensive defects or lesions. Considering our protocol for collecting five milliliters of blood to produce a platelet-rich fibrin clot sufficient to cover an average of 2.0–2.5 cm^2 of the lesion area, it is evident that extensive lesions would require a large volume of blood to be collected for exclusive PRF treatment [3, 26, 55].

On the other hand, non-autologous PRF therapy, which involves allogenic and xenogenic application, requires the screening of donor animals, detailing the screening of blood-borne agents, in the same way as those carried out in the context of transfusion medicine. In these circumstances, the biosafety criteria involved in obtaining blood products for veterinary clinical applications must be followed, always considering the potential risk of transmission of infectious agents in periods of subclinical disease, which is generally not identified by the clinician [1, 79].

7. Anticipating the future of PRF therapy in veterinary regenerative dermatology

Recently and in a similar way, human medicine has also used PRFs for the treatment of complicated wounds, such as those recurrent in diabetic patients, burns, and varicose venous ulcers [49, 84, 85]. PRF therapy has been used for corneal lesions, such as ulcers, in humans with an autologous approach [3, 86, 87].

As researchers and clinicians, we recommend PRF therapy as an adjunct to medical and surgical treatments, especially for skin defects or wounds that require second healing soft tissue closure, requiring induction of granulation tissue (**Figure 8**).

Autologous methodology should be considered limited in small-sized dogs and in cats, especially in the treatment of wounds, where several PRF clots are required, at different timepoints. Moreover, autologous PRFS combined with precision medicine strategies may be suitable to achieve. We have described an innovative surgical approach for the correction of recurrent oronasal fistula in a senior cat in 2018, in which the

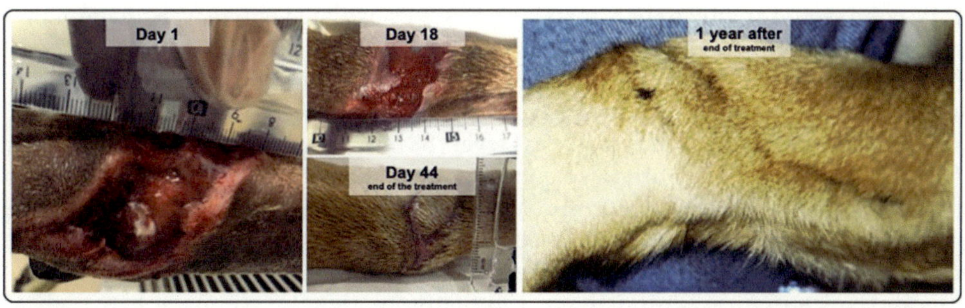

Figure 8.
Scarring evolution documented during autologous PRF therapy, in a female canine, 1 year and 8 months old. Wound resulting from being run over, right anterior limb. On day 1, the lesion appears, before starting regenerative therapy. Until the 18th, three treatments with PRFs were carried out, from which date PRF therapy was suspended, as it was no longer considered necessary. Complete closure was reached on the 44th day. The owner provided a photograph of the region, 1 year after the end of the PRF treatments.

application of autologous PRF was combined with bone marrow aspirate, leading to the formation of a matrix rich in cells and molecules with regenerative action [25]. In this case, PRF was used as a strategy associated with tissue engineering. A polycaprolactone implant, obtained by 3D printing, was completely adapted to the animal's defect in a precision regenerative medicine approach. In autologous PRF therapy, it is important to assess (a) the extension and depth of the injury; (b) estimate how many treatments may be required (two or certainly more?); (c) the collaboration of the patient regarding the blood the blood collections; (d) the absence of hematological abnormalities or the administration of pharmaceutical drugs that may result in impaired platelet or leucocyte concentrations.

When not all the requirements of the autologous method are met, allogenic (from other canine donor) or xenogenic PRFs (from canine origin for feline patients) are advocated for wound therapy in patients for whom autologous methodology is not suitable due to co-morbidities or other reasons that prevent blood collection, such as low body weight or non-cooperation for venous collection [26].

The clinical application of PRFs in wounds leads to the rapid formation and proliferation of granulation tissue, which is characterized by intense red color and exuberant vascularization, with a peripheral-to-the-center healing pattern being observed in all wounds. This is particularly important in lesions with extensive tissue deficit. We also observed a significant contraction of the treated traumatic injuries, especially in larger wounds, with subsequent re-epithelialization and crust formation. All treatments carried out by us resulted in minimal esthetic scarring [75].

8. The boundaries of platelet therapy: mandatory use of standardized treatment protocols

In clinical practice, studies focusing standardized and optimized protocols for platelet-rich hemoderivatives arrived only after its clinical use. In veterinary medicine, some PDPs are administered based solely on the patient's platelet composition and clinical response, which can be a limiting factor [1]. Furthermore, the clinical application of platelet-based formulations is associated with uncertainties due to the lack of a standard protocols, doses, or therapeutic procedures for various lesions and species in which they have been used. For instance, degenerative joint disease is one of the conditions for which the clinical use of PDPs has been extensively documented in both human and animal patients, even prior to the biochemical characterization of the PDPs used [1, 5, 82]. This provides evidence for the growing need to fully and clearly characterize the products used in regenerative strategies. This is essential for the advancement of the field at a clinical level [88]. In addition to these critical points of standardization, these works also question other subjects such as the composition of the PDPs. It is not always described, and the methodology and diversity of clinical studies that use PDPs are obtained through non-standardized protocols. Often, they do not follow similar therapeutic regimens nor they apply similar number of applications and concentration administered, and therefore, they are comparable to each other [89–91]. This diversity is evident in the studies conducted on both human and animal patients.

As occurring in PRP, different protocols to prepare the PRF are reported in human patients. In fact, one of the most boundaries is the lack of critical evaluation of the different studies by comparative meta-analysis [21]. There are still few reports of PRF therapy in veterinary area compared with human field, and it is important that newcomer researchers apply standardized protocols, in order to allow the comparison between studies, avoiding the heterogenicity of results such as those observed in the report of PRP clinical documentation in the literature. This has been the main propose of our research group, where the same PRF protocol is applied in all clinical cases, after its optimization and biochemical characterization. To increase objectivity, several studies are using nomenclature for the PDPs that is not universally recognized [92].

It is imperative to promote well-characterized veterinary PDPs such as PRF, using standardizing methods, in both clinical and research scenarios (**Figure 9**). Also, comparative research based on consistent and well-defined criteria, using representative numbers of participants and with long-term follow-up periods, should be carried out to better understand the benefits of this biomaterial [1, 8].

The rise of several human-sourced PDPs such as PRP and PRF, and even other derived formulations, has promoted misperception and debate among the scientific community once that different formulations were indistinctly cited in the literature. In 2009, the working group of Dohan Eherenfest suggested four categories of platelet concentrates (P-PRP, L-PRP, P-PRF, and L-PRF), as an attempt to use categorized and standardized PDPs. Furthermore, this claim promoted scientific research to understand and explain the intrinsic biochemical proprieties of PDPs, assuming the demanding need to validate their use, in clinical settings [93]. In 2012, the group of DeLong presented their classification PAW system, based on the report of three constituents in PRP preparation: number of platelets, platelet activation method, and the presence or absence of white blood cells [94]. Until the present, there are no consensual documents in veterinary setting proposing key parameters for the preparation of characterized PDPs, and the only scientific document addressing this issue was published in 2021, by Soares et al. [1].

In summary (**Table 2**), the use of key parameters to prepare and document well-characterized PDPs is strongly demanded, to avoid dubious and incomparable scientific data related to platelet therapy.

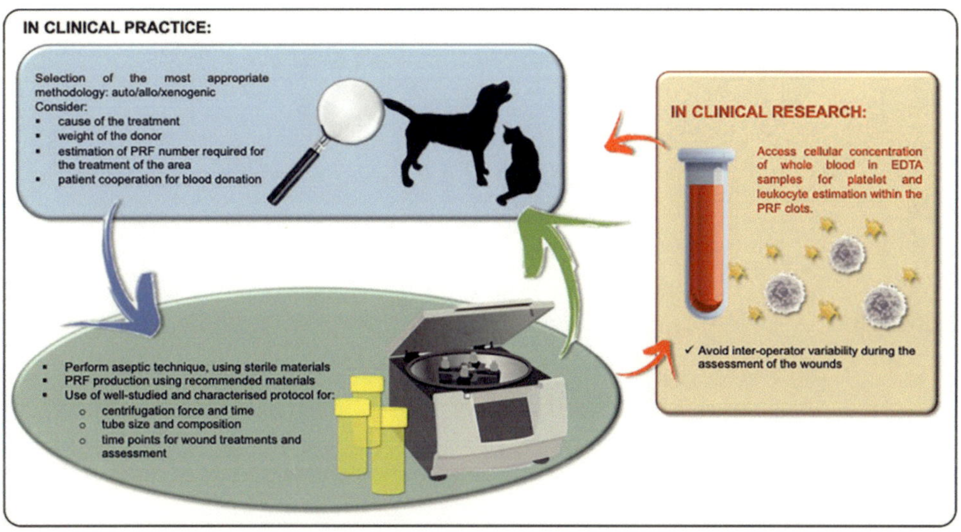

Figure 9.
Suggested criteria to consider when implementing PRF therapy, both in clinical practice and research.

Author, year	Aim, Area	Division/Parameter	Subdivision
Eherenfest et al. [9]	Platelet concentrate classification, human area	A: Material, preparation kits, and centrifuges	(A1) Size and weight of the centrifuge required for the method (A2) Duration of the procedure (from blood harvest to surgical application) (A3) Budget (initial cost of equipment and repeated costs for reagents and kits) (A4) Technicity of the kit (including required manipulations) and complexity of the procedure
		B: Platelets and leukocytes	(B1) Final volume of platelet gel material (relative to initial blood harvest) (B2) Platelet recovery efficiency (B3) Leucocyte recovery efficiency (B4) Preservation of the platelets and leucocytes
		C: Fibrin matrix	(C1) Fibrinogen concentration and fibrin density (C2) Fibrin polymerization typology
DeLong et al. [94]	PAW system: classification of platelet-rich plasma formulations, human area	P: PLT concentration	Subdivision in four groups, according to PLT concentration present: (P1) Above baseline values (P2) Between baseline and 750,000 platelets/μL (P3) Between 750,000 and 1,250,000 platelets/μL (P4) Superior to 1,250,000 platelets/μL
		A: Activation system	Exogenous activator used/ or not used
		W: WBC existence	Subdivision in two groups, according to WBC concentration present: a. Above baseline b. Below baseline Sectioning according to neutrophil concentration: (α) Above baseline (β) Below baseline

DOI: http://dx.doi.org/10.5772/intechopen.1004700

Author, year	Aim, Area	Division/Parameter	Subdivision
Soares et al. [1]	Classification for platelet-based products, veterinary area	A. Source	• Autologous • Allogenic • Xenogenic (or heterologous)
		B. Preparation technique	Subdivision in five sections: • Addition of anticoagulant solution • Centrifugation process • Methodology applied • Platelet presence • Leucocyte presence
		C. Utilization-related	Subdivision in three sections: • Physical form • Activation state • Cytokine and growth factor content

PLT, platelet; WBC, white blood cell or leukocytes.

Table 2.
Review of main publications suggesting key parameters to document on the preparation protocol of well-characterized PDPs.

9. Concluding remarks

PRF is an environmentally sustainable biomaterial as it is biodegradable and obtained through blood centrifugation promoting platelets and leucocytes concentration in a specific region of the matrix. This forms a natural and biocompatible matrix containing higher than physiological concentrations of cells (platelets and leukocytes) with regenerative activity, mimicking the natural healing process. Studies evaluating the kinetics of the cytokines and growth factors released by the PRF biomaterial have proven that this occurs actively and progressively over time. Autologous, allogenic, and xenogenic PRF therapy can be considered as an effective therapeutic strategy in the veterinary clinic. It constitutes an alternative biological regenerative treatment, suitable for wound regeneration in veterinary practice, accelerating wound healing by second intention mechanism.

The PRF enhances the mechanism of local tissue regeneration through the sustained release of molecules that signal the systems involved in the skin healing cascade. However, further clinical studies are required for complete validation, particularly for the xenogenic methodology. In this sense, chronic or critical injuries that are inaccessible or unresponsive to surgical reconstruction, even if infected or contaminated, such as burns, abscesses, and/or skin trauma involving deep structures, are appropriate candidates for PRF therapy, considering that, in these cases of wound regeneration by second intention, it is the appropriate therapeutic decision.

Acknowledgements

This present work was supported by the Ph.D. grant SFRH/BD/118871/2016 and by the project UIDB/00772/2020 (Doi:10.54499/UIDB/00772/2020) funded by the Portuguese Foundation for Science and Technology (FCT).

Conflict of interest

Pedro P. Carvalho is the C.E.O. of the biotechnology company, Vetherapy, which commercializes veterinary regenerative therapies.

The authors declare that there are no other conflicts of interest.

Notes/thanks/other declarations

The authors thank the Laboratory of Histology and Anatomic Pathology and the Centre for Veterinary and Animal Research (CECAV), both at the University of Trás-os-Montes E Alto Douro.

Appendices and nomenclature

DAMPs	damage associated molecular patterns
EGF	epidermal growth factor
FGF	fibroblast growth factor
g	g-force or gravitational force equivalent

H&E	hematoxylin and eosin stain
IFN-gamma	interferon gamma
IL	interleukin
LPS	lipopolysaccharides
PC	platelet concentrate
PDGF-BB	platelet-derived growth factor, subunit BB
PLT	platelet
PPP	platelet-poor plasma
PRF	platelet-rich fibrin
PRP	platelet-rich plasma
PDP	platelet-derived products
Rpm	rotations per minute
SIRS	inflammatory response syndrome
TNF-alpha	tumor necrosis factor alpha
TNR	toll-like receptors (TLR)
TGF-β1	transforming growth factor beta 1
VEGF-A	vascular endothelial growth factor A
μL	microliter
WBC	white blood cells, or leukocytes

Author details

Carla S. Soares[1,2,3]*, Pedro P. Carvalho[4] and Maria dos Anjos Pires[1]

1 Center for Animal and Veterinary Science (CECAV), AL4AnimaLS, Department of Veterinary Sciences, School of Veterinary Sciences, University of Trás-os-Montes and Alto Douro (UTAD), Vila Real, Portugal

2 VetLamaçães, Veterinary Clinic, Braga, Portugal

3 CIVG, Vasco da Gama Research Center/EUVG – Vasco da Gama University School, Coimbra, Portugal

4 Vetherapy – Research and Development in Biotechnology, Coimbra, Portugal

*Address all correspondence to: carlasoares.medvet@gmail.com

References

[1] Soares CS, Babo PS, Reis RL, Carvalho PP, Gomes ME. Platelet-derived products in veterinary medicine: A new trend or an effective therapy? Trends in Biotechnology. 2021;**39**:225-243. DOI: 10.1016/j.tibtech.2020.07.011

[2] Webb TL, Spaas JH, Guest DJ. Editorial: One health and veterinary regenerative medicine: Translational applications. Frontiers in Veterinary Science. 2022;**9**:9-11. DOI: 10.3389/fvets.2022.959564

[3] Soares CS, Babo PS, Faria S, Pires MA, Carvalho PP. Standardized platelet-rich fibrin (PRF) from canine and feline origin: An analysis on its secretome pattern and architectural structure. Cytokine. 2021;**148**:155695. DOI: 10.1016/j.cyto.2021.155695

[4] Barrett JG. A set of grand challenges for veterinary regenerative medicine. Frontiers in Veterinary Science. 2016;**3**:1-4. DOI: 10.3389/fvets.2016.00020

[5] Canapp SO, Canapp DA, Ibrahim V, Carr BJ, Cox C, Barrett JG. The use of adipose-derived progenitor cells and platelet-rich plasma combination for the treatment of supraspinatus tendinopathy in 55 dogs: A retrospective study. Frontiers in Veterinary Science. 2016;**3**:61. DOI: 10.3389/fvets.2016.00061

[6] Andia I, Rubio-Azpeitia E, Martin JI, Abate M. Current concepts and translational uses of platelet rich plasma biotechnology. In: Biotechnology. London, UK: InTechOpen; 2015. p. 13. DOI: 10.5772/59954

[7] Bogers SH. Cell-based therapies for joint disease in veterinary medicine: What we have learned and what we need to know. Frontiers in Veterinary Science. 2018;**5**. DOI: 10.3389/fvets.2018.00070

[8] Ehrenfest DMD, Sammartino G, Shibli JA, Wang H, Zou D, Bernard J. Guidelines for the publication of articles related to platelet concentrates (platelet-rich plasma - PRP, or platelet-rich fibrin - PRF): The international classification of the POSEIDO. POSEIDO Journal. 2013;**1**:17-27

[9] Dohan Ehrenfest DM, Rasmusson L, Albrektsson T. Classification of platelet concentrates: From pure platelet-rich plasma (P-PRP) to leucocyte- and platelet-rich fibrin (L-PRF). Trends in Biotechnology. 2009;**27**:158-167. DOI: 10.1016/j.tibtech.2008.11.009

[10] Bielecki T, Ehrenfest DMD, Everts PA, Wiczkowski A. The role of leukocytes from L-PRP/L-PRF in wound healing and immune defense: New perspectives. Current Pharmaceutical Biotechnology. 2012;**13**:1153-1162. DOI: 10.2174/138920112800624373

[11] Lana JF, Huber SC, Purita J, Tambeli CH, Santos GS, Paulus C, et al. Leukocyte-rich PRP versus leukocyte-poor PRP - The role of monocyte/macrophage function in the healing cascade. Journal of Clinical Orthopaedics and Trauma. 2019;**10**:S7-S12. DOI: 10.1016/j.jcot.2019.05.008

[12] Mościcka P, Przylipiak A. History of autologous platelet-rich plasma: A short review. Journal of Cosmetic Dermatology. 2021;**20**:2712-2714. DOI: 10.1111/jocd.14326

[13] Anitua E, Sánchez M, Orive G. The importance of understanding what is platelet-rich growth factor (PRGF) and what is not. Journal of Shoulder

and Elbow Surgery. 2011;**20**:23-24. DOI: 10.1016/j.jse.2010.07.005

[14] Martínez CE, Smith PC, Palma Alvarado VA. The influence of platelet-derived products on angiogenesis and tissue repair: A concise update. Frontiers in Physiology. 2015;**6**:290. DOI: 10.3389/fphys.2015.00290

[15] Naik B, Karunakar P, Jayadev M, Marshal VR. Role of platelet rich fibrin in wound healing: A critical review. Journal of Conservative Dentistry. 2013;**16**:284. DOI: 10.4103/0972-0707.114344

[16] Choukroun J, Adda F, Schoeffler C, Vervelle A. Une opportunité en paro-implantologie: Le PRF. Implantodontie. 2001;**42**:55-62

[17] Dohan DM, Choukroun J, Diss A, Dohan SL, Dohan AJJ, Mouhyi J, et al. Platelet-rich fibrin (PRF): A second-generation platelet concentrate. Part I: Technological concepts and evolution. Oral Surgery, Oral Medicine, Oral Pathology, Oral Radiology, and Endodontology. 2006;**101**:e37-44. DOI: 10.1016/j.tripleo.2005.07.008

[18] Farghali HA, AbdElKader NA, AbuBakr HO, Ramadan ES, Khattab MS, Salem NY, et al. Corneal ulcer in dogs and cats: Novel clinical application of regenerative therapy using subconjunctival injection of autologous platelet-rich plasma. Frontiers in Veterinary Science. 2021;**8**:1-17. DOI: 10.3389/fvets.2021.641265

[19] Perego R, Spada E, Moneta E, Baggiani L, Proverbio D. Use of autologous leucocyte- and platelet-rich plasma (L-PRP) in the treatment of aural hematoma in dogs. Veterinary Sciences. 2021;**8**:172. DOI: 10.3390/vetsci8090172

[20] Carr BJ, Canapp SO. Regenerative medicine for soft tissue injury and osteoarthritis. Today's Vet Paractice. 2016;**53**:53-60

[21] de Carvalho CKL, Fernandes BL, de Souza MA. Autologous matrix of platelet-rich fibrin in wound care settings: A systematic review of randomized clinical trials. Journal of Functional Biomaterials. 2020;**11**:31. DOI: 10.3390/jfb11020031

[22] Jo CH, Shin JS, Lee SY, Shin S. Allogeneic platelet-rich plasma for rotator cuff repair. Acta Ortopedica Brasileira. 2017;**25**:38-43. DOI: 10.1590/1413-785220172501163417

[23] Greppi N, Mazzucco L, Galetti G, Bona F, Petrillo E, Smacchia C, et al. Treatment of recalcitrant ulcers with allogeneic platelet gel from pooled platelets in aged hypomobile patients. Biologicals. 2011;**39**:73-80. DOI: 10.1016/j.biologicals.2011.01.002

[24] Zhang Z-Y, Huang A-W, Fan JJ, Wei K, Jin D, Chen B, et al. The potential use of allogeneic platelet-rich plasma for large bone defect treatment: Immunogenicity and defect healing efficacy. Cell Transplantation. 2013;**22**:175-187. DOI: 10.3727/096368912X653183

[25] Soares CS, Barros LC, Saraiva V, Gomez-Florit M, Babo PS, Dias IR, et al. Bioengineered surgical repair of a chronic oronasal fistula in a cat using autologous platelet-rich fibrin and bone marrow with a tailored 3D printed implant. Journal of Feline Medicine and Surgery. 2018;**20**:835-843. DOI: 10.1177/1098612X18789549

[26] Soares CS, Dias IR, Pires MA, Carvalho PP. Canine-origin platelet-rich fibrin as an effective biomaterial for wound healing in domestic cats: A preliminary study. Veterinary Sciences. 2021;**8**:213. DOI: 10.3390/vetsci8100213

[27] Chung T, Baek D, Kim N, Park J, Park C. Topical allogeneic platelet-rich plasma treatment for a massive cutaneous

lesion induced by disseminated intravascular coagulation in a toy breed dog. Irish Veterinary Journal. 2015;**68**:4. DOI: 10.1186/s13620-015-0032-7

[28] Kim SE, Lee M-K, Seo K. Clinical application of serum eye drops for herpetic keratitis in cats: A pilot. International Journal of Applied Research in Veterinary Medicine. 2018;**16**:221-225

[29] Ghoshal K, Bhattacharyya M. Overview of platelet physiology: Its hemostatic and nonhemostatic role in disease pathogenesis. Scientific World Journal. 2014;**2014**:1-16. DOI: 10.1155/2014/781857

[30] Ratajczak J, Vangansewinkel T, Gervois P, Merckx G, Hilkens P, Quirynen M, et al. Angiogenic properties of 'leukocyte- and platelet-rich fibrin'. Scientific Reports. 2018;**8**:1-10. DOI: 10.1038/s41598-018-32936-8

[31] Englar RE. Common Clinical Presentations in Dogs and Cats. Wiley; 2019. DOI: 10.1002/9781119414612

[32] Souci L, Denesvre C. 3D skin models in domestic animals. Veterinary Research. 2021;**52**:21. DOI: 10.1186/s13567-020-00888-5

[33] Holt DE, Griffin G. Bite wounds in dogs and cats. The Veterinary Clinics of North America. Small Animal Practice. 2000;**30**:669-679. DOI: 10.1016/S0195-5616(00)50045-X

[34] Bowler PG, Duerden BI, Armstrong DG. Wound microbiology and associated approaches to wound management. Clinical Microbiology Reviews. 2001;**14**:244-269. DOI: 10.1128/CMR.14.2.244-269.2001

[35] Kožár M, Hamilton H, Koščová J. Types of wounds and the prevalence of bacterial contamination of wounds in the clinical practice of small animals. Folia Veterinaria. 2018;**62**:39-47. DOI: 10.2478/fv-2018-0036

[36] Ishii JB, Freitas JC, Arias MVB. Resistência de bactérias isoladas de cães e gatos no Hospital Veterinário da Universidade Estadual de Londrina (2008-2009). Pesquisa Veterinaria Brasileira. 2011;**31**:533-537. DOI: 10.1590/S0100-736X2011000600013

[37] Nolff MC, Reese S, Fehr M, Dening R, Meyer-Lindenberg A. Assessment of wound bio-burden and prevalence of multi-drug resistant bacteria during open wound management. The Journal of Small Animal Practice. 2016;**57**:255-259. DOI: 10.1111/jsap.12476

[38] Bosco J. Principles of wound Care & Bandaging Techniques. Today's Veterinary Practice. 2012;**2**:61-67. DOI: 10.7748/ns.3.38.52.s69

[39] Tobias K. Basic wound care. NAVC Clinician's Brief. 2012:74-78

[40] Gupta V, Bains VK, Singh GP, Mathur A, Bains R. Regenerative potential of platelet rich fibrin in dentistry: Literature review. Asian Journal of Oral Health & Allied Sciences. 2011;**1**:23

[41] Castilho MS, Rahal SC, das Dias Neto RN, Pereira AC, de Francia CCDA, dos Mesquita LR, et al. Preparation and characterization of leukocyte- and platelet-rich fibrin membrane derived from cats' blood. Microscopy Research and Technique. 2021:jemt.23737. DOI: 10.1002/jemt.23737

[42] Dohan DM, Choukroun J, Diss A, Dohan SL, Dohan AJJ, Mouhyi J, et al. Platelet-rich fibrin (PRF): A second-generation platelet concentrate. Part III:

Leucocyte activation: A new feature for platelet concentrates? Oral Surgery, Oral Medicine, Oral Pathology, Oral Radiology, and Endodontology. 2006;**101**:e51-e55. DOI: 10.1016/j.tripleo.2005.07.010

[43] Kobayashi E, Flückiger L, Fujioka-Kobayashi M, Sawada K, Sculean A, Schaller B, et al. Comparative release of growth factors from PRP, PRF, and advanced-PRF. Clinical Oral Investigations. 2016;**20**:2353-2360. DOI: 10.1007/s00784-016-1719-1

[44] Fitzpatrick J, Bulsara MK, McCrory PR, Richardson MD, Zheng MH. Analysis of platelet-rich plasma extraction: Variations in platelet and blood components between 4 common commercial kits. Orthopaedic Journal of Sports Medicine. 2017;**5**:1-8. DOI: 10.1177/2325967116675272

[45] Marx RE. Platelet-rich plasma (PRP): What is PRP and what is not PRP? Implant Dentistry. 2001;**10**:225-228. DOI: 10.1097/00008505-200110000-00002

[46] Kornsuthisopon C, Pirarat N, Osathanon T, Kalpravidh C. Autologous platelet-rich fibrin stimulates canine periodontal regeneration. Scientific Reports. 2020;**10**:1850. DOI: 10.1038/s41598-020-58732-x

[47] Jansen EE, Braun A, Jansen P, Hartmann M. Platelet-therapeutics to improve tissue regeneration and wound healing—Physiological background and methods of preparation. Biomedicine. 2021;**9**:869. DOI: 10.3390/biomedicines9080869

[48] Nasirzade J, Kargarpour Z, Hasannia S, Strauss FJ, Gruber R. Platelet-rich fibrin elicits an anti-inflammatory response in macrophages in vitro. Journal of Periodontology. 2020;**91**:244-252. DOI: 10.1002/JPER.19-0216

[49] Somani A, Rai R. Comparison of efficacy of autologous platelet-rich fibrin versus saline dressing in chronic venous leg ulcers: A randomised controlled trial. Journal of Cutaneous and Aesthetic Surgery. 2017;**10**:8-12. DOI: 10.4103/JCAS.JCAS_137_16

[50] Miron RJ, Fujioka-Kobayashi M, Bishara M, Zhang Y, Hernandez M, Choukroun J. Platelet-rich fibrin and soft tissue wound healing: A systematic review. Tissue Engineering. Part B, Reviews. 2017;**23**:83-99. DOI: 10.1089/ten.teb.2016.0233

[51] Jiménez-Aristazábal RF, Carmona JU, Prades M. Changes on the structural architecture and growth factor release, and degradation in equine platelet-rich fibrin clots cultured over time. Journal of Equine Veterinary Science. 2019;**82**:102789. DOI: 10.1016/j.jevs.2019.102789

[52] Dohan Ehrenfest DM, Bielecki T, Jimbo R, Barbé G, Del Corso M, Inchingolo F, et al. Do the fibrin architecture and leukocyte content influence the growth factor release of platelet concentrates? An evidence-based answer comparing a pure platelet-rich plasma (P-PRP) gel and a leukocyte- and platelet-rich fibrin (L-PRF). Current Pharmaceutical Biotechnology. 2012;**13**:1145-1152. DOI: 10.2174/138920112800624382

[53] Pavlovic V, Ciric M, Jovanovic V, Trandafilovic M, Stojanovic P. Platelet-rich fibrin: Basics of biological actions and protocol modifications. Open Medicine. 2021;**16**:446-454. DOI: 10.1515/med-2021-0259

[54] Dohan Ehrenfest DM, Del Corso M, Diss A, Mouhyi J, Charrier J-B.

Three-dimensional architecture and cell composition of a Choukroun's platelet-rich fibrin clot and membrane. Journal of Periodontology. 2010;**81**:546-555. DOI: 10.1902/jop.2009.090531

[55] Soares C, Dias I, Pires MA, Carvalho P. Autologous platelet-rich fibrin (PRF) in canine regenerative wound therapy: A natural haemostasis mimetic. Journal of Comparative Pathology. 2022;**191**:60. ISSN 0021-9975. DOI: 10.1016/j.jcpa.2021.11.138. Available from: https://www.sciencedirect.com/science/article/pii/S002199752100284X

[56] Zinder R, Cooley R, Vlad LG, Molnar JA. Vitamin A and wound healing. Nutrition in Clinical Practice. 2019;**34**:839-849. DOI: 10.1002/ncp.10420

[57] Lin P-H, Sermersheim M, Li H, Lee P, Steinberg S, Ma J. Zinc in wound healing modulation. Nutrients. 2017;**10**:16. DOI: 10.3390/nu10010016

[58] Burnouf T, Chou M-L, Wu Y-W, Su C-Y, Lee L-W. Antimicrobial activity of platelet (PLT)-poor plasma, PLT-rich plasma, PLT gel, and solvent/detergent-treated PLT lysate biomaterials against wound bacteria. Transfusion. 2013;**53**:138-146. DOI: 10.1111/j.1537-2995.2012.03668.x

[59] Feng M, Wang Y, Zhang P, Zhao Q, Yu S, Shen K, et al. Antibacterial effects of platelet-rich fibrin produced by horizontal centrifugation. International Journal of Oral Science. 2020;**12**:1-8. DOI: 10.1038/s41368-020-00099-w

[60] Shariati A, Moradabadi A, Azimi T, Ghaznavi-Rad E. Wound healing properties and antimicrobial activity of platelet-derived biomaterials. Scientific Reports. 2020;**10**:1-9. DOI: 10.1038/s41598-020-57559-w

[61] Maddah HA. Polypropylene as a promising plastic: A review. American Journal of Polymer Science. 2016;**6**:1-11. DOI: 10.5923/j.ajps.20160601.01

[62] Albilia J, Herrera-Vizcaíno C, Weisleder H, Choukroun J, Ghanaati S. Liquid platelet-rich fibrin injections as a treatment adjunct for painful temporomandibular joints: Preliminary results. Cranio. 2020;**38**:292-304. DOI: 10.1080/08869634.2018.1516183

[63] Al-Hamed FS, Tawfik MA-M, Abdelfadil E. Clinical effects of platelet-rich fibrin (PRF) following surgical extraction of lower third molar. Saudi Journal of Dental Research. 2017;**8**:19-25. DOI: 10.1016/j.sjdr.2016.05.002

[64] Park J, Hwang S, Yoon I-S. Advanced growth factor delivery systems in wound management and skin regeneration. Molecules. 2017;**22**:1259. DOI: 10.3390/molecules22081259

[65] Nurden AT. Platelets, inflammation and tissue regeneration. Thrombosis and Haemostasis. 2011;**105**:13-33. DOI: 10.1160/THS10-11-0720

[66] Crisci A, Manfredi S, Crisci M. The L-PRF membrane (fibrin rich in platelets and leukocytes) and its derivatives useful as a source of stem cells in wound surgery. Journal of Stem Cell Reports. 2019;**1**:1-11

[67] Ghanaati S, Booms P, Orlowska A, Kubesch A, Lorenz J, Rutkowski J, et al. Advanced platelet-rich fibrin: A new concept for cell-based tissue engineering by means of inflammatory cells. The Journal of Oral Implantology. 2014;**40**:679-689. DOI: 10.1563/aaid-joi-D-14-00138

[68] Mariani E, Roffi A, Cattini L, Pulsatelli L, Assirelli E, Krishnakumar GS, et al. Release kinetic of pro- and anti-inflammatory biomolecules from platelet-rich plasma and functional study

on osteoarthritis synovial fibroblasts. Cytotherapy. 2020;**22**:344-353. DOI: 10.1016/j.jcyt.2020.02.006

[69] Ellis S, Lin EJ, Tartar D. Immunology of wound healing. Current Dermatology Reports. 2018;**7**:350-358. DOI: 10.1007/s13671-018-0234-9

[70] Lee KY. M1 and M2 polarization of macrophages: A mini-review. Medical Biological Science and Engineering. 2019;**2**:1-5. DOI: 10.30579/mbse.2019.2.1.1

[71] Orekhov AN, Orekhova VA, Nikiforov NG, Myasoedova VA, Grechko AV, Romanenko EB, et al. Monocyte differentiation and macrophage polarization. Vessel Plus. 2019;**3**:10. DOI: 10.20517/2574-1209.2019.04

[72] McGrath MH. Peptide growth factors and wound healing. Clinics in Plastic Surgery. 1990;**17**:421-432

[73] Tottoli EM, Dorati R, Genta I, Chiesa E, Pisani S, Conti B. Skin wound healing process and new emerging technologies for skin wound care and regeneration. Pharmaceutics. 2020;**12**:735. DOI: 10.3390/pharmaceutics12080735

[74] Jiménez-Aristizabal RF, López C, Álvarez ME, Giraldo C, Prades M, Carmona JU. Long-term cytokine and growth factor release from equine platelet-rich fibrin clots obtained with two different centrifugation protocols. Cytokine. 2017;**97**:149-155. DOI: 10.1016/j.cyto.2017.06.011

[75] Soares CS, Barros LC, Dias IR, Pires MA, Carvalho PP. Clinical insights of platelet-rich fibrin (PRF) as an active biomaterial for wound regeneration. In: 17th Montenegro International Veterinary Congress Santa Maria da Feira, Portugal. 2021

[76] Soares CS, Barros LC, Dias IR, Pires MA, Carvalho PP. Platelet-rich fibrin in regenerative wound therapy: Preliminary outcomes in canine patients. In: South. Eur. Vet. Conf., Barcelona, Spain. 2020

[77] Gemignani F, Perazzi A, Iacopetti I. Use of canine sourced platelet-rich plasma in a feline contaminated cutaneous wound. The Canadian Veterinary Journal. 2017;**58**:141-144

[78] Karina Gomes Barros A, Bruno Nascimento B, Inara Guastini D, Eliane Szücs Dos S, Cecília Braga L, Gisele Alborghetti N, et al. Effects of heterologous platelet-rich plasma gel on standardized dermal wound healing in rabbits. Acta Cirúrgica Brasileira. 2015;**30**:209-215. DOI: 10.1590/S0102-865020150030000008

[79] Wardrop KJ, Birkenheuer A, Blais MC, Callan MB, Kohn B, Lappin MR, et al. Update on canine and feline blood donor screening for blood-borne pathogens. Journal of Veterinary Internal Medicine. 2016;**30**:15-35. DOI: 10.1111/jvim.13823

[80] Gibson G. Transfusion medicine. In: King L, Boag A, editors. BSAVA Man. Canine Feline Emerg. Crit. Care. 2nd ed. Quedgeley, Gloucs United Kingdom: British Small Animal Veterinary Association; 2007. pp. 215-227

[81] Hamed MA, Abouelnasr KS, El-Adl M, Abo Elfadl EA, Farag A, Lashen S. Effectiveness of allogeneic platelet-rich fibrin on second-intention wound healing of experimental skin defect in distal limb in donkeys (Equus asinus). Journal of Equine Veterinary Science. 2019;**73**:131-138. DOI: 10.1016/j.jevs.2018.12.014

[82] Catarino J, Carvalho P, Santos S, Martins Â, Requicha J. Treatment of

canine osteoarthritis with allogeneic platelet-rich plasma: Review of five cases. Open Veterinary Journal. 2020;**10**:226-231. DOI: 10.4314/ovj.v10i2.12

[83] Ozgul O, Senses F, Er N, Tekin U, Tuz HH, Alkan A, et al. Efficacy of platelet rich fibrin in the reduction of the pain and swelling after impacted third molar surgery: Randomized multicenter split-mouth clinical trial. Head & Face Medicine. 2015;**11**:37. DOI: 10.1186/s13005-015-0094-5

[84] Ozer K, Colak O. Leucocyte- and platelet-rich fibrin as a rescue therapy for small-to-medium-sized complex wounds of the lower extremities. Burn Trauma. 2019;7:11. DOI: 10.1186/s41038-019-0149-0

[85] Pinto NR, Ubilla M, Zamora Y, Del Rio V, Dohan Ehrenfest DM, Quirynen M. Leucocyte- and platelet-rich fibrin (L-PRF) as a regenerative medicine strategy for the treatment of refractory leg ulcers: A prospective cohort study. Platelets. 2018;**29**:468-475. DOI: 10.1080/09537104.2017.1327654

[86] Arnalich F, Rodriguez AE, Luque-Rio A, Alio JL. Solid platelet rich plasma in corneal surgery. Ophthalmology and Therapy. 2016;**5**:31-45. DOI: 10.1007/s40123-016-0051-9

[87] Alio JL, Rodriguez AE, WróbelDudzińska D. Eye platelet-rich plasma in the treatment of ocular surface disorders. Current Opinion in Ophthalmology. 2015;**26**:325-332. DOI: 10.1097/ICU.0000000000000169

[88] Mariani E, Pulsatelli L. Platelet concentrates in musculoskeletal medicine. International Journal of Molecular Sciences. 2020;**21**:1328. DOI: 10.3390/ijms21041328

[89] Anitua E, Alkhraisat MH, Orive G. Perspectives and challenges in regenerative medicine using plasma rich in growth factors. Journal of Controlled Release. 2012;**157**:29-38. DOI: 10.1016/j.jconrel.2011.07.004

[90] McNamee MJ, Coveney CM, Faulkner A, Gabe J. Ethics, evidence based sports medicine, and the use of platelet rich plasma in the English premier league. Health Care Analysis. 2018;**26**:344-361. DOI: 10.1007/s10728-017-0345-7

[91] Dohan Ehrenfest DM, Bielecki T, Mishra A, Borzini P, Inchingolo F, Sammartino G, et al. In search of a consensus terminology in the field of platelet concentrates for surgical use: Platelet-rich plasma (PRP), platelet-rich fibrin (PRF), fibrin gel polymerization and leukocytes. Current Pharmaceutical Biotechnology. 2012;**13**:1131-1137. DOI: 10.2174/138920112800624328

[92] Mautner K, Malanga GA, Smith J, Shiple B, Ibrahim V, Sampson S, et al. A call for a standard classification system for future biologic research: The rationale for new PRP nomenclature. Journal of Physical Medicine and Rehabilitation. 2015;7:S53-S59. DOI: 10.1016/j.pmrj.2015.02.005

[93] Marín, Fermín T, Calcei JG, Della Vedova F, Martinez Cano JP, Arias Calderon C, Imam MA, et al. Classification of platelet concentrates: From pure platelet-rich plasma (P-PRP) to leucocyte- and platelet-rich fibrin (L-PRF). Journal of ISAKOS. 2023;S2059-7754(23)00545-X. DOI: 10.1016/j.jisako.2023.07.010

[94] Delong JM, Russell RP, Mazzocca AD. Platelet-rich plasma: The PAW classification system. Arthroscopy: The Journal of Arthroscopic & Related Surgery. 2012;**28**:998-1009. DOI: 10.1016/j.arthro.2012.04.148

Chapter 4

Amniotic Membrane in the Treatment of Hard-to-Heal Wounds

Febe Antoinette Bruwer

Abstract

Chronic or hard to heal wounds result in protracted healing trajectories that place a significant burden on both the patient and the society. Wounds that are classified as hard to heal often result in management challenges for which adjunctive therapies are indicated to assist in the healing process. Adjunctive therapy in wound management refers to additional treatment methods that are used to support or enhance the effectiveness of the primary wound therapy. Several types of adjunctive therapies are available, each with its own merit. Adjunctive therapy is used in conjunction with standard wound care practices to promote healing and assist in preventing complications. In the race against increasing costs, an aging population and increased incidence and prevalence of debilitating co-morbid conditions like diabetes, clinicians need to be innovative in the utilization of recourses that could assist in improving outcomes for patients that suffer from chronic or hard to heal wounds. The use of adjunctive therapy like amniotic membrane (AM) is supported by elevated levels of evidence in that this therapy could, when incorporated into an evidence-based standard of care regime, support or enhance the effectiveness of care and improve outcomes for patients suffering with chronic or hard to heal wounds. The following sections will give an overview of chronic wound healing, where in the treatment algorithm an adjunctive therapy like amniotic membrane could be utilized as well as the practical application of amniotic membrane.

Keywords: chronic wounds, hard to heal, wound bed preparation, amniotic membrane, placenta, adjunctive therapy

1. Introduction

Chronic or hard-to-heal wounds include lower leg ulcers, diabetic foot ulcers (DFU), pressure injuries (PI), atypical wounds, and both burns or surgical wounds that have complicated [1]. These wounds represent a huge socioeconomic burden to both the patient suffering from it and the community at large [2].

In the United States and Europe, the cost of treating these ulcers amounts to 1–2% of the annual healthcare resources [3, 4]. Chronic wounds have protracted healing trajectories and require advanced interdisciplinary management for a successful outcome, and even then, about 2% of the wounds will never heal [5, 6]. Chronic wounds furthermore result in reduced quality of life due to pain and suffering [1].

Within the spectrum of interdisciplinary management, adjunctive therapies are considered a valuable resource in the management of these challenging wounds. Adjunctive therapies could aid the healing process by augmenting or supporting the treatment when wounds are not responding to the standard of care [1].

Historically, the amniotic membrane was first used in the early 1900s as "skin transplantation" for burns and other wounds [7]. Later, it was used as a graft to promote healing and reduce inflammation in cases of corneal ulcers and ocular surface reconstruction. It can be used to repair damaged or diseased ocular surfaces, such as in cases of chemical burns, Stevens-Johnson syndrome, or other traumatic injuries [8]. Amniotic membranes are also used in the treatment of dry eye syndrome and limbal stem cell deficiency, as well as conjunctival reconstruction and ocular surgery. It can also be used to reduce inflammation and promote tissue repair in various ocular conditions, such as uveitis or scleritis [8].

Some of the benefits of amniotic membranes includes the promotion of epithelialization by providing a structure for cellular migration and proliferation [9]. This could contribute to reduced time to healing and reduced costs [10]. Several studies have shown that the use of AM with standard-of-care treatment significantly improves healing times in both venous leg ulcers and diabetic foot ulcers [11, 12]. Tettelbach et al. [11] showed significantly improved healing times in the group of patients with diabetic foot ulcers that were treated with dehydrated human amnion/chorion membrane, which supported the findings of Snyder et al. [13]. A systematic review by Lakmal et al. [14] furthermore concluded that healing time is reduced with the use of AM when compared to only standard of care. Amniotic membrane (AM) is thus one such adjunctive therapy that could be beneficial in the treatment of hard-to-heal wounds.

Adjunctive therapies have the best potential to promote healing when patient factors, the underlying cause of the wound, potential for healability, and resource limitations are accounted for in hard-to-heal wounds [5].

2. Defining a chronic or hard-to-heal wound

The wound-healing cascade has four distinct but overlapping phases, which are described as hemostasis, inflammation, proliferation, maturation, and remodeling [15]. This cascade is coordinated and usually happens within a certain time frame, i.e., 4–6 weeks.

Chronic wounds, unlike acute wounds, do not follow the expected healing cascade and often develop due to underlying issues that have not or could not be addressed [4]. These underlying issues furthermore contribute to failure to heal and chronicity of the wound [3, 16].

A chronic wound is thus a wound that has not healed within the expected time frame, typically lasting longer than 6 weeks [3, 6]. These wounds often occur as a result of underlying health conditions, such as diabetes, vascular disease (arterial or venous), or other comorbidities, and often require specialized treatment and care to achieve healing. Chronic wounds can be painful, complicate due to infections, and have a significant impact on a person's quality of life [5, 17]. Chronic wounds are often stalled within the inflammatory phase of wound healing due to local wound bed issues like the presence of devitalized tissue, local infection, and the presence of increased levels of proteolytic enzymes, which, if not modulated by an intrinsic immune response, could, contribute to chronicity [4].

For healing to occur, this tissue microenvironment requires sufficient levels of bioactive proteins, such as growth factors and other soluble mediators of cell signaling, functional fibroblasts, keratinocytes, and vascular endothelial cells [18]. Furthermore, this process also needs controlled levels of proteases and bacteria in an environment that supports the healing process through the presence of adequate blood supply and favorable conditions for healing [16, 19, 20].

The presence of persistent inflammation, cell senescence, growth factor deficiencies, high levels of bioburden, elevated concentrations of destructive proteases, and stem cell deficiencies are typically found in chronic wounds [21].

Chronic wounds could furthermore be classified as hard to heal, maintenance, or non-healable wounds due to either patient or system factors that could not be addressed or treated [5].

These factors include intrinsic and extrinsic factors like infection, hypoxia, underlying diseases, and several other pathophysiological events, which result in prolonged inflammation, increased bioload, cell senescence, and an inability to heal [6]. Comorbidities like hypertension, diabetes, malnutrition, autoimmune diseases, and respiratory or kidney disease could influence healing [22]. Coexistent issues such as peripheral vascular disease, neuropathy, poor glycemic control, or anemia could furthermore contribute to the slow healing rates and high recurrence rates of these wounds. Lifestyle choices like smoking or obesity or a sedentary lifestyle could additionally increase the risk of delayed healing [3].

System factors could include health system challenges which might involve a lack of resources, limited access to care, and limited skill or expertise of the health care practitioner [5].

Wound size reduction is seen as a measure of healing, and a reduction in size of 40% in 4 weeks is a significant predictor of a healing outcome at 12 weeks [16]. A wound that has not reduced in size by 40–50% at week four with standard of care being delivered could thus be classified as hard to heal. Re-assessment by an interdisciplinary team and the use of adjunctive therapies are then indicated to assist the healing process [5, 16].

However, without maintenance debridement and normalization of proteases and the inflammatory process, an effective extracellular matrix cannot be restored, and healing is unlikely to progress [16, 23]. Prior to using amniotic membranes, a thorough initial assessment of the patient and the wound is necessary, which includes a comprehensive history [24]. Gather information on the history of the wound, including the duration of the wound, what treatments have been tried, and the patient's comorbidities. Once this is done, the next step should involve wound bed preparation.

3. Wound bed preparation

Wound bed preparation is described as a "structured approach" to wound management in that the focus is shifted from only treating the wound to treating the patient with a wound by addressing underlying causes and determining healability before addressing local wound care issues [16].

Standard of care with regard to wound management include debridement, infection control, and proper wound dressing, as well as treatment of the underlying cause, to enhance the healing process and improve patient outcomes. It is important to note that these therapies should be used under the supervision of healthcare professionals who specialize in wound management.

Wound bed preparation principles involve assessing and treating the underlying cause determining healability, after which appropriate local wound management includes debridement of devitalized tissue, treating infection, managing moisture, and promoting epithelial advancement [16]. The wound bed should be clear of any necrotic tissue and should not have any signs of infection to facilitate the effective application of AM. The application of AM is described in Section 5.

3.1 Debridement

Debridement is the removal of any foreign material from the wound bed to facilitate the healing process. This includes devitalized tissue, foreign bodies, senescent cells, and bacteria or biofilm. The presence of the foreign material could result in a state of chronic inflammation and prevent healing. Adequate debridement is vital for the application of adjunctive therapies like AM. Prior to choosing a debridement method, it is essential that the patient's healing ability, i.e., blood supply to the area, be assessed and confirmed as being adequate.

Methods of debridement are outlined in **Table 1**.

When choosing a debridement method, it is imperative that the clinician establish if the blood supply to the area is adequate, after which the best possible option should

Type of debridement	Method	Considerations and contraindications
Autolytic	Facilitated through the application of occlusive dressings. Endogenous enzymes break down devitalized tissue.	Safe and easy but can protracted and has a risk of peri-wound maceration. Contraindicated with inadequate blood supply (arterial insufficiency) or when the wound is infected.
Enzymatic	Requires the application of a proteolytic enzyme.	Safe and easy but requires daily application. It could be costly.
Biological	Medical-grade maggots secrete a proteolytic enzyme and liquefy devitalized tissue.	Fast and effective but contraindicated in ischemic wounds. Patient preference should be considered as growing maggots could cause pain and anxiety.
Sharp	The use of surgical instruments to remove devitalized tissue. It could also include hydro surgery, ultrasound, or laser debridement).	Fast and effective, it requires skill and the use of local anesthetic and could cause bleeding. Contra is indicated when arterial supply is not adequate or malignancies.
Surgical	Done in the operating room under anesthesia.	Although fast and effective, it is invasive and could be costly, and all risks associated with surgery should be considered.
Mechanical	Removal of necrotic tissue by mechanical force. This includes "wet-to-dry," pulse lavage, or monofilament pads.	Although easy, this method could be painful and cause damage to granulation tissue, resulting in bleeding.

Table 1.
Debridement methods (adapted from [1, 3]).

be discussed with the patient with regard to accessibility, cost, and outcome. Written consent is often required.

3.2 Wound infection

Although all chronic wounds have a high probability of being contaminated with bacteria, the presence of wound infection is one of the most significant contributors to delayed healing. Current guidelines and consensus advocate for early diagnosis and appropriate treatment in line with antimicrobial stewardship principles.

Link to the Internationl Wound Infection Institute Consensus document: https://doi.org/10.12968/jowc.2022.31.Sup12.S10

AM does have some antimicrobial properties but for effective use, it is advisable to treat wound infection prior to the application thereof.

3.3 Other types of adjunctive therapies

Adjuvant or adjunctive therapy in wound management refers to additional treatment methods that are used to support or enhance the effectiveness of the primary wound therapy. Adjunctive therapies are indicated when wounds become stalled or "hard to heal" [1]. Some common adjunctive therapies in wound management include:

Negative Pressure Wound Therapy (*NPWT*) involves applying a vacuum to a wound dressing to create negative pressure, which helps to remove excess fluid, reduce swelling, and promote tissue granulation and healing [25]. The use of NPWT in the treatment of non-ischemic DFUs is supported by high levels of evidence but less so for venous lower leg ulcers and pressure injuries [25, 26].

Hyperbaric Oxygen Therapy (*HBOT*) involves exposing the patient to pure oxygen at higher than atmospheric pressure, which can improve oxygen delivery to tissues, reduce inflammation, and promote wound healing, especially in acute injuries [1, 27]. Some studies suggest the use of HBOT in conjunction with the standard of care may have some benefits and improved healing outcomes [28].

Electrical stimulation involves the application of electrical currents to the wound site, which could stimulate cell growth and possibly promote healing [29]. Current evidence suggests that *electrical stimulation* could possibly be utilized as adjunctive therapy [30]. More evidence seems to be needed to support its use.

Several other adjunctive therapies are in the process of being evaluated, and some evidence supports the use of modalities like *biological dressings* that are made from materials such as collagen, hyaluronic acid, or other biologically active substances that could promote tissue repair, but more robust evidence is needed [26]. Another adjunctive therapy is *autologous blood clots* made from the patient's own blood, and a variety of studies, both in vitro and human trials does, suggest that the use thereof could accelerate tissue repair [31].

The application of *growth factor*-containing gels or creams to the wound site also seems to have some merit, but more evidence is required [32]. Advanced biological therapies including platelet-rich plasma (PRP), bioengineered cell-based therapies, and recombinant growth factors (r-GF) may be of benefit in enhancing healing and quality of life in patients with recalcitrant foot ulcers [33]. The use of these modalities is currently only supported by low-level evidence and is not routinely recommended [1].

Autologous platelet-rich plasma (*PRP*) is derived from a sample of blood taken from the patient, and then separated by utilizing a centrifuge; the plasma is then applied to the wound locally. A Cochrane review done in 2016 has, however, concluded that the use of PRP is only supported by low-level evidence, and the results were not conclusive as to the efficacy of enhancing wound healing in chronic wounds [34].

Low-level laser therapy has been shown to enhance tissue repair, reduce inflammation, and relieve pain in certain types of wounds [1, 29, 35]. Moreover, the use of therapeutic ultrasound in the treatment of lower leg ulcers is thus far only supported by low-level evidence [26].

Amniotic membrane (AM), which in obtained from human placenta is an adjunctive therapy with much potential as it can be utilized as an adjunctive therapy to aid wound healing and supported by several levels of evidence [12, 36]. Amniotic membrane contains growth factors (GFs), cytokines, and stem cells that could stimulate the regeneration of tissue and even inhibit infection [8]. Amniotic membrane has gained significant attention in wound healing and tissue regeneration due to its unique properties and benefits [8]. A meta-analysis done by Haugh et al. [36] found significant improvement in healing rates in DFUs, whereas Serena et al. reported improved healing rates in venous lower leg ulcers treated with AM and compression when compared to wounds only treated with compression [21].

4. Amniotic membrane

4.1 Structure and function of amniotic membrane

Amniotic membrane is the innermost part of the placenta collected or harvested post birth from human donors, as illustrated in **Figure 1**.

The amnion consists of three basic layers adjacent to the chorion. These layers are the inner epithelial layer, the basement membrane, and the stromal layer, which also has three layers, namely the compact, fibroblast, and reticular layers [37]. Within this scaffold, an array of regulatory proteins are found that could assist in tissue modulation and promote healing [18, 37].

The layers contain growth factors, prostaglandins, cytokines and extracellular proteins as well as proteoglycans, collagen and elastin. These components contribute to the AM's unique properties [8].

Figure 2 is an illustration of the layers within the amniotic membrane.

The introduction and use of AM seem to have had a slow evolution, which could possibly be attributed to the initial concerns about disease transmission or other immunologic concerns, but the improved harvesting and preservation techniques have contributed to expanded utilization and availability [8]. Several proprietary methods are utilized to harvest, process, and preserve the membranes for use.

The placental membrane is recovered aseptically from donated placental membranes through elective cesarean section. All donors are routinely screened for infectious, malignant, neurological, and autoimmune diseases to determine whether they are suitable for donation. The donor blood is usually assessed by an independent certified laboratory at the time of delivery. Only donor tissue of donors that have tested negative for the minimum serological tests is used to produce AM. Tests conducted include HIV PCR qualitative, HIV I & II ELISA, hepatitis B surface antigen (HBsAg), hepatitis B surface antibodies (HBsAb), hepatitis B core antibody (HBcAb), hepatitis C antibody (HCVAb), HTLV I & II antibodies, syphilis (RPR), treponema pallidum IgG, treponema pallidum IgM, CMV IgG, CMV IgM, and IgG antibodies [38].

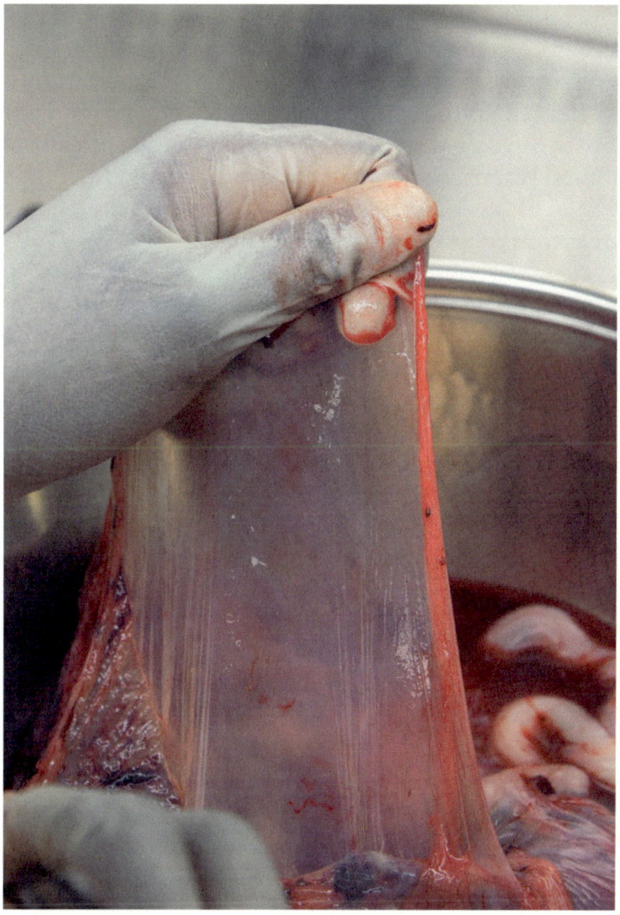

Figure 1.
Image of placental membrane (supplied by Next Bioscences).

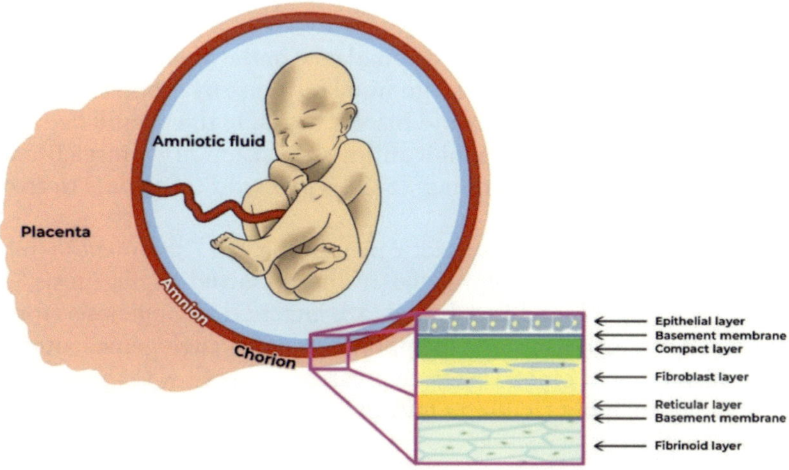

Figure 2.
Snapshot illustration of the layers within the amniotic membrane.

The placental membrane layer is mechanically separated from the placenta under aseptic conditions before being enzymatically treated to remove epithelial cells from the membrane surface. The membrane is also photochemically cross-linked. The membrane is oriented epithelial side down and laid onto a specifically designed polyester net before being dehydrated for packing. Once aseptically packaged, the dehydrated membrane is sterilized by gamma irradiation.

4.2 Mechanism of action of amniotic membrane

The proposed mechanism of action of amniotic membrane is creating an environment rich in growth factors and cytokines and reducing levels of proteases [12]. The amniotic membrane furthermore has several properties which could contribute to healing. The properties of AM include:

- Anti-inflammatory properties
- Immune modulating properties
- Promotion of angiogenesis
- Extra cellular matrix support
- Antimicrobial properties
- Pain reduction

Figure 3 is a schematic of the properties and associated biomarkers identified within the AM. Used with permission from both Elkhenany et al. [9] and Springer Publishing.

Amniotic membrane contains various anti-inflammatory molecules such as cytokine inhibitors, growth factors, and immunomodulatory factors [8]. These components help reduce inflammation in chronic wounds, which is crucial for initiating the healing process and preventing further tissue destruction typical to chronic wound healing [4].

Chronic wounds often suffer from an imbalance in the immune response [1, 4]. Amniotic membrane helps regulate the immune response by modulating the activity of immune cells, such as neutrophils and macrophages, in the wound bed. Amniotic membranes contain proteins that exhibit antimicrobial action against a broad spectrum of bacteria, viruses, and even fungi [8, 9]. This could contribute to an optimized environment for healing.

Within the second layer of the amniotic membrane, the "basement membrane," several macro molecules regulate epithelial proliferation and angiogenesis. Chronic wounds often lack proper blood supply and face impaired angiogenesis (formation of new blood vessels). Amniotic membrane contains angiogenic factors and promotes the formation of blood vessels, increasing blood flow to the wound area. This enhanced blood supply facilitates nutrient and oxygen delivery to the wound, promoting healing [8].

Amniotic membrane furthermore serves as a natural scaffold, providing structural support and acting as a physical barrier to prevent infection. It contains proteins like

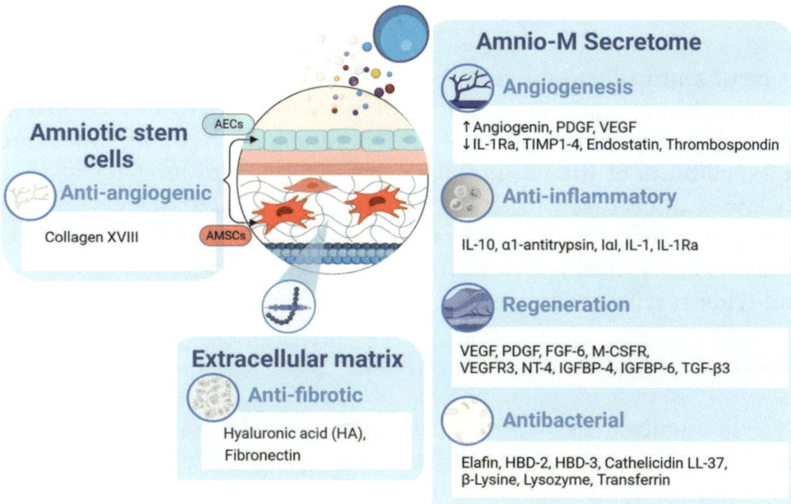

Figure 3.
Schematic of the effects of amniotic membrane (used with permission [9]).

collagen, fibronectin, and laminin within the stromal layer, which help in the formation of new tissue and enhance the migration and proliferation of cells involved in wound healing [8].

Chronic wounds are more inclined to infections [39]. Wound infection is one of the single most frequent contributors to delayed healing [39]. Amniotic membrane exhibits antimicrobial activity against several bacteria and fungi, reducing the risk of infections and promoting an environment for optimal healing.

Debilitating pain that influences the patient's quality of life is often associated with chronic wounds [4, 40]. The use of amniotic membrane has been shown to alleviate pain by reducing inflammation, promoting healing, and providing a barrier to external stimuli [41]. Overall, the unique combination of anti-inflammatory, immune modulating, angiogenic, antimicrobial, and scaffold properties makes amniotic membranes a promising option to accelerate the healing process of chronic wounds. Its natural origin, ease of application, and effectiveness make it an attractive treatment modality in wound care [11, 12, 41].

4.3 Types of amniotic membrane

There are basically three types of amniotic membranes available, and the main difference lies in the method of preservation and the resulting properties for medical use.

4.3.1 Dehydrated amniotic membrane

This type of amniotic membrane is processed to remove water content, resulting in a dehydrated, thin, and translucent membrane that can be stored at room temperature. It is commonly used in the treatment of wounds, burns, and surgical procedures. **Figure 2** is an image of a dehydrated amniotic membrane.

4.3.2 Cryopreserved amniotic membrane

This type of amniotic membrane is processed and preserved using cryopreservation techniques to maintain its biological properties and integrity. Cryopreserved amniotic membrane is preserved using a freezing process to maintain the viability of the tissue. This method allows for long-term storage at extremely low temperatures, typically in liquid nitrogen, to preserve the tissue for an extended period of time. It is typically stored at ultra-low temperatures and can be used for various clinical applications, including ophthalmic surgeries, soft tissue repair, and regenerative medicine.

4.3.3 Hypothermically stored amniotic membrane

This type of membrane is preserved at an extremely low temperature in a solution that maintains its structural and biological integrity. Hypothermically, it is stored at low temperatures, but not frozen. It is typically kept at temperatures just above freezing to maintain the viability of the tissue for a shorter period of time compared to cryopreserved tissue. This type of preservation is designed to maintain the native properties of the amniotic membrane and is typically used for surgical applications such as wound healing and tissue repair.

Figure 4 is an image of a dehydrated amniotic membrane.

4.4 Contraindications for the use of amniotic membrane

For the application of amniotic membrane to be effective, the wound bed needs to be sufficiently debrided and clean of debris. There should also be no clinical signs of infection. Please follow the manufacturer's instructions as some products utilized in the preservation process might cause allergic reactions.

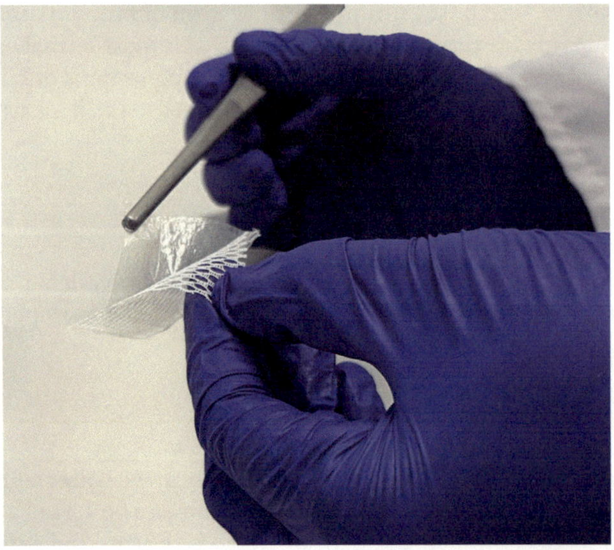

Figure 4.
Image of dehydrated amniotic membrane (supplied by Next Biosciences).

4.5 Economic considerations

It is difficult to definitively determine whether AM is more cost-effective that some of the other adjunctive therapies available as there are many variables that can affect the cost of each option. With regard to AM, costs to consider may include the initial cost of processing and preparing the amniotic membrane, the cost of storage and transportation, the shelf life of diverse types of amniotic membrane, and the specific requirements of the medical procedure for which the amniotic membrane will be used.

Additionally, the specific needs and preferences of the healthcare provider and patient may also influence the cost-effectiveness of each option. Therefore, it is important to consider all of these factors when comparing the cost-effectiveness of adjunctive therapies.

According to NICE guidance on the use of allografts, there is currently no published economic evidence on the use of amniotic membrane, but several studies have concluded that the use of AM in hard-to-heal wounds does reduce time to healing when compared to standard of care [13, 14, 21]. From this data, one could deduce that a reduction in time to healing could have a favorable economic outcome; improved healing would lead to fewer hospital visits for people with chronic wounds and reduced risk of infection and limb amputation, leading to significant quality-of-life improvements. Glat et al. compared the cost of treatment of AM to tissue-engineered human skin and concluded that healing time is significantly reduced with the use of AM but also the cost of treatment [10].

4.6 Ethical use of amniotic membrane

Amniotic membrane is harvested from discarded amnions after giving birth, and thus, "medical waste and the procurement is not affiliated with ethical issues when compared to for instance embryonic stem cells" [37].

Amnion-derived stem cells have been found to be non-tumorigenic and have low immunogenicity [37]. Patient-centered concerns should be assessed as some patients might object to the use of AM due to religious or cultural beliefs. The procurement of AM has developed to such an extent that the product is more readily available and has a longer shelf life [8].

5. Application of amniotic membrane

Amniotic membrane can be applied to a wound in several ways, which include:

Surgical placement: A surgeon can apply amniotic membrane directly to the wound during a surgical procedure. The membrane is carefully positioned over the wound and secured in place, typically with sutures or surgical adhesive.

Transplantation: In this method, the amniotic membrane is placed over the wound and carefully secured using medical dressings and bandages. Over time, the membrane incorporates into the wound.

Injections: Amniotic membrane can also be processed into a liquid or gel form for injection directly into the wound site. This method is typically used for smaller, less severe wounds.

Regardless of the method used, the amniotic membrane acts as a biological dressing that provides a protective barrier for the wound, promotes tissue regeneration, and reduces inflammation and scarring. It can also be customized to match the size and shape of the wound, making it a versatile option for wound care.

The images in **Table 2** illustrate how dehydrated amniotic membrane is removed from the packaging and net and then applied directly onto a cleansed prepared wound bed.

Amniotic membrane sterile packaging	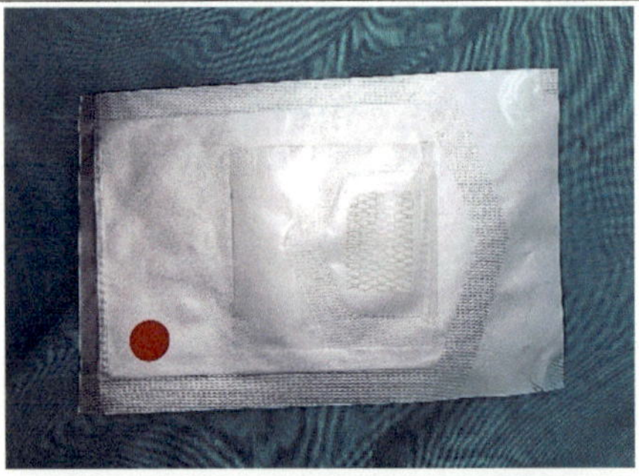
Amniotic membrane being removed from net backing	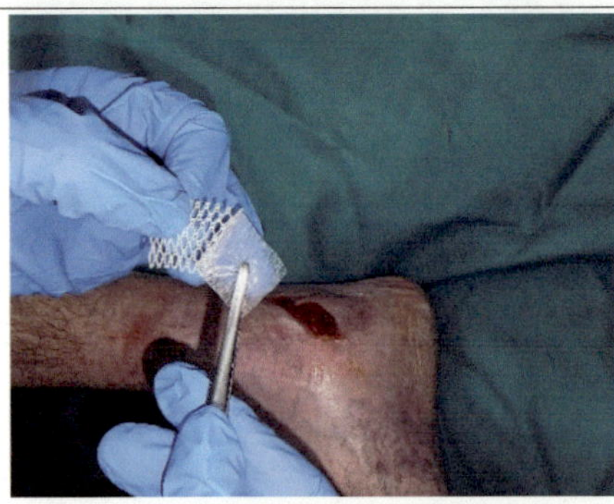
Amniotic membrane removed from net, ready for application	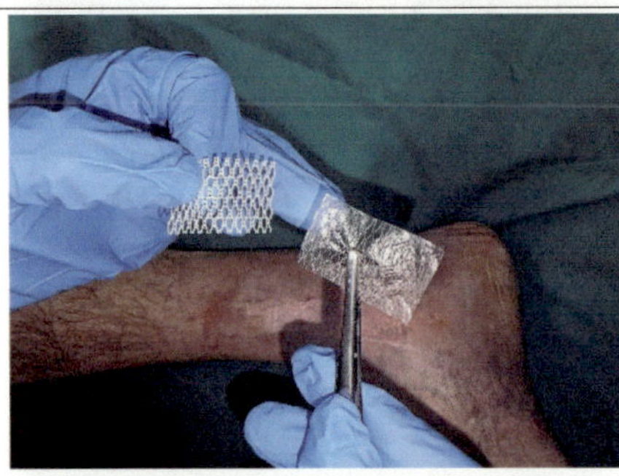
Amniotic membrane being applied on prepared wound bed	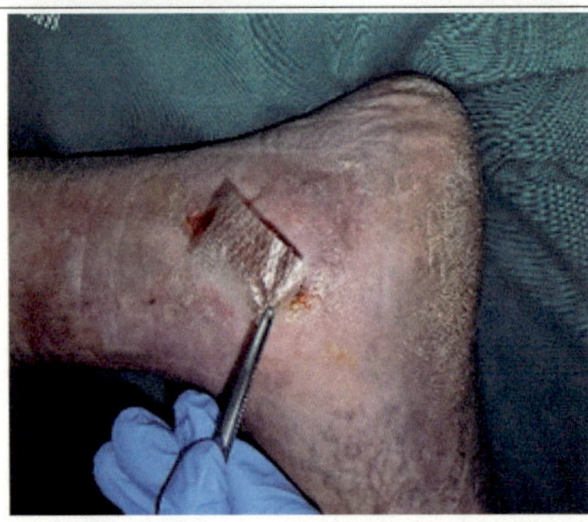

Table 2.
The application of AM to a prepared wound bed.

The AM is usually packed in a sterile container that should be stored according to the manufacturer's instructions.

AM is easy to apply, painless, and requires very little resources, i.e., hospital or theater. Most patients are treated in an outpatient setting.

6. Clinical application of amniotic membrane

Amniotic membrane has an array of applications. Several publications over the last 5–7 years have concluded that the use of amniotic membranes in hard-to-heal wounds like diabetic foot ulcers, lower leg ulcers, and pressure injuries could result in reduced time to healing and recurrence [13, 21, 42].

Lakmal et al. concluded in a systematic review of the available evidence on the use of AM in the treatment of diabetic foot ulcers that the evidence does confirm a reduction in healing time when compared with the standard of care [14].

Data from a Randomized control trial (RCT) done by Tettelbach et al. [11] showed results of complete healing with the use of AM in 70% of the patients with DFUs when compared to 50% of complete healing in the control group receiving standard of care. For the treatment of venous lower leg ulcers, Bianchi et al. [43] found a 60% healing rate at 12 weeks with patients treated with AM when compared to a 35% healing rate in patients treated with standard of care i.e. compression.

A review of different types of chronic wounds concluded that treatment efficacy were between 86-89% when using amniotic membrane with standard of care in chronic wounds [44].

The following illustrates two examples of its utilization in hard to heal wounds.

6.1 Case 1

This case is an 87-year-old female patient who was bitten by a dog. This resulted in a very large laceration with tissue loss over the right calf. The patient was treated conservatively as she did not have medical funding. Wound cleansing and debridement were done in an outpatient wound center. Comorbidities identified that might influence healing are outlined in **Table 3**.

Standard of care included wound cleansing with hypochlorous acid and autolytic debridement. The wound exudate was furthermore managed with a hydrofiber dressing, and compression therapy was applied using the "African Bandaging System," which comprises two 150 mm knitted crepe and orthopedic wool [45]. This was a more cost-effective option when considering the patient's lack of resources.

The patient gave written consent for the utilization of images. Images courtesy of FA Bruwer (the author). **Figure 5** is an image of the wound shortly after injury on 10 August 2023.

Intrinsic	Extrinsic
Age	Location of the wound
Hypertension	Size and severity of the wound
Cardiac disease	Limited resources

Table 3.
Comorbidities identified in patient 1.

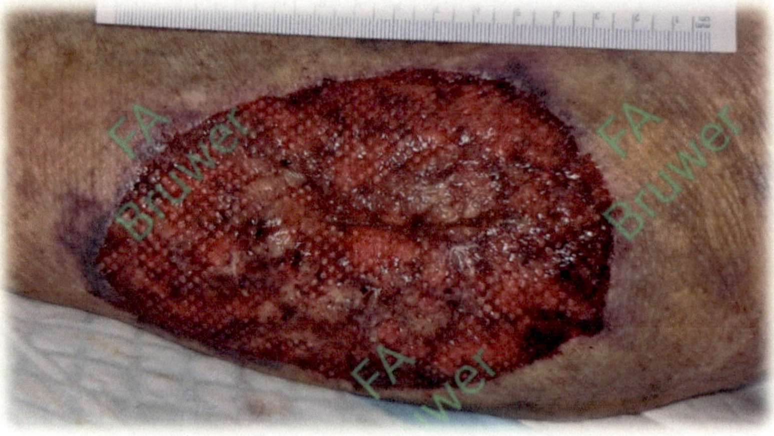

Figure 5.
Image of the wound shortly after the injury on 10 August 2023.

Although there was progress, the wound size has decreased from 96 cm^2 to about 76 cm^2, which calculates to a 20% reduction in size at 6 weeks post-injury. This is seen as a slower than expected rate and could indicate a protracted healing trajectory [16]. The suggested treatment was a split-thickness skin graft, but that would imply hospitalization and cost, which the patient declined. Due to the patient's comorbidities, which included age and hypertension, this was also not a favorable option. The wound bed was prepared, and an amniotic membrane was applied. The application did not require any special procedures. **Figure 6** shows the wound about 6 weeks after the initial injury.

Figure 7 shows the wound 2 weeks after the first application of AM. AM was applied weekly. The standard of care remained the same. One of the challenges of care was the fact that the patient had advanced dementia and kept on removing the compression bandage.

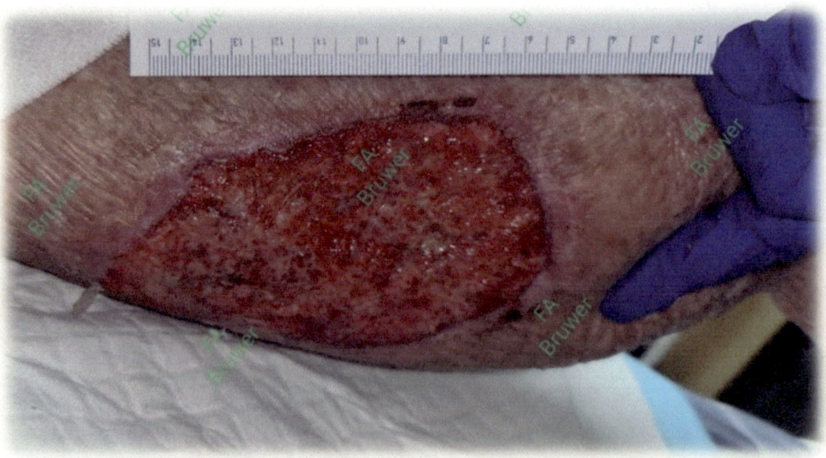

Figure 6.
Image of the wound about 6 weeks after initial injury.

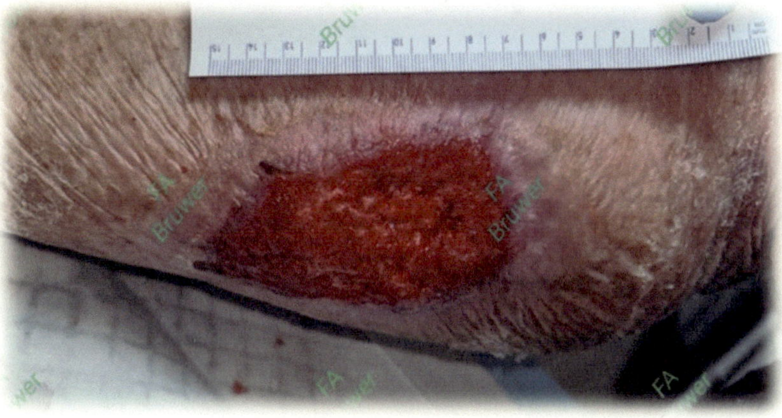

Figure 7.
Image of the wound 2 weeks after initial application.

Figure 8 shows the wound 4 weeks after the initial application of amniotic membrane.

Figure 9 shows wound 6 weeks after initial application. Dressing change frequency could be reduced to weekly. Only a very basic wound contact layer was required, and compression continued.

Figure 10 was taken 14 weeks after the initial injury, but 8 weeks after the application of the first AM. Wounds on the lower leg tend to have extended healing trajectories of between 12 and 24 weeks with standard of care.

At this stage, the patient could be stepped down to compression hosiery to prevent recurrence [40].

Injuries on the lower leg often result in chronic non-healing wounds that are both debilitating to the patient and very costly to treat. On average, lower leg ulcers take 12–24 weeks to heal when all underlying issues are addressed, and the patient is receiving standard of care, i.e., compression therapy [5].

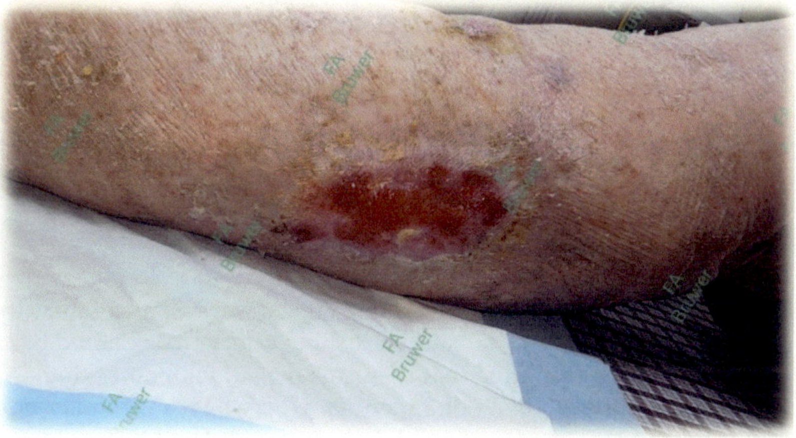

Figure 8.
Four weeks after initial application.

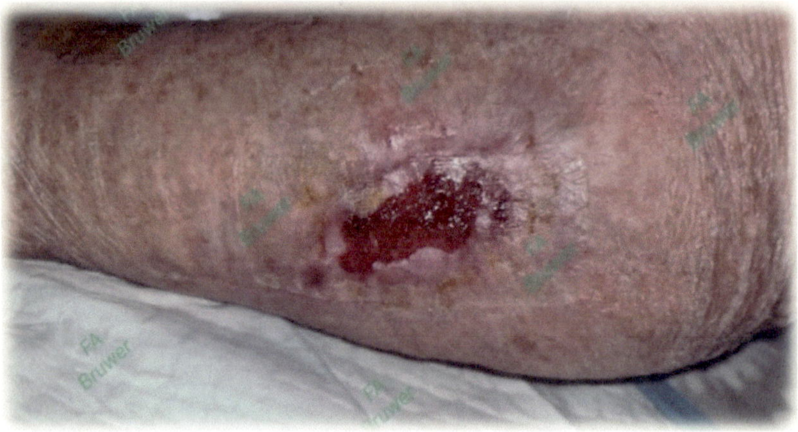

Figure 9.
Image of the wound 6 weeks after initial application.

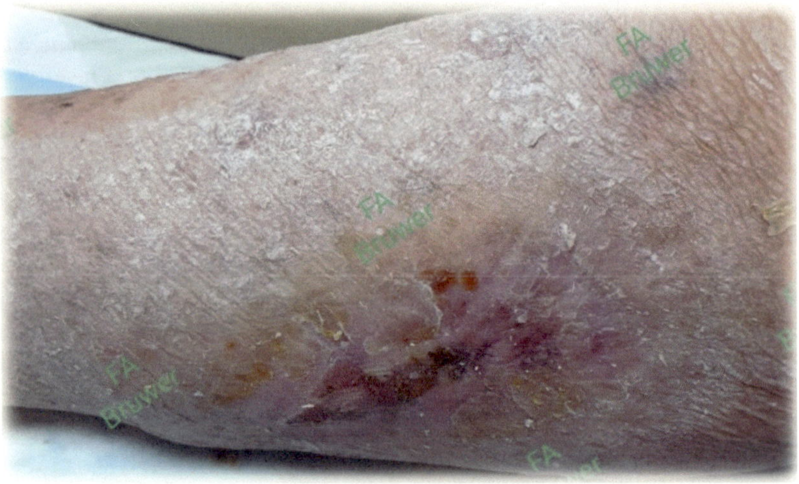

Figure 10.
Complete healing by week 14.

In this specific case, the patient did not require a skin graft, and at 3 months follow-up, the wound was still healed, as illustrated in **Figure 11**.

6.2 Case 2

This is a case of a 64-year-old male who sustained a work-related injury to his right foot. A steel beam fell on his foot, causing a crushing injury that resulted in a forefoot amputation. The skin was so injured that the surgeon could not do a skin flap to cover the bone. The patient was on NPWT of 3 months, after which a section of bone was still exposed (**Figure 12**). The patient was hypertensive and had high cholesterol. In an attempt to salvage the remaining part of his foot/heel, AM was applied to aid in granulation tissue formation over the bone.

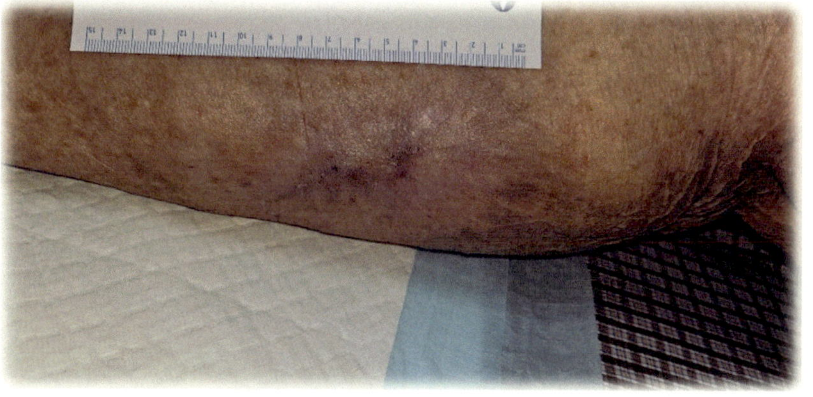

Figure 11.
Three-month follow-up—skin still healed.

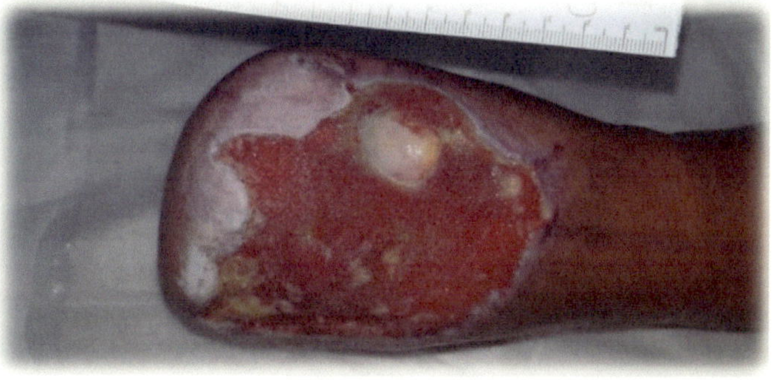

Figure 12.
Three months post-NPWT showing exposed bone.

Figure 13 shows the wound only 4 days after application of AM over the exposed bone. Granulation tissue is visible.

Figure 14 was taken after the second application; more than 70% of the exposed bone is covered. The surgeon grafted the patient within a week after this image was taken, and **Figure 15** shows the wound post-grafting.

In this case, the utilization of AM reduced treatment time, resulting in granulation tissue formation over the exposed bone and enhancing the efficacy of the split-skin graft. Adhesions and complications thereof were also avoided as the skin was soft and pliable with increased tensile strength when compared to scar tissue.

6.3 Case 3

An 83-year-old male, NIDDM, patient had an open tib/fib fracture about 40 years ago, and the bone union was abnormal, which resulted in deformity. Calf muscle functioning was limited, and the patient then developed a wound within the scar (left lower leg). HbA1C was 6.5.

Patient has had the wound for 6 years prior to referral. Various topical applications were applied prior to initial assessment. Wound was debrided with an enzymatic

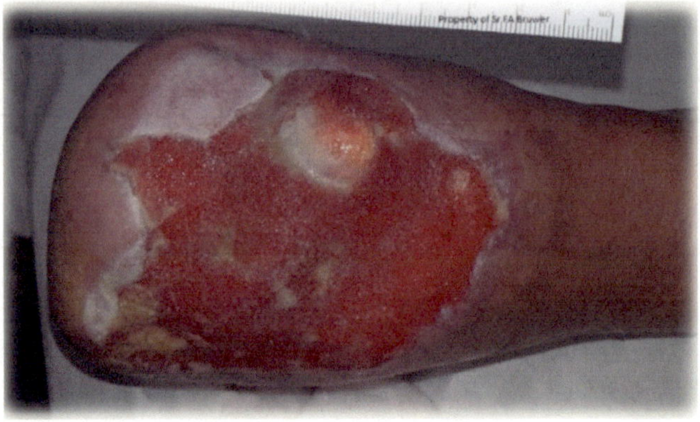

Figure 13.
Granulation tissue formation visible over exposed bone 4 days after initial application.

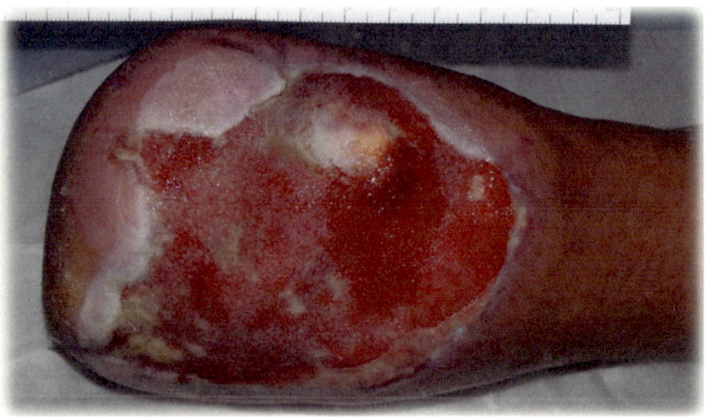

Figure 14.
Image of the wound 1 week after initial application.

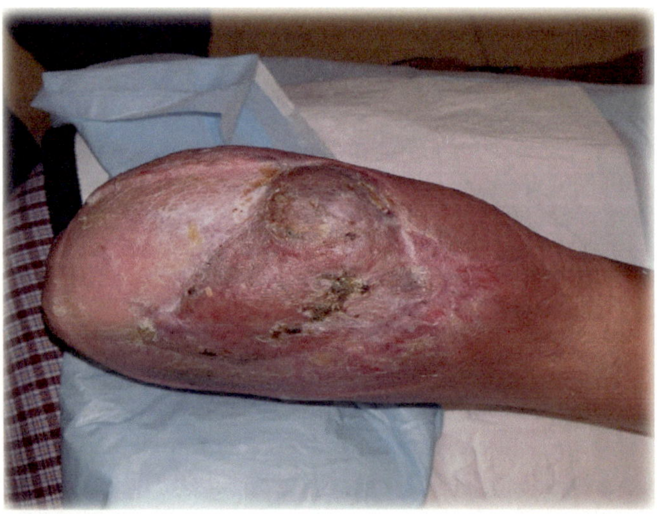

Figure 15.
Image of the leg 4 weeks post-split-skin graft.

debrider to prepare wound bed. The infection was treated with a silver-impregnated dressing. The wound initially had extremely high exudate levels that were managed with a superabsorber and compression.

Although ankle brachial pressure index (ABPI) was within normal range, modified compression was applied due to leg deformity. Pain assessment 9/10 (Wong Baker).

Image at initial assessment: 08 April 2023 (**Figure 16**).

Comorbidities listed in **Table 4**.

Figure 17 was taken almost 3 months later 14 June 2023. The wound had not decreased in size by 30% at week 4, and progress was slow regardless of the standard of care, which included maintenance debridement and modified compression. The application of amniotic membrane (AM) was discussed with the patient, and he consented. AM was applied, and a non-adherent contact layer was applied to prevent the AM from adhering to the foam dressing and foam to manage exudate. Modified compression continued. The size was measured at 5.5 × 3.5 cm (small area at the 12 o'clock position has not granulated up to epithelial level and measures about 0.2 cm deep). Wound was treated weekly. Pain assessment 8/10.

The second and third applications were made on 21 June 2023 and 28 June 2023, as illustrated in **Figures 18** and **19**. The wound has already shown marked improvement with size reduction. The size is 3.5 × 2.1 cm (small cavity has granulated up

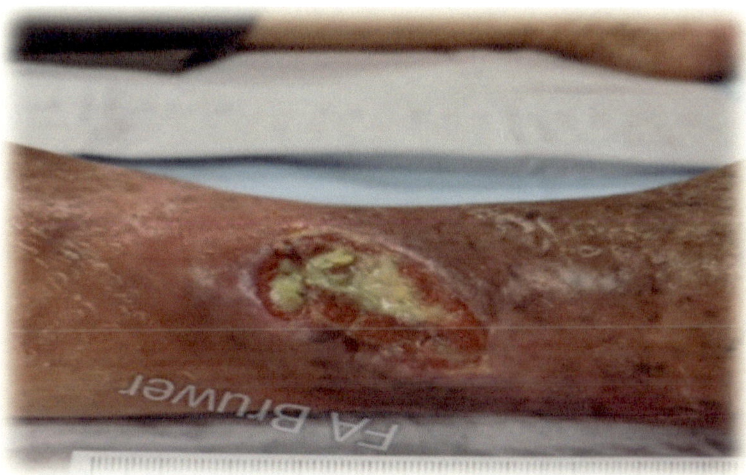

Figure 16.
Image of wound on initial assessment 08 April 2023.

Intrinsic	Extrinsic
Age	Location of the wound
Diabetes	Size and severity of the wound
Hypertension	Chronicity of the wound
Cardiac disease	Presence of devitalize tissue
Calf muscle dysfunction	
Leg deformity due to trauma	

Table 4.
Comorbidities identified in case 3.

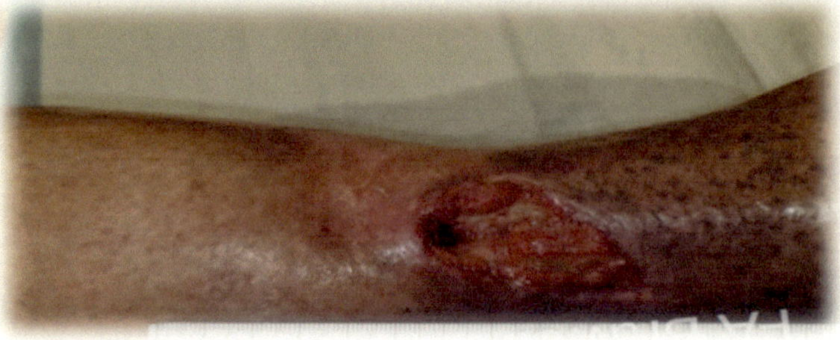

Figure 17.
Inage of the wound 3 months later.

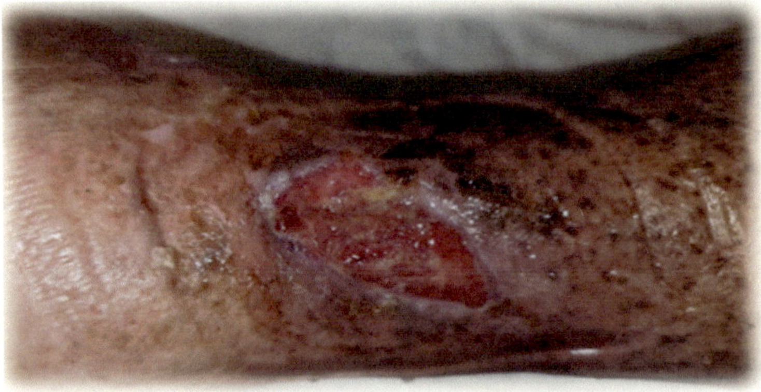

Figure 18.
The wound on 21 June 2023 with second application of AM.

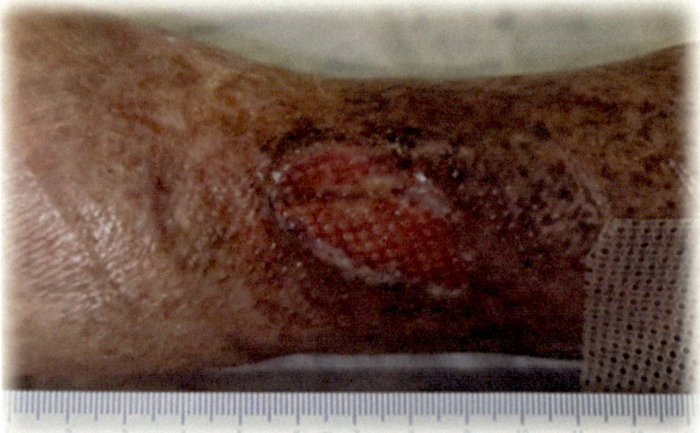

Figure 19.
The wound on 28 June 2023 (third application).

to epithelial level). Wound edges seemed more viable. Pain reduced 5/10. Second amniotic membrane application applied. Non-adherent contact layer changed to silicon-based.

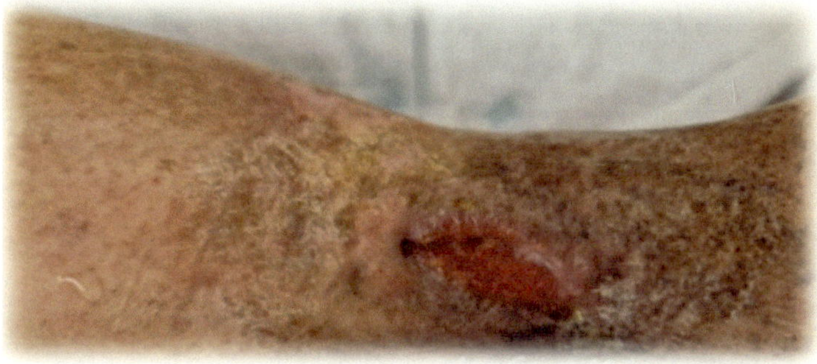

Figure 20.
Wound image four weeks after initial application.

Third application: Size 3.2 × 1.9 cm. Pain reduced 3/10.

Figure 20 shows the wound 4 weeks after initial application (13 July 2023); 50% reduction in size (2.5 × 1.5 cm) exudate has reduced. Final application was done. Only a foam dressing and modified compression. The patient verbalized that he had no pain.

Figure 21 shows the wound 2 weeks after the last application. The wound was 20% of the initial size (02 August 2023). At this stage only a silicon contact layer was applied with modified compression. The patient verbalized that he had no pain.

Figure 22 shows the final photo that was taken in the second week of August 2023, which was about 8 weeks post-initial application. The wound is completely epithelialized. Patient could be stepped down to compression stockings and scar management initiated.

Wound pain reduced immediately after application. Wound bed preparation is key, and wound infection needs to be addressed before application [11]. The time to complete healing 8 weeks; as the exudate reduced, the topical application could be adjusted, which reduced cost even further.

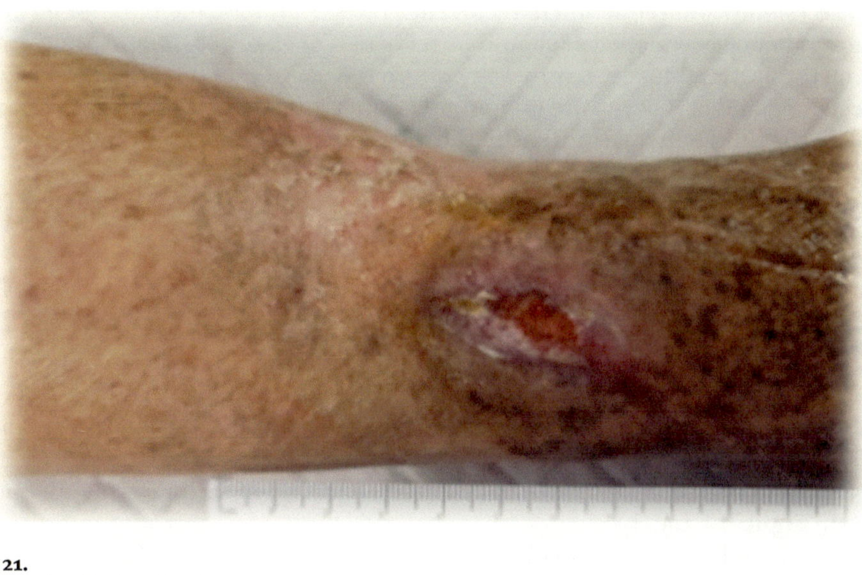

Figure 21.
Two weeks after final application.

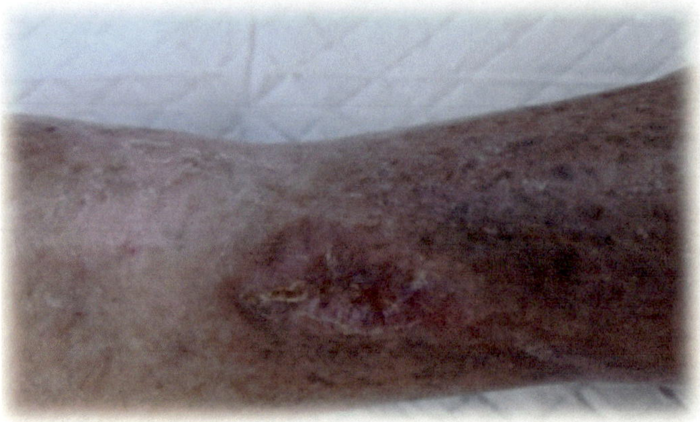

Figure 22.
Final image of the wound on 10 August 2023.

7. Conclusion

The use of AM as an adjunctive therapy with standard of care in hard-to-heal wounds is supported by a high level of evidence with significantly higher healing rates when compared to only standard-of-care treatments. Improved healing rates directly correlate with a reduced risk of infection and associated complications like amputation and death.

With reference to the socioeconomic burden of chronic and hard-to-heal wounds, the use of adjunctive therapies that are accessible and affordable and could result in a potential cost and lifesaving outcome for the patient should be considered when managing these wounds. Future studies could possibly evaluate the economic value of adjunctive therapies like AM.

The available data strongly favor the use of amniotic membranes to improve wound healing with potentially significant cost savings in the overall treatment cost as well as a significant reduction in recurrence rates. Amniotic membrane and amnion itself are valuable products that should be revisited for their regenerative and antibacterial properties. More recently, a review on the use of amniotic fluid containing stem cells concluded that the use of amniotic fluid requires further research as to how the cell in the fluid will differentiate in the microenvironment of a wound as well as possible therapeutic applications [46].

Reduced healing times could result in improved quality of life as well as a reduced burden on the patient suffering from the wound and society.

Acknowledgements

The author would like to acknowledge Dr. Hoda Elkhanary of The Center of Excellence for Stem Cells and Regenerative Medicine (CESC), Zewail City of Science and Technology, October Gardens, Giza, Egypt, for granting permission to utilize **Figure 4** and for the South African company, Next Biosciences for supplying the images in **Figures 1** and **3**.

Mr. Johannes Botma of Botma Designs is acknowledged for the illustration of **Figure 2**.

The author would also like to acknowledge the patients' that consented to the use of the images.

Conflict of interest

The author declares no conflict of interest.

Author details

Febe Antoinette Bruwer
Nianwi Healthcare, Johannesburg, South Africa

*Address all correspondence to: febebruwer@gmail.com

References

[1] Atkin L, Bućko Z, Montero EC, Cutting K, Moffatt C, Probst A, et al. Implementing TIMERS: The race against hard-to-heal wounds. Journal of Wound Care. 2019;**23**(3):S1-S52

[2] Woo KY, Botros M, Kuhnke J, Evans R, Alavi A. Best practices for the management of foot ulcers in people with diabetes. Advances in Skin and Wound Care. 2013;**26**(11):512-524

[3] Gupta S, Andersen C, Black J, de Leon J, Fife C, Lantis JC, et al. Management of chronic wounds: Diagnosis, preparation, treatment, and follow-up. Wounds-A Compendium of Clinical Research and Practice. 2017;**29**(9):S19-S36

[4] Murphy C, Atkin L, Swanson T. Consensus document defying hard-to-heal wounds with an early antibiofilm intervention strategy : Wound hygiene. Journal of Wound Care. 2020;**29**(3b):S1-S28

[5] Boersema G, Smart H, Giaquinto-Cilliers MGC, Mulder M, Weir G, Bruwer FA. Management of nonhealable and maintenance wounds: A systematic integrative review and referral pathway. Advances in Skin and Wound Care. 2021;**2021**:11-22

[6] Han G, Ceilley R. Chronic wound healing: A review of current management and treatments. Advances in Therapy. 2017;**34**(3):599-610

[7] Davis JS. Skin transplantation with a review of 550 cases at the Johns Hopkins Hospital. Johns Hopkins Medical Journal. 1910;**14**:542-549. Available from: https://www.ncbi.nlm.nih.gov/pmc/articles/PMC1407162/pdf/annsurg00889-0033.pdf

[8] Jay RM, Huish JP, Wray JH. Amniotic membrane in clinical medicine: History, current status, and future use. In: Mooradian DL, editor. Extracellular Matrix-Derived Implants in Clinical Medicine [Internet]. Woodhead: Elsevier Ltd; 2016. pp. 151-176. DOI: 10.1016/B978-0-08-100166-0.00009-8

[9] Elkhenany H, El-Derby A, Abd Elkodous M, Salah RA, Lotfy A, El-Badri N. Applications of the amniotic membrane in tissue engineering and regeneration: The hundred-year challenge. Stem Cell Research & Therapy. 2022;**13**(1):1-19

[10] Glat P, Orgill DP, Galiano R, Armstrong D, Serena T, Didomenico LA, et al. Placental membrane provides improved healing efficacy and lower cost versus a tissue-engineered human skin in the treatment of diabetic foot ulcerations. Plastic and Reconstructive Surgery—Global Open. 2019;**7**(8):1-8

[11] Tettelbach W, Cazzell S, Reyzelman AM, Sigal F, Caporusso JM, Agnew PS. A confirmatory study on the efficacy of dehydrated human amnion/chorion membrane dHACM allograft in the management of diabetic foot ulcers: A prospective, multicentre, randomised, controlled study of 110 patients from 14 wound clinics. International Wound Journal. 2019;**16**(1):19-29

[12] Serena TE, Yaakov R, Moore S, Cole W, Coe S, Snyder R, et al. A randomized controlled clinical trial of a hypothermically stored amniotic membrane for use in diabetic foot ulcers. Journal of Comparative Effectiveness Research. 2020;**9**(1):23-34

[13] Snyder RJ, Shimozaki K, Tallis A, Kerzner M, Reyzelman A, Lintzeris D, et al.

A prospective, randomized, multicenter, controlled evaluation of the use of dehydrated amniotic membrane allograft compared to standard of care for the closure of chronic diabetic foot ulcer. Wounds. 2016;**28**(3):70-77

[14] Lakmal K, Basnayake O, Hettiarachchi D. Systematic review on the rational use of amniotic membrane allografts in diabetic foot ulcer treatment. BMC Surgery. 2021;**21**(1):1-8. DOI: 10.1186/s12893-021-01084-8

[15] Young A, McNaught CE. The physiology of wound healing. Surgery in the United Kingdom [Internet]. 2014;**32**(9):445-450. DOI: 10.1016/j.mpsur.2011.06.011

[16] Sibbald RG, Elliott JA, Persaud-Jaimangal R, Goodman L, Armstrong DG, Harley C, et al. Wound bed preparation 2021. Advances in Skin & Wound Care. 2021;**34**(4):183-195

[17] Moffatt C, Vowden P. Hard-to-heal wounds : A holistic approach. European Wound Management Association (EWMA). 2008;**1**:1-19

[18] Piaggesi A, Läuchli S, Bassett. Cells and tissue-based therapies, physical and bio-physical therapies, smart and it-based technologies health economics and regulatory issues advanced therapies in wound management. Journal of Wound Care. 2018;**27**(6):6. Available from: https://www.markallengroup.com

[19] Zelen CM, Serena TE, Denoziere G, Fetterolf DE. A prospective randomised comparative parallel study of amniotic membrane wound graft in the management of diabetic foot ulcers. International Wound Journal. 2013;**10**(5):502-507

[20] Weir GR, Smart H, Van Marle J, Cronje FJ. Arterial disease ulcers, part 1: Clinical diagnosis and investigation. Advances in Skin and Wound Care. 2014;**27**(9):421-428

[21] Serena TE, Carter MJ, Le LT, Sabo MJ, Dimarco DT, Lullove E, et al. A multicenter, randomized, controlled clinical trial evaluating the use of dehydrated human amnion/chorion membrane allografts and multilayer compression therapy vs. multilayer compression therapy alone in the treatment of venous leg ulcers. Wound Repair and Regeneration. 2014;**22**(6):688-693

[22] Stotts N, Wipke-Tevis D, Hopf H. Cofactors in impaired wound healing. In: Krasner DL, Rodeheaver GT, Sibbald RG, Woo KY, editors. Chronic Wound Care 5: A Clinical Source Book for Healthcare Professionals. Vol. 15. 5th ed. Malvern: HMP Communications; 2012. pp. 199-206

[23] Zhao R, Liang H, Clarke E, Jackson C, Xue M. Inflammation in chronic wounds. International Journal of Molecular Sciences. 2016;**17**(12):2085. Available from: http://www.ncbi.nlm.nih.gov/pubmed/27973441%0Ahttp://www.mdpi.com/1422-0067/17/12/2085

[24] Hess CT. Practice Points Comprehensive Patient and Wound Assessments Practice Points. 2019;(June):287-288

[25] Bruwer FA, Kairinos N, Adams K, Weir G, Sander J. The use of negative pressure wound therapy: Recommendations by the wound healing Association of Southern Africa. Wound Healing Southern Africa [Internet]. 2021;**14**(2):40-51. Available from: https://www.proquest.com/scholarly-journals/use-negative-pressure-wound-therapy/docview/2612819258/se-2%0Ahttps://media.proquest.com/media/hms/PFT/1/YzirL?_a= ChgyMDIyMDgy

MTE2MTMyNDc0NTox
NDU5OTQSBTc4OTI2Ggp
PTkVfU0VBUkN IIgwy MTAuNTcu
MjE2LjQ qBzUxNTUyNDMyCjI2M

[26] Team V, Chandler PG, Weller CD. Adjuvant therapies in venous leg ulcer management: A scoping review. Wound Repair and Regeneration. 2019;**27**(5):562-590

[27] Weir GR, Smart H, Van Marle J, Cronje FJ, Gary Sibbald R. Arterial disease ulcers, part 2: Treatment. Advances in Skin and Wound Care. 2014;**27**(10):462-476

[28] Waniczek D, Kozowicz A, Muc-Wierzgoń M, Kokot T, Świętochowska E, Nowakowska-Zajdel E. Adjunct methods of the standard diabetic foot ulceration therapy. Evidence-Based Complementary and Alternative Medicine. [Internet]. 2013;**1**:1-12. DOI: 10.1155/2013/243568

[29] Aleksandrowicz H, Owczarczyk-Saczonek A, Placek W. Venous leg ulcers: Advanced therapies and new technologies. Biomedicine. 2021;**9**(11):1-12

[30] Rajendran SB, Challen K, Wright KL, Hardy JG. Electrical stimulation to enhance wound healing. Journal of Functional Biomaterials. 2021;**12**(2):1-17

[31] Richter DM, Ku JC, Keckler KE, Burke LR, Abd GM, Li Y. Autologous blood clots: A natural biomaterial for wound healing. Frontiers in Materials. 2023;**10**(July):1-7

[32] Braun LR, Fisk WA, Lev-Tov H, Kirsner RS, Isseroff RR. Diabetic foot ulcer: An evidence-based treatment update. American Journal of Clinical Dermatology. 2014;**15**(3):267-281

[33] Kiliçoglu ÖI, Demirel M, Aktas S. New trends in the orthopaedic management of diabetic foot. EFORT Open Reviews. 2018;**3**(5):269-277

[34] Martinez-Zapata MJ, Martí-Carvajal AJ, Solà I, Expósito JA, Bolíbar I, Rodríguez L, et al. Autologous platelet-rich plasma for treating chronic wounds. Cochrane Database of Systematic Reviews. 2016;**2016**

[35] Nguyen HM, Ngoc Le TT, Nguyen AT, Thien Le HN, Pham TT. Biomedical materials for wound dressing: Recent advances and applications. RSC Advances. 2023;**13**(8):5509-5528

[36] Haugh AM, Witt JG, Hauch A, Darden M, Parker G, Ellsworth WA, et al. Amnion membrane in diabetic foot wounds: A meta-analysis. Plastic and Reconstructive Surgery—Global Open. 2017;**5**(4):1-6

[37] Kang NH, Hwang KA, Kim SU, Kim YB, Hyun SH, Jeung EB, et al. Potential antitumor therapeutic strategies of human amniotic membrane and amniotic fluid-derived stem cells. Cancer Gene Therapy. 2012;**19**(8):517-522

[38] Dehghani M, Azarpira N, Karimi VM, Mossayebi H, Esfandiari E. Grafting with cryopreserved amniotic membrane versus conservative wound care in treatment of pressure ulcers: A randomized clinical trial. Bulletin of Emergency and Trauma. 2017;**5**(4):249-258

[39] Swanson T, Angel D. International Wound Infection Institute wound infection in clinical practice update principles of best practice. Wounds International. 2022;**24**(8):1-59

[40] Harding K, Dowsett C, Fias L, Jelnes R, Mosti G. Concensus recommendations: Simplifying venous

leg ulcer management. Wounds International. 2015;**72**

[41] DiDomenico LA, Orgill DP, Galiano RD, Serena TE, Carter MJ, Kaufman JP, et al. Use of an aseptically processed, dehydrated human amnion and chorion membrane improves likelihood and rate of healing in chronic diabetic foot ulcers: A prospective, randomised, multi-centre clinical trial in 80 patients. International Wound Journal. 2018;**15**(6):950-957

[42] Zelen CM, Serena TE, Gould L, Le L, Carter MJ, Keller J, et al. Treatment of chronic diabetic lower extremity ulcers with advanced therapies: A prospective, randomised, controlled, multi-centre comparative study examining clinical efficacy and cost. International Wound Journal. 2016;**13**(2):272-282

[43] Bianchi C, Cazzell S, Vayser D, Reyzelman AM, Dosluoglu H, Tovmassian G. A multicentre randomised controlled trial evaluating the efficacy of dehydrated human amnion/chorion membrane (EpiFix®) allograft for the treatment of venous leg ulcers. International Wound Journal. 2018;**15**(1):114-122

[44] Schmiedova I, Dembickaja A, Kiselakova L, Nowakova B, Slama P. Using of amniotic membrane derivatives for the treatment of chronic wounds. Membranes (Basel). 2021;**11**(12):1-14

[45] Smart H. The Africa bandage system and application technique - bringing compression science to resource-restrained environments. WCET Journal. 2014;**34**(1):8-15

[46] Luo H, Wang Z, Qi F, Wang D. Applications of human amniotic fluid stem cells in wound healing. Chinese Medical Journal. 2022;**135**(19):2272-2281

Chapter 5

Molecular Hydrogen and Its Effect on Wound Healing and Tissue Regeneration

Mikhail Yu. Artamonov, Tyler W. LeBaron, Felix A. Pyatakovich and Inessa A. Minenko

Abstract

Chronic, non-healing wounds represent a major clinical challenge with substantial economic burden. Impaired wound healing stems from excessive inflammation, infection, ischemia, and oxidative stress. Molecular hydrogen has recently emerged as a therapeutic medical gas with antioxidant, anti-inflammatory, and cytoprotective properties through selective free radical scavenging, activating antioxidant enzymes, reducing pro-inflammatory cytokines, and potentially modulating cell signaling. Arly preclinical evidence shows hydrogen therapy may promote wound healing through accelerated closure, decreased inflammation, and mitigated tissue injury. Initial small-scale human pilots and case reports demonstrate feasibility and apparent safety of administering hydrogen via inhalation, ingestion, topical application, or baths. However, rigorous clinical trials validating therapeutic efficacy are lacking. Further research should optimize delivery, dose, timing, and tissue bioavailability to translate promising preclinical findings into effective clinical hydrogen treatments for wound care. Definitive large-scale studies are critical next steps.

Keywords: molecular hydrogen, wound healing, oxidative stress, antioxidant therapy, inflammation, hydrogen gas, hydrogen water, topical delivery, medical gases

1. Introduction

Wound healing is a complex physiological process that involves coordinated cellular, molecular, and biochemical events leading to tissue repair and restoration of function after injury. This dynamic process can be categorized into four overlapping phases: hemostasis, inflammation, proliferation, and tissue remodeling. While ideal wound healing results in restored tissue integrity without scar formation, this orchestrated process can be impaired by both intrinsic and extrinsic factors, leading to chronic non-healing wounds [1].

Upon tissue injury, the first response is hemostasis, which stops bleeding and limits blood loss. Vascular constriction induced by localized reflexes and circulating catecholamines achieves initial hemostatic control. This is further reinforced by platelet aggregation and fibrin clot formation, with cross-linked fibrin serving as a temporary matrix [2]. The hemostatic plug also contains various growth factors and cytokines released by degranulating platelets that help initiate the inflammatory phase.

Inflammation begins shortly after injury with the extravasation and chemotaxis of immune cells, particularly neutrophils followed by macrophages, to the wound site. Neutrophils phagocytose and destroy bacteria and debris, while macrophages debride dead tissue and continue phagocytosis in the later stages of inflammation [3]. Macrophages also release a variety of growth factors and cytokines that promote fibroblast proliferation, extracellular matrix synthesis, and angiogenesis. Key pro-inflammatory cytokines released include tumor necrosis factor α (TNF-α), interleukins 1 and 6 (IL-1 and IL-6), and transforming growth factor β (TGF-β) [1].

After approximately 48–72 h, the proliferation phase commences which involves several processes to restore tissue integrity. A provisional extracellular matrix formed during inflammation is enhanced as fibroblasts proliferate and deposit collagen, fibronectin, glycosaminoglycans and proteoglycans [2]. Angiogenesis stimulated by factors like vascular endothelial growth factor (VEGF) supplies the healing tissue with nutrients and oxygen. Keratinocytes also proliferate and migrate across the wound bed to re-epithelialize the surface. The final phase of wound healing is remodeling, which can last for months to years. Matrix metalloproteinases (MMPs) degrade excess collagen to remodel scar tissue and increase tensile strength [4]. Myofibroblasts contract wound edges together while collagen fibers become organized along tension lines. Remodeling gradually returns the injured tissue to a pre-wound architecture and functional state, although the resulting scar tissue only regains approximately 80% of its original strength [5].

While this phased wound healing process allows the efficient repair of injured tissue. Advanced age is associated with delayed healing, likely due to reduced growth factor production and angiogenesis [1]. Wounds in the elderly also exhibit diminished collagen accumulation and remodeling [6]. Obesity can also impair healing through chronic inflammation and vascular dysfunction. Diabetes strongly inhibits healing due to hyperglycemia, reduced growth factors, deficient angiogenesis and collagen accumulation, immune dysfunction, and susceptibility to infection (**Figure 1**) [7].

Chronic non-healing wounds are also characterized by prolonged inflammation and elevated pro-inflammatory cytokines like TNF-α and IL-1β [8]. This prevents transition to the proliferative phase. Immune dysfunction due to illness, stress or medications like steroids also impedes normal healing. Ionizing radiation generates reactive oxygen species that damage cells and lead to poorly vascularized tissue with abnormal extracellular matrix [9]. Wound infections need to be controlled to allow progression beyond the inflammatory stage. Compromised circulation in conditions like peripheral arterial disease or venous insufficiency results in ischemia and hypoxia that impair healing [1]. Finally, nutritional deficits including protein, vitamins C and A, and zinc can delay healing by inhibiting cell proliferation and collagen synthesis (**Figure 2**) [10].

Inflammation is a critical part of the normal wound healing response. During the inflammatory phase, various cytokines, chemokines, and growth factors are released to recruit immune cells like neutrophils and macrophages to the wound [11]. These inflammatory cells defend against infection, debride damaged tissue, and release additional signals to activate tissue repair processes like angiogenesis and fibroplasia. However, uncontrolled inflammation driven by elevated pro-inflammatory cytokines like TNF-α and IL-1 can also impair healing. Chronic wounds often exhibit prolonged inflammation that prevents transition to the proliferative phase [12]. Therefore,

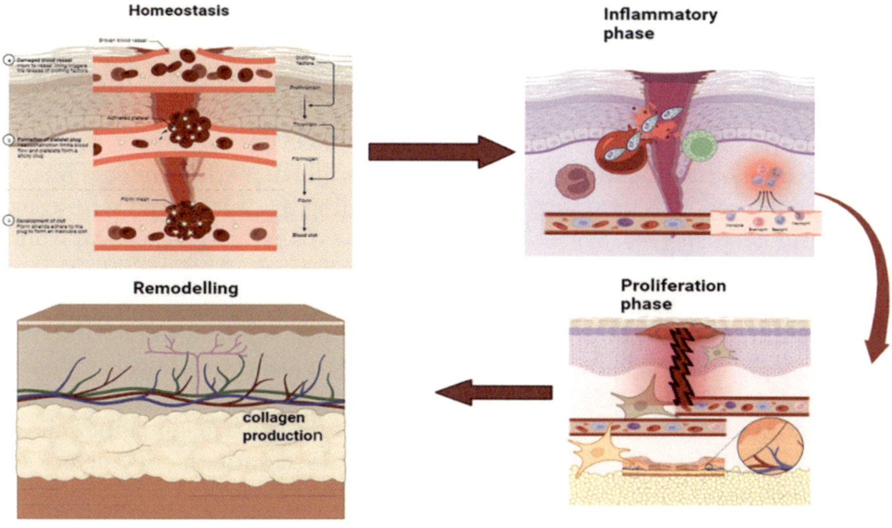

Figure 1.
Phases of wound healing as depicted in the given figure. Hemostasis occurs immediately after injury to halt bleeding. Inflammation follows to clean the wound by recruiting immune cells. Proliferation phase involves processes like re-epitheliallization (1), fibroblast proliferation (2), angiogenesis (3), and matrix deposition (4) to cover the wound site. Remodeling then strengthens the wound over months/years via collagen remodeling and apoptosis. This coordinated process effectively closes the wound and restores the epithelial barrier.

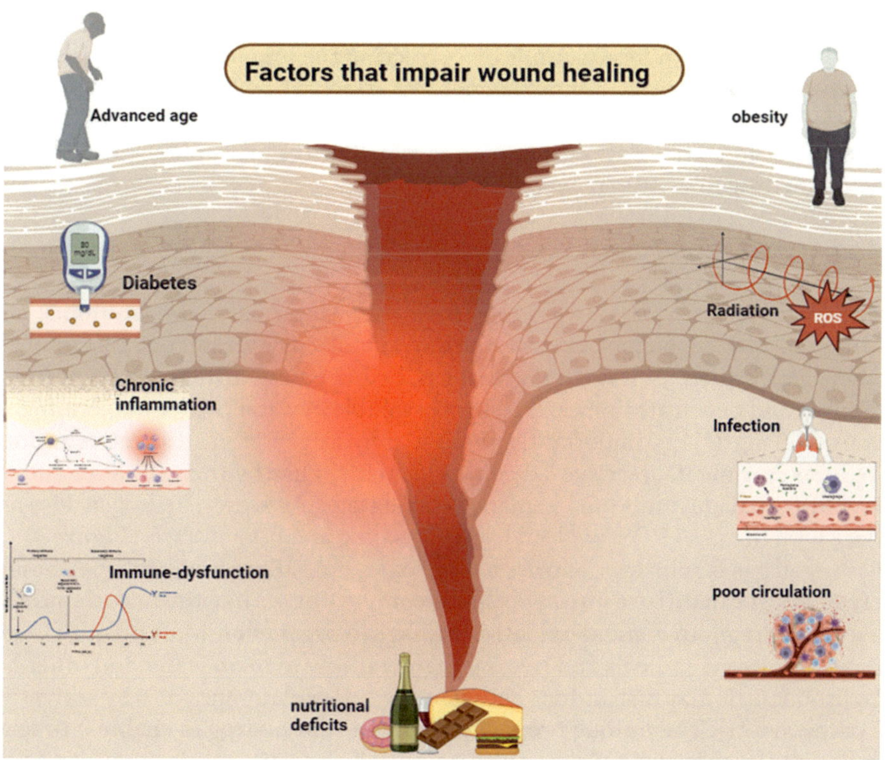

Figure 2.
Barriers to wound healing: unraveling the complex factors that inhibit the regenerative journey.

inflammation is necessary for healing but its careful regulation is equally important. Reactive oxygen species (ROS) are generated as a consequence of aerobic metabolism and inflammatory cell activation during wound healing. At low concentrations, ROS facilitate defense against microbes and act as signaling molecules to promote cell proliferation and migration [13]. However, excessive ROS damage lipids, proteins, nucleic acids and extracellular matrix components while depleting endogenous antioxidant defenses. This oxidative stress stalls healing by causing cell senescence, apoptosis, and necrosis [14]. Systemic conditions like diabetes and the local wound environment can both contribute to disrupted redox balance. Antioxidants that scavenge ROS and boost endogenous antioxidant capacity may help correct oxidative stress and facilitate wound healing. Topical antioxidants including curcumin, honey, and alpha-tocopherol have shown promise in animal models but clinical evidence in humans remains limited [15]. Other antioxidant therapies like ebselen and zinc have demonstrated efficacy in diabetic wound models but also need further clinical evaluation [16]. A key challenge is effective and sustained antioxidant delivery to heal chronic wounds in patients.

2. Molecular hydrogen

Molecular hydrogen (H2) has recently emerged as a physiological inert gas with antioxidant, anti-inflammatory, and cytoprotective effects in animal models [17]. As the smallest molecule, hydrogen can readily diffuse and accumulate in subcellular compartments to reduce localized oxidative stress. Administering hydrogen in either inhaled gas, dissolved saline or water, or topical formulations may have therapeutic potential for difficult to heal wounds by correcting the underlying redox imbalance. Early preclinical studies have shown beneficial effects of hydrogen in rodent models of skin flap ischemia, burns, radiation injury, and diabetic wounds. However, rigorous clinical investigations are still needed to translate these promising findings with molecular hydrogen to human wound healing.

2.1 Mechanisms of molecular hydrogen

Molecular hydrogen (H_2) is a gas consisting of two attached hydrogen atoms. This stable diatomic hydrogen molecule has the lowest molecular weight of 2.02 g/mol and is physiologically inert [18]. As the lightest gas, hydrogen can diffuse rapidly across cell membranes and penetrate tissues. It is slightly soluble in water, with a maximum solubility around 1.6 mg/L [19]. Importantly, molecular hydrogen acts as a selective antioxidant that reduces detrimental reactive oxygen species (ROS) like hydroxyl radicals and peroxynitrite that are implicated in many disease states. However, hydrogen does not interfere with essential ROS involved in cell signaling and homeostasis (**Figure 3**) [20].

Hydrogen gas is colorless, odorless, non-toxic, non-allergenic, and environmentally friendly. It can diffuse into subcellular compartments like the mitochondria and nucleus, enabling it to combat oxidative damage in organelles. Molecular hydrogen eliminates hydroxyl radicals and peroxynitrite rapidly to form water and other harmless byproducts. It may also induce endogenous antioxidant enzymes by activating the Nrf2 pathway [21]. The unique properties of molecular hydrogen enable it to selectively decrease cytotoxic ROS while also potentially boosting endogenous antioxidant defenses. This makes hydrogen a promising therapeutic agent for clinical applications targeting oxidative stress like difficult to heal wounds.

DOI: http://dx.doi.org/10.5772/intechopen.1004921

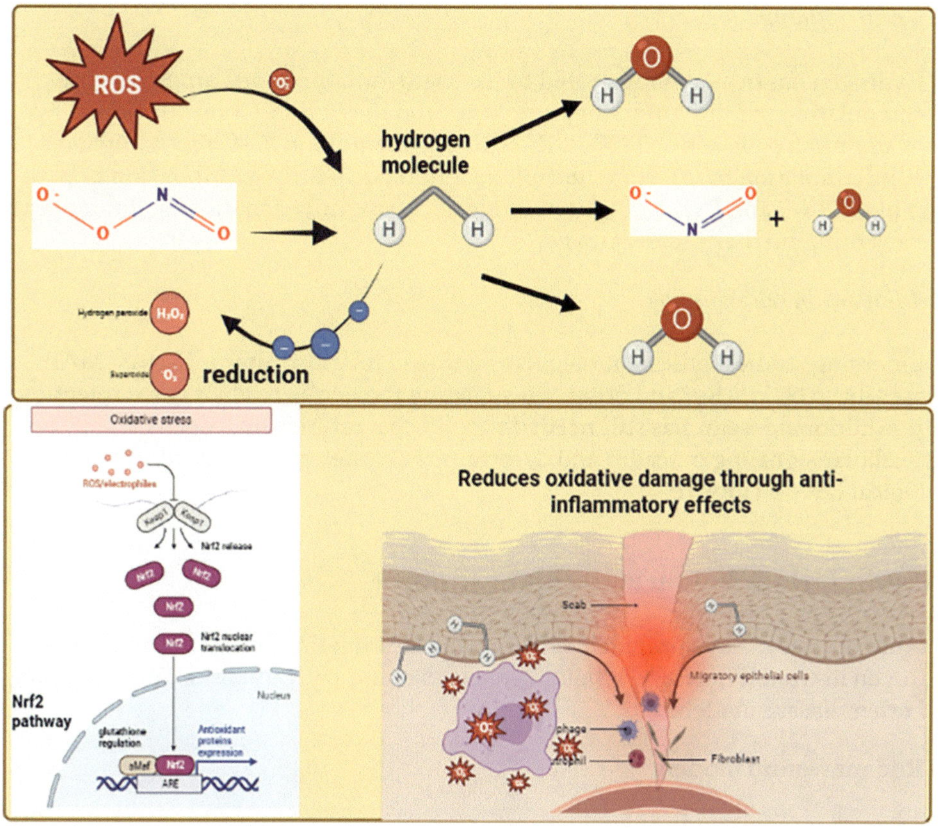

Figure 3.
Direct and indirect antioxidant mechanisms of molecular hydrogen. Direct effects include scavenging hydroxyl radicals (−OH) to form water, eliminating peroxynitrite (ONOO−) by converting it to nitrite and water, and reducing hydrogen peroxide (H_2O_2) and superoxide radicals. Indirect effects include activating the Nrf2 pathway to upregulate antioxidant genes like glutathione, and reducing oxidative damage through anti-inflammatory effects. Together, these direct radical-scavenging activities and indirect modulation of signaling pathways and inflammation confer the antioxidant benefits of molecular hydrogen.

2.1.1 Radical scavenging

The primary mechanism of action of hydrogen is through direct scavenging of cytotoxic reactive oxygen species (ROS), particularly hydroxyl radicals and peroxynitrite [18]. Molecular hydrogen reacts extremely rapidly with hydroxyl radicals, even faster than with superoxide, to generate water and prevent propagation of free radical damage [22]. Hydrogen also reduces peroxynitrite to form nitrite and water, eliminating this highly reactive nitrogen species [23].

2.1.2 Activation of antioxidant enzymes

Studies in rodent models have shown that molecular hydrogen activates the Nrf2 transcription factor, which induces expression of several endogenous antioxidant enzymes [24]. Hydrogen upregulates antioxidants like glutathione, superoxide dismutase, catalase, NADPH quinone oxidoreductase-1, and heme oxygenase-1 through Nrf2 nuclear translocation and activation of the antioxidant response element [25]. Boosting these intrinsic antioxidants enhances the cell's own defense capacity against oxidative damage.

2.1.3 Anti-inflammatory effects

Hydrogen has been demonstrated to have anti-inflammatory properties by downregulating pro-inflammatory cytokines and mediators. Consumption of hydrogen water reduced levels of TNF-α, IL-6, IL-1β, chemokine (C-C motif) ligand 2, and other inflammation markers in multiple rodent models through inhibition of pathways like NF-kB and JNK [26]. Attenuating excessive inflammation facilitates healing by preventing further tissue damage.

2.1.4 Impact on cell signaling

Emerging studies indicate molecular hydrogen may also alter miRNAs, MAP kinases like p38, PPARγ, and other cell signaling molecules to elicit cytoprotection [27]. Additional research is still needed to fully characterize hydrogen's effects on intracellular signaling cascades and determine how they might contribute to its biological effects (**Figure 4**).

3. Preclinical studies on molecular hydrogen

Animal studies have provided evidence for the beneficial effects of molecular hydrogen in wound healing, ischemia-reperfusion injury, radiation-induced damage, and other disease models.

3.1 Rodent wound models

Multiple studies in diabetic and non-diabetic mice have shown molecular hydrogen improves wound closure and healing [28]. Hydrogen administered

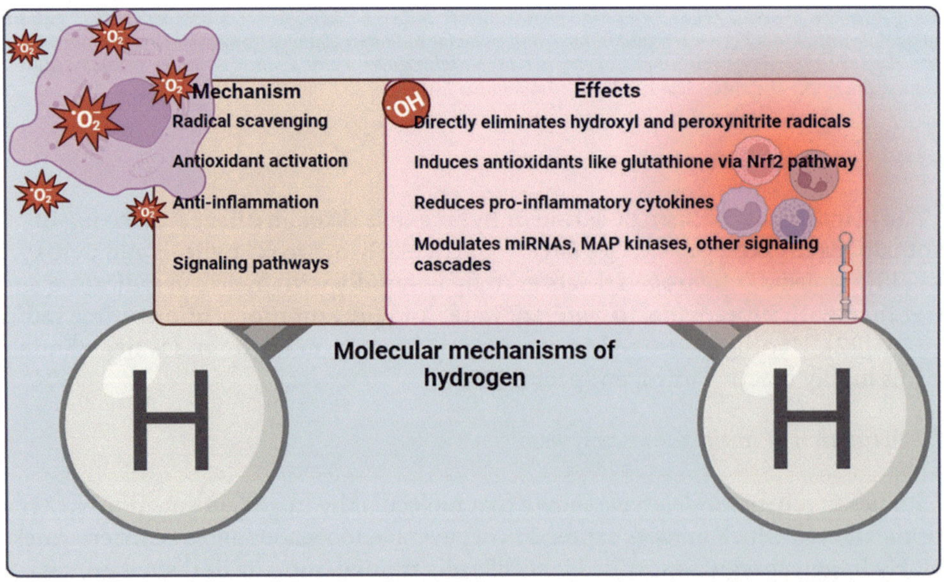

Figure 4.
Diagram illustrating some of the key mechanisms through which Hydrogen exerts its beneficial health effects, including radical scavenging, antioxidant activation, anti-inflammation, and modulation of signaling pathways.

through ingestion of hydrogen water accelerated wound closure in both normal and diabetic mice compared to control. Topical application of a hydrogen gel also improved wound healing in diabetic mice by preserving viable dermal tissue. In rats, hydrogen gel reduced wound size and facilitated earlier recovery [29]. The benefits are mediated through reduction of oxidative stress and inflammation (**Figure 5**).

3.2 Skin flap models

Ischemia-reperfusion injury is a significant impediment to skin flap survival post-transplantation. Molecular hydrogen treatment has been shown to reduce tissue necrosis and apoptosis in rat skin flap models [30]. Hydrogen inhalation improved skin flap viability by upregulating vascular endothelial growth factor (VEGF) expression and increasing neovascularization in the ischemic tissue. It also decreased malondialdehyde and increased superoxide dismutase levels, indicating reduced oxidative damage.

3.3 Radiation injury models

Exposure to ionizing radiation generates substantial oxidative stress and cell damage. Studies in mice and rats demonstrate hydrogen treatment mitigates radiation-induced injury in skin and other tissues by neutralizing oxidation and apoptosis [31]. Drinking hydrogen water ameliorated radiation-impaired wound healing in mice by preserving proliferating cells [29]. The radioprotective effects likely involve regulation of pro-inflammatory cytokines and cell cycle proteins.

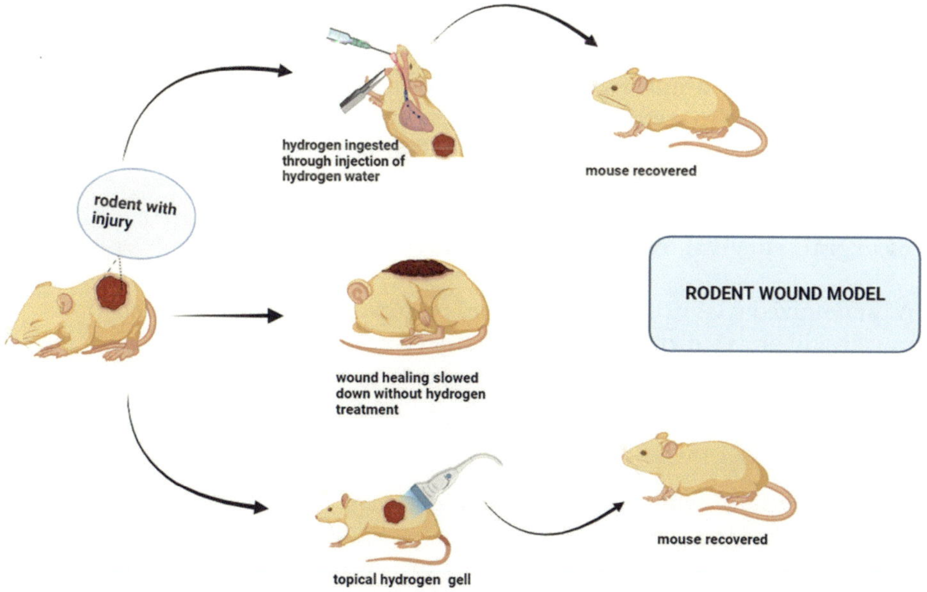

Figure 5.
Molecular hydrogen improves wound healing in both diabetic and non-diabetic mice. Ingestion of hydrogen water speeds wound closure compared to controls. Topical hydrogen gel also facilitates wound healing, especially in diabetic mice, by reducing oxidative stress and inflammation. Rats treated with a hydrogen gel showed smaller wound size and faster recovery.

3.4 Burn wound models

Hydrogen therapy has also shown efficacy in burn wound models. Inhalation of hydrogen gas attenuated inflammation and oxidative stress in burn-injured rats [32]. This was accompanied by increased VEGF and granulation tissue formation. Topical hydrogen treatment also improved healing of second-degree burns in rats. The benefits were mediated through reducing tissue edema, neutrophil infiltration, and apoptosis.

While molecular hydrogen has demonstrated efficacy in rodent wound models, larger animal studies are still limited. Ongoing research is needed to evaluate its clinical potential for improving problematic wound healing in patients.

4. Clinical studies on molecular hydrogen

4.1 Early pilot studies on hydrogen for wound healing

While animal studies have provided promising results, only limited clinical research exists evaluating molecular hydrogen for wound healing applications. However, early pilot studies have explored the feasibility and potential therapeutic effects of hydrogen therapy in patients with skin graft surgery, radiation injury, diabetic ulcers, and other problematic wounds. In one study, drinking hydrogen-rich water improved grafted skin viability and reduced oxidative stress in five patients undergoing surgical reconstruction for head and neck tumors [28]. Plasma markers for oxidation like 8-OHdG were lower in patients ingesting hydrogen water.

Inhalation of hydrogen gas was also found to be feasible and well-tolerated in 13 patients undergoing radiotherapy for malignant pelvic tumors [33]. This small study suggested possible benefits for radiation-induced dermatitis. Topical application of electrolyzed hydrogen saline helped improve ulcer area and ischemia in five diabetic patients, though the sample size was limited [34]. While these early pilot studies are inconclusive due to low patient numbers, they provide preliminary evidence for the safety and potential efficacy of molecular hydrogen delivery through ingestion, inhalation, and topical routes.

4.2 Skin graft survival, radiation tissue injury

A randomized trial in 40 patients found perioperative hydrogen inhalation improved skin graft survival after Mohs surgery compared to control [35]. Another trial reported hydrogen bathing three times weekly decreased radiation dermatitis severity and improved quality of life in patients undergoing radiotherapy for breast cancer [36].

4.3 Meta-analysis of wound healing trials

A recent meta-analysis combined data from 8 clinical trials and found hydrogen therapy significantly improved wound healing by facilitating granulation and epithelialization [37].

In addition to small trials, case reports have shown beneficial outcomes with hydrogen treatment for certain conditions related to problematic wound healing. For example, drinking hydrogen water led to rapid improvement of radiation-induced oral mucositis in a patient with tongue cancer [33]. Hydrogen was also reported to diminish radiation dermatitis in two patients undergoing cranial radiation therapy [38].

4.4 Safety, tolerability in humans

Safety data from clinical studies indicates molecular hydrogen is well tolerated with no major adverse effects observed. Ingestion of hydrogen water and inhalation of hydrogen gas up to 4–5% concentration appear to be safe intervention methods. Topical hydrogen preparations also seem not to irritate skin or wounds [39]. While clinical data remain limited, existing evidence suggests hydrogen therapy is a safe, feasible adjunct treatment that may benefit wound healing and related conditions through antioxidant and anti-inflammatory mechanisms. More rigorously designed trials are warranted to fully evaluate efficacy in patients.

5. Practical use of molecular hydrogen

5.1 Inhalation of hydrogen gas

Inhalation of hydrogen gas is an efficient delivery method that allows rapid uptake into the systemic circulation [18]. However, precautions must be taken before administering hydrogen gas to patients. Pulmonary function tests should be performed to assess lung capacity and identify patients with severe respiratory disease who may not be suitable candidates for hydrogen inhalation [40]. Patients receiving hydrogen gas should be closely monitored for adverse effects with continuous pulse oximetry [41]. The hydrogen/air mixture must be properly diluted and regulated to less than 4–5% hydrogen to prevent flammability risk [42]. This treatment should be administered in specialized clinical settings with staff experienced in handling medical gases [24]. Patients inhale the hydrogen/air mixture through a face mask, nasal cannula, or ventilation circuit [20]. The hydrogen is detected in the blood within minutes and reaches tissues throughout the body. However, the specialized equipment and training required to safely prepare and deliver regulated concentrations of hydrogen gas may limit its feasibility to specialized research centers or hospitals [43].

5.2 Topical administration

Topical preparations like gels, creams, and solutions allow direct application of molecular hydrogen to the skin and surface wounds. These topical formulations can be prepared on-site or obtained commercially pre-made. Penetration depth of topical molecular hydrogen is limited, so strategies to improve delivery and absorption are being studied. These include occlusive dressings, cyclodextrin carriers, liposomal vesicles, and nanoparticles. The dressings themselves are not directly "impacted with hydrogen." Rather, the formulations applied underneath are designed to better transmit or carry hydrogen.

Sustained-release antioxidant hydrogel systems containing dissolved hydrogen have also been developed to enable prolonged topical delivery. The specific polymers, crosslinkers, plasticizers, and hydrogen donors/carriers would depend on the desired viscosity, adhesion, flexibility, and hydrogen release kinetics. Overall, advanced topical delivery systems with carriers and sustained-release capacities can improve tissue absorption compared to simple ointments and solutions, but reaching deeper tissues remains challenging.

5.3 Optimizing dose, timing, delivery route

While different methods for delivering molecular hydrogen have been investigated, protocols still need to be optimized for factors such as dosage, timing, and route of administration. Establishing the ideal effective doses is important, as both very low and very high doses of hydrogen may be less effective. Ingestion of hydrogen water typically aims to provide ~0.5–1 mM hydrogen concentration in blood. Higher hydrogen inhalation doses around 2–4% by volume have been used as well [44].

Administration frequency and duration should also be optimized. Continual daily dosing may be required to maintain therapeutic levels, especially with shorter-acting delivery modes like ingestion. Prolonged hydrogen treatment over weeks or months is likely necessary for wound healing [20]. The route of delivery should be tailored based on the target condition and practical considerations. For example, topical administration makes sense for localized skin wounds, while systemic delivery via ingestion or inhalation may be preferable for internal ulcers [45]. Optimization of dose, timing, and route of delivery is an important current research focus for translation of hydrogen therapies. Carefully designed clinical studies are needed to help establish standardized dosing protocols.

5.4 Prototypes of H2 generating wound dressings

Several research groups have created prototype wound dressings that generate and release hydrogen gas directly into the tissue microenvironment [46]. These active wound dressings contain hydrogen-producing compounds that allow sustained localized hydrogen release when hydrated (**Figure 6**).

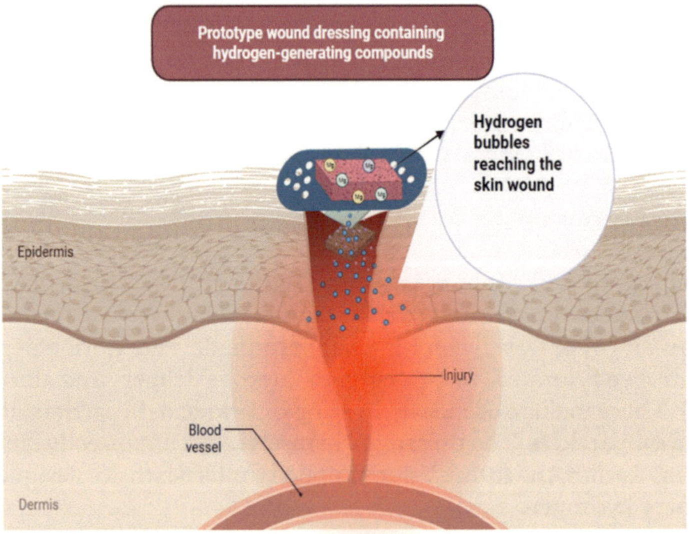

Figure 6.
Hydrogen-releasing wound dressing prototype: a visual overview of sustained antioxidant effects in chronic skin ulcers.

6. Design of future clinical trials

Well-designed clinical trials are now needed to rigorously evaluate molecular hydrogen therapies for wound treatment. Challenges include selecting appropriate outcome measures like wound closure rate and quality of life metrics. Blinding may be difficult for modalities like inhaled hydrogen. Optimal dosing parameters and delivery methods should be assessed. Multicenter trials with larger sample sizes will be key to provide high-quality evidence on the efficacy of hydrogen for healing impairments.

7. Conclusion

Chronic non-healing wounds represent a major and growing clinical challenge, especially among aging, diabetic, and vascular disease populations. The impaired healing is driven by pathological inflammation, infection, ischemia, and oxidative stress. Molecular hydrogen is an emerging therapeutic agent that combats these underlying drivers through its antioxidant, anti-inflammatory, and cytoprotective mechanisms.

Animal studies have provided promising evidence supporting the benefits of hydrogen in accelerating wound closure, increasing skin flap viability, mitigating radiation injury, and improving healing in other models. However, clinical research remains limited thus far. Early pilot studies and case reports have shown feasibility and potential efficacy of various hydrogen delivery methods including inhaled gas, drinking hydrogen water, topical preparations, and hydrogen baths. Small trials point to possible benefits of hydrogen therapy for skin graft survival, radiation dermatitis, and chronic ulcers.

While current clinical data is insufficient to confirm efficacy, molecular hydrogen remains a promising adjuvant therapy to overcome healing impairments by regulating oxidation, inflammation, apoptosis, and growth factor expression. Ongoing studies are optimizing protocols for dose, timing, and route of administration. Topical formulations, transdermal carriers, and hydrogen-generating wound dressings may enable more efficient localized delivery.

High-quality randomized controlled trials with larger sample sizes are warranted to properly evaluate molecular hydrogen therapies for wound treatment. Multicenter studies assessing inhaled hydrogen, drinking hydrogen water, topical preparations, and combination protocols are needed. Appropriate outcome measures like wound closure rate, quality of life, and biomarker levels should be determined. If efficacy is established, molecular hydrogen could become part of standard of care to improve healing outcomes and reduce patient suffering.

Hydrogen is a safe, economically feasible adjunctive therapy that preclinical evidence suggests may benefit problematic wound healing through its multifaceted mechanisms. Rigorously designed clinical trials will determine if molecular hydrogen lives up to its promise as an effective intervention for intractable wounds. Bringing hydrogen therapy into clinical practice could impact patient lives and reduce health care costs. Further research will clarify the future trajectory of molecular hydrogen for wound treatment.

Author details

Mikhail Yu. Artamonov[1*], Tyler W. LeBaron[2,3], Felix A. Pyatakovich[1] and Inessa A. Minenko[1]

1 MJA Research and Development, Inc., East Stroudsburg, PA, USA

2 Department of Kinesiology and Outdoor Recreation, Southern Utah University, Cedar City, UT, USA

3 Molecular Hydrogen Institute, Enoch, UT, USA

*Address all correspondence to: drmike@mjahealthcare.com

References

[1] Guo SA, Dipietro LA. Factors affecting wound healing. Journal of Dental Research. 2010;**89**(3):219-229

[2] Velnar T, Bailey T, Smrkolj V. The wound healing process: An overview of the cellular and molecular mechanisms. Journal of International Medical Research. 2009;**37**(5):1528-1542

[3] Eming SA, Krieg T, Davidson JM. Inflammation in wound repair: Molecular and cellular mechanisms. Journal of Investigative Dermatology. 2007;**127**(3):514-525

[4] Lazaro J et al. Elevated levels of matrix metalloproteinases and chronic wound healing: An updated review of clinical evidence. Journal of Wound Care. 2016;**25**(5):277-287

[5] Gurtner GC et al. Wound repair and regeneration. Nature. 2008;**453**(7193):314-321

[6] Keylock KT et al. Exercise accelerates cutaneous wound healing and decreases wound inflammation in aged mice. American Journal of Physiology-Regulatory, Integrative and Comparative Physiology. 2008;**294**(1):R179-R184

[7] Schreml S et al. Oxygen in acute and chronic wound healing. British Journal of Dermatology. 2010;**163**(2):257-268

[8] Zhao R et al. Inflammation in chronic wounds. International Journal of Molecular Sciences. 2016;**17**(12):2085

[9] Zhao W, Robbins ME. Inflammation and chronic oxidative stress in radiation-induced late normal tissue injury: Therapeutic implications. Current Medicinal Chemistry. 2009;**16**(2):130-143

[10] Russell L. The importance of patients' nutritional status in wound healing. British Journal of Nursing. 2001;**10**(Sup. 1):S42-S49

[11] Adamson R. Role of macrophages in normal wound healing: An overview. Journal of Wound Care. 2009;**18**(8):349-351

[12] Sindrilaru A et al. An unrestrained proinflammatory M1 macrophage population induced by iron impairs wound healing in humans and mice. The Journal of Clinical Investigation. 2011;**121**(3):985-997

[13] Schäfer M, Werner S. Oxidative stress in normal and impaired wound repair. Pharmacological Research. 2008;**58**(2):165-171

[14] Redza-Dutordoir M, Averill-Bates DA. Activation of apoptosis signalling pathways by reactive oxygen species. Biochimica et Biophysica Acta (BBA)-Molecular Cell Research. 2016;**1863**(12):2977-2992

[15] Comino-Sanz IM et al. The role of antioxidants on wound healing: A review of the current evidence. Journal of Clinical Medicine. 2021;**10**(16):3558

[16] Zhang W et al. Antioxidant therapy and antioxidant-related bionanomaterials in diabetic wound healing. Frontiers in Bioengineering and Biotechnology. 2021;**9**:707479

[17] Ohta S. Molecular hydrogen as a novel antioxidant: Overview of the advantages of hydrogen for medical applications. Methods in Enzymology. 2015;**555**:289-317

[18] Ohsawa I et al. Hydrogen acts as a therapeutic antioxidant by selectively

reducing cytotoxic oxygen radicals. Nature Medicine. 2007;**13**(6):688-694

[19] Li F-Y et al. Consumption of hydrogen-rich water protects against ferric nitrilotriacetate-induced nephrotoxicity and early tumor promotional events in rats. Food and Chemical Toxicology. 2013;**61**:248-254

[20] Ichihara M et al. Beneficial biological effects and the underlying mechanisms of molecular hydrogen-comprehensive review of 321 original articles. Medical Gas Research. 2015;**5**(1):1-21

[21] Tian Y et al. Hydrogen, a novel therapeutic molecule, regulates oxidative stress, inflammation, and apoptosis. Frontiers in Physiology. 2021;**12**:789507

[22] Hanaoka T et al. Molecular hydrogen protects chondrocytes from oxidative stress and indirectly alters gene expressions through reducing peroxynitrite derived from nitric oxide. Medical Gas Research. 2011;**1**(1):1-9

[23] Hayashida K et al. Inhalation of hydrogen gas reduces infarct size in the rat model of myocardial ischemia–reperfusion injury. Biochemical and Biophysical Research Communications. 2008;**373**(1):30-35

[24] Itoh T et al. Molecular hydrogen inhibits lipopolysaccharide/interferon γ-induced nitric oxide production through modulation of signal transduction in macrophages. Biochemical and Biophysical Research Communications. 2011;**411**(1):143-149

[25] Zhao M et al. Hydrogen-rich water improves neurological functional recovery in experimental autoimmune encephalomyelitis mice. Journal of Neuroimmunology. 2016;**294**:6-13

[26] Chen H-G et al. Heme oxygenase-1 mediates the anti-inflammatory effect of molecular hydrogen in LPS-stimulated RAW 264.7 macrophages. International Journal of Surgery. 2013;**11**(10):1060-1066

[27] Iuchi K et al. Molecular hydrogen regulates gene expression by modifying the free radical chain reaction-dependent generation of oxidized phospholipid mediators. Scientific Reports. 2016;**6**(1):18971

[28] Kawasaki H, Guan J, Tamama K. Hydrogen gas treatment prolongs replicative lifespan of bone marrow multipotential stromal cells in vitro while preserving differentiation and paracrine potentials. Biochemical and Biophysical Research Communications. 2010;**397**(3):608-613

[29] Kawamura T et al. Hydrogen gas reduces hyperoxic lung injury via the Nrf2 pathway in vivo. American Journal of Physiology-Lung Cellular and Molecular Physiology. 2013;**304**(10):L646-L656

[30] Xie K et al. Protective effects of hydrogen gas on murine polymicrobial sepsis via reducing oxidative stress and HMGB1 release. Shock. 2010;**34**(1):90-97

[31] Qian L et al. Radioprotective effect of hydrogen in cultured cells and mice. Free Radical Research. 2010;**44**(3):275-282

[32] Guo SX et al. Beneficial effects of hydrogen-rich saline on early burn-wound progression in rats. PLoS One. 2015;**10**(4):e0124897

[33] Kang K-M et al. Effects of drinking hydrogen-rich water on the quality of life of patients treated with radiotherapy for liver tumors. Medical Gas Research. 2011;**1**(1):1-8

[34] Yuniati R et al. Application of topical sucralfate and topical

platelet-rich plasma improves wound healing in diabetic ulcer rats wound model. Experimental Pharmacology. 2021;**13**:797-806

[35] Dong Z et al. Concurrent CCR7 overexpression and RelB knockdown in immature dendritic cells induces immune tolerance and improves skin-graft survival in a murine model. Cellular Physiology and Biochemistry. 2017;**42**(2):455-468

[36] Nakao A et al. Effectiveness of hydrogen rich water on antioxidant status of subjects with potential metabolic syndrome—An open label pilot study. Journal of Clinical Biochemistry and Nutrition. 2010;**46**(2):140-149

[37] Zhang L et al. A systematic review and meta-analysis of clinical effectiveness and safety of hydrogel dressings in the management of skin wounds. Frontiers in Bioengineering and Biotechnology. 2019;**7**:342

[38] Chuai Y et al. A possible prevention strategy of radiation pneumonitis: Combine radiotherapy with aerosol inhalation of hydrogen-rich solution. Medical Science Monitor: International Medical Journal of Experimental and Clinical Research. 2011;**17**(4):HY1

[39] Kurokawa R et al. Convenient methods for ingestion of molecular hydrogen: Drinking, injection, and inhalation. Medical Gas Research. 2015;**5**:1-8

[40] Nakao A et al. Amelioration of rat cardiac cold ischemia/reperfusion injury with inhaled hydrogen or carbon monoxide, or both. The Journal of Heart and Lung Transplantation. 2010;**29**(5):544-553

[41] Huang C-S et al. Hydrogen inhalation ameliorates ventilator-induced lung injury. Critical Care. 2010;**14**(6):1-15

[42] Zhai Y et al. Hydrogen-rich saline ameliorates lung injury associated with cecal ligation and puncture-induced sepsis in rats. Experimental and Molecular Pathology. 2015;**98**(2):268-276

[43] Saitoh Y et al. Neutral pH hydrogen-enriched electrolyzed water achieves tumor-preferential clonal growth inhibition over normal cells and tumor invasion inhibition concurrently with intracellular oxidant repression. Oncology Research Featuring Preclinical and Clinical Cancer Therapeutics. 2008;**17**(6):247-255

[44] Huang C-S et al. Recent advances in hydrogen research as a therapeutic medical gas. Free Radical Research. 2010;**44**(9):971-982

[45] Ohta S. Molecular hydrogen as a preventive and therapeutic medical gas: Initiation, development and potential of hydrogen medicine. Pharmacology & Therapeutics. 2014;**144**(1):1-11

[46] Liu H et al. Hydrogen-rich saline reduces cell death through inhibition of DNA oxidative stress and overactivation of poly (ADP-ribose) polymerase-1 in retinal ischemia-reperfusion injury. Molecular Medicine Reports. 2015;**12**(2):2495-2502

Chapter 6

Rationale for Discrete Light Treatment Approaches in Wound Care

Ridham Varsani, Victoria Oliveira, Rodrigo Crespo Mosca, Mahmud Amin, Moiz Khan, Nimisha Rawat, Jonathan Kaj and Praveen Arany

Abstract

Wound healing is a multifaceted and sequential process influenced by both local and systemic conditions. Chronic wounds can lead to functional impairments, persistent pain, and reduced quality of life posing a significant burden on the healthcare system. In the US, approximately 6.5 million patients suffer from chronic wounds annually, costing the healthcare system over $25 billion. Given these substantial costs, there is an urgent need for innovative and effective wound management approaches. Historically, light therapy has been utilized to treat various skin diseases. There has been tremendous recent progress in light treatment approaches. This chapter outlines the fundamentals of wound healing and examines how different types of light can modulate specific stages of wound healing. These treatments can be broadly categorized based on their biological tissue interactions as photothermal therapy (PTT), photodynamic therapy (PDT), and photobiomodulation (PBM). Each treatment has a discrete mechanism of action evoking directed biological responses to promote wound healing. Additionally, appreciating the fundamental premise of each approach enables rationalized combinations for optimal therapeutic clinical benefits. Light treatments offer an additional innovative approach to effective wound management.

Keywords: wound healing, photothermal therapy, photodynamic therapy, photobiomodulation, lasers, laser therapy

1. Introduction

Wound healing is an extraordinarily dynamic and complex process. There are three overlapping phases of wound healing: inflammation, proliferation, and remodeling (maturation). A wound is defined as a break in the skin or other body tissues, usually due to mechanical injury. As most wound healing processes are examined post-injury, the earliest stage of healing usually involves hemostasis, which is often considered the initial phase of a four-stage process [1, 2]. There are other wound scenarios where the bleeding phase may not be discretely apparent, such as contusions, pressure or crush injuries, chemotherapeutic agents, and ionizing radiation-induced injuries, among others. The individual phases occur in a concurrent, organized manner, and the duration of each stage can vary depending on several extrinsic (presence of biofilms, moisture, etc.) and intrinsic (nutrition, blood flow, etc.) factors. Early stage post-injury, extravasation of blood that fills the injured area with plasma and cellular elements, mainly platelets. This initial scaffold serves as a provisional matrix necessary for cell migration and a reservoir of cytokines and growth factors [1, 3].

The inflammatory response, therefore, starts with vasodilation and increased vascular permeability, promoting the migration of neutrophils to the wound site [4–6]. The inflammatory cells namely, neutrophils, macrophages and lymphocytes are recruited by chemotactic substances released by platelets that adhere to the endothelial-lined vessel walls and transmigrate to the site of injury [7]. The activated macrophage is a key player responsible for removing microbes and damaged tissues [8–10]. These cells also secrete cytokines and growth factors that contribute to angiogenesis, fibroplasia, and extracellular matrix synthesis, including initial granulation tissue. The next stage is the proliferative phase, which involves new tissue formation and wound contraction involving concurrent proliferation of the epithelial, fibroblasts, and endothelial cells [11, 12]. Concurrent co-migration of fibroblasts and endothelial cells contributes to angiogenesis and fibroplasia. The new tissue forms a new network of blood vessels called the granulation tissue, providing increased perfusion and nutrition to the healing tissues. The leakiness of these early vessels is responsible for the clear wound fluid and creates a fluid microenvironment for cells to migrate and reorganize. Angiogenesis is characterized by migrating endothelial cells buddings, and maturing into tubular capillaries driven by platelet-derived growth factor (PDGF), vascular endothelial growth factor (VEGF) and transforming growth factor-beta (TGF-β) that also promotes matrix secretion, wound contraction, and angiogenesis [7, 11, 13].

The final phase of wound healing is remodeling and resolution, where the anatomical structures are functionally restored. During this phase, the wound contracts and becomes stronger, and collagen deposition occurs that is initially thinner (Type III) and oriented parallel to the skin. This is subsequently remodeled into thicker (Type I) collagen and reoriented along the lines of tension, increasing tensile strength. Successful completion of the healing process necessitates a balance between the synthesis of the new matrix and turnover of provisional healing matrix [7, 11, 14]. Excessive collagen synthesis due to an imbalance of either mechanical forces or biochemical factors, such as persistent inflammation, can result in scars such as keloids (skin or mucosa) or adhesions (internal organs).

2. Factors affecting wound chronicity

The return of injured tissue to its normal anatomical structure and function within a reasonable period is considered successful wound healing. However, some wounds do not heal in a timely and orderly manner. Clinically, a chronic wound is defined as a full-thickness skin defect that fails to heal after 3 months of standard care [15]. Various factors (systemic and local) may impede the finely balanced repair processes, resulting in chronic, non-healing wounds [16]. The differential diagnosis of chronic wounds is broad, with the main causes being chronic venous insufficiency of the lower limbs, peripheral vascular and neuropathic changes associated with diabetes mellitus, and related ulcers with pressure mechanisms. This may result from lower mitogenic activity, premature aging of fibroblasts, and greater activity of matrix metalloproteinases (MMP), leading to greater extracellular matrix (ECM) degradation and persistent inflammatory mechanisms [15, 17]. As an example, diabetic hyperglycemia contributes to a diverse systemic complication, causing an array of local pathologies manifesting within the wound microenvironment, including chronic inflammation, dysregulated angiogenesis, and hypoxia-induced oxidative stress, among others. As a result, diabetic patients develop wounds characterized by impaired healing, prolonged inflammation, and reduced epithelization. Around 15% of patients suffering from type II diabetes will develop ulcers localized on the lower limbs, named diabetic foot ulcers (DFUs), a severe form of diabetic wounds that may lead to lower limb amputation or death [15]. Wound chronicity implies important functional limitations, decreased quality of life, chronic pain, and associated complications that have psychosocial repercussions on patients, as well as a significant increase in health care costs [17]. Managing non-healing wounds, specifically modulating individual healing phases, represent a significant wound management strategy [14].

3. Fundamental therapeutic premise of laser-biological tissue interactions

Biological responses to laser energy is based on photon interaction with biomolecules [18]. Laser energy is a coherent, collimated, and monochromatic energy source [18]. Incident laser energy can be transformed depending on the rate and total dose into biokinetic (thermal), biophysical (conformational), biochemical (fluorescence, redox) or their combinations within the exposed tissue environment (**Figure 1**) [20]. Incident laser energy is absorbed by the characteristic tissue chromophores defined as a chemical group that absorbs light, and if present in the visible region of the electromagnetic spectrum, imparts color to the substance [21]. Another form of energy transfer, especially with low-dose laser energy, in non-homogenous biological tissues is inelastic scattering. In ablative high-power laser-tissue interaction, incident laser energy is absorbed by the chromophores, which eventually raises the temperature, resulting in a process known as *photothermolysis* or *photoablation* [22]. The laser

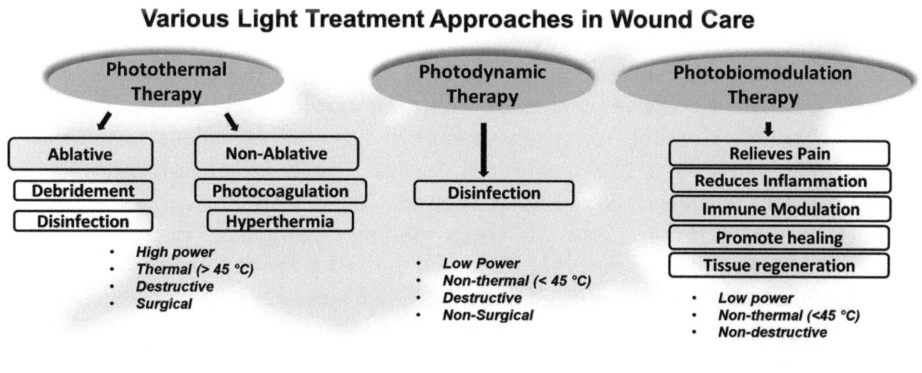

Figure 1.
Outlines the three main categories of phototherapy and their subcategories based on the mechanisms of action and effects. Photothermal therapy is divided into ablative techniques like debridement and disinfection, which involve thermal effects above 45°C and are destructive/surgical, versus non-ablative techniques like photocoagulation and hyperthermia, which are non-surgical. Photodynamic therapy involves disinfection through non-thermal (below 45°C) and destructive but non-surgical means. Photobiomodulation therapy encompasses non-thermal (below 45°C) and non-destructive, non-surgical applications such as relieving pain, reducing inflammation, modulating the immune system, promoting healing, and facilitating tissue regeneration. Modified from Arany [19].

energy can be confined temporally by pulsing the beam into micro- to femtoseconds. This results in the development of high electromagnetic fields (plasma) around the interaction, eventually resulting in tissue degradation or vaporization [23]. Lower powers can be employed for photocoagulation or hypothermia that have additional benefits in wound care. As the major outcome of these interactions is based on heat generation, we will refer to the former high-power as *ablative* PTT and the latter as *non-ablative* Photothermal Therapy (PTT). In contrast to these high-dose photon interactions, lower-dose photons can incite non-thermal photochemical responses employed by discrete forms of light treatments, namely photodynamic therapy (PDT, destructive) and photobiomodulation (PBM) [19]. The remaining chapter outlines the utility of each of these discrete approaches in wound management.

4. Photothermal therapy

The primary use of surgical lasers is to surgically remove damaged or necrotic tissues while additionally assisting with dysbiotic biofilm disinfection. Lasers can also be used for hemostasis, such as its use after surgical excisions or debridement. In contrast, using light devices, especially near-infrared lamps, offers discrete non-ablative benefits in promoting wound healing. This latter field is more popularly termed hyperthermia therapy, where body temperature is elevated in a controlled manner. Both approaches are further discussed in the following sections.

4.1 High-power, ablative PTT (A-PTT) for surgical wound debridement and disinfection

The spatial precision of a laser, perhaps best evidenced with LASIK in ophthalmology with its depth and width control, offers exquisite advantages over surgical curettes and blades. Further, the concurrent photocoagulation (bloodless surgical field) provides superior field visualization, reducing inadvertent tissue damage. The use of lasers for wound debridement has been examined in various contexts, including burns, Sulfur mustard injuries, chronic wounds, infected wounds, and diabetic wounds [24–29]. Research indicates that serial debridement of wounds results in a decreased infection rate and faster healing compared to infrequent or no debridement [30]. These effects have been ascribed to debridement reducing bacterial bioburden, relieving excessive pressure, promoting cytokine release, and facilitating drainage. Laser debridement is a largely unexplored wound debridement method limited to burn wounds and oral, periodontal contexts [31–33]. Despite restricted usage, it possesses numerous advantages, such as accuracy and consistency of tissue ablation (thereby minimizing injury to the wound site), enhanced patient comfort, and potential facilitation of wound healing. Particularly, the development of the erbium-doped yttrium-aluminum-garnet (Er: YAG) laser (2940 nm) and the erbium, chromium-doped yttrium-scandium-gallium-garnet (Er, Cr: YSGG) laser (2780 nm), which can be used on hard tissues with minimal thermal effect when combined with water cooling, make treatment of periodontal tissues (such as gingiva, tooth roots and bone tissue), as well as titanium implant, surfaces possible with lasers [34].

The efficacy and safety of using lasers for the treatment of chronic wounds has been clearly demonstrated by a few recent studies, one of which investigated these aspects in fully ablative CO_2 laser debridement and compared it to conventional surgical debridement when treating chronic wounds [26]. Guan et al. observed in a retrospective matched cohort trial that fully ablative CO_2 laser debridement had several advantages over routine sharp surgical debridement. Superior improvement in the wound's condition and reduced wound area were observed; patients treated with CO_2 laser debridement also showed reduced healing time for chronic wounds without any adverse events. Similar results were observed by Gaur et al. when using a diode laser in conjugation with conventional surgical biopsy for the treatment and sterilization of the biopsy site [35]. Overall, the efficacy of laser debridement has shown to be more conservative, less painful, reduced microbial loads, and improved perfusion and healing. This approach has been advocated in refractory or complex wounds with dehiscence or bone exposures [36–38]. Some investigators have examined initial full-field ablation versus fractal resurfacing for maintenance [39]. This direct ablative approach must be distinguished from the laser-induced shockwaves for agitation of antimicrobial solutions that improve wound disinfection [40, 41].

4.2 Lower-power, non-ablative PTT (*N*A-PTT) or hypothermia treatments

This non-invasive treatment strategy utilizes either light alone or additional photothermal transduction agents (PTAs) to convert increased kinetic photonic energy into thermal energy. This therapy aims to achieve a controlled temperature elevation from 37°C to 39.5°C or 40.5°C (range 41.8–44°C) [42]. PTAs absorb photon energy under the effect of near-infrared radiation and induce conditions of local hyperthermia. As most of these agents also generate photochemical reactions, *NA*-PTT with PTAs are discussed under the PDT section. This part only elaborates on the light-alone approach that generates non-ablative heating in target tissues. Among all the wavelengths typically used, near-infrared radiation (650–900 nm) is favored for its simplicity of application, capacity for precise targeting, and minimal absorption by neighboring tissues and skin, facilitating noninvasive penetration to relatively deeper tissue layers [43]. *NA*-PTT can be performed locally, regionally or whole body with light devices, ultrasounds, shockwaves, radiofrequency, and magnetic fields. *NA*-PTT has several advantages: low drug resistance, high efficacy, limited complications, and non-invasiveness.

Exposure to mild local heat (41–43°C) can assist in cell proliferation, angiogenesis, wound healing, and bone regeneration [44]. Moderate heat ranging from 45°C to 50°C can rapidly destroy tumor cells while minimal damage to normal cells. Hyperthermia temperatures (>50°C) have been shown to be effective in inhibiting bacterial proliferation. Rapid cell death due to protein denaturation and damage to the cell membrane is induced using relatively high light intensity at sub-coagulative (43–55°C) or coagulative (55–100°C) temperatures. Alternatively, a state of hyperthermia can be induced using milder temperatures (41–43°C); however, these temperature settings do not result in cell death unless applied for a prolonged duration (>1 h) [45]. Cell death due to *NA*-PTT can result from two different signaling pathways in cells exposed to temperatures greater than 42°C: apoptosis and necrosis. While necrosis has been reported as the conventional cellular response for *NA*-PTT, a few studies highlight apoptosis as the principal cell death mechanism for specific irradiation conditions [46]. Typically, it has been seen that high-energy irradiation induces necrosis while low-energy irradiation promotes apoptosis. Duration of treatment and presence of external photoabsorbers (such as nanoparticles) also influence cell death. Additionally, necroptosis is a cell death mechanism that has been recently reported in *NA*-PTT [47]. Heat-induced protein denaturation is the central mechanism of *NA*-PTT cytotoxicity, where higher temperatures result in faster and more effective cell death. Exposure to temperatures over 42°C results in irreversible tissue damage, further leading to necroptosis and apoptosis at 46°C [47]. Heating tissue at temperatures over 49°C causes disruption of the cell membrane and results in leakage of cytoplasmic matter, leading to inflammation and necrosis [48].

4.3 Non-ablative PTT (*NA*-PTT) or hypothermia to promote wound healing

Several challenges exist that can affect normal wound healing, including bacterial infection, chronic wounds, and excessive wound healing [2]. To combat these, *NA*-PTT has been proposed as a treatment that imparts negligible damage to normal tissues and selectively eliminates bacteria to promote wound healing. While the efficiency of therapy can be countered by the elevation of heat shock proteins that assist cell survival (leading to cellular thermal resistance), numerous studies have affirmed that mild hyperthermia can increase the susceptibility of cancer cells and bacteria to therapeutic methods used in conjugation with *NA*-PTT [49]. Light (typically within the near-infrared region) is absorbed by the agent, which is stimulated to an excited singlet state. It then undergoes nonradiative vibrational relaxation to return to its ground state, which results in a collision between the excited PTA and surrounding molecules, heating up the environment due to increased kinetic energy to achieve local photocoagulation [45, 50]. Among the various PTAs available, organic nanomaterials have shown good biocompatibility and biodegradability; however, low photothermal conversion efficiency, poor photothermal stability, and complicated synthesis limit their widespread usage. Contrastingly, inorganic nanomaterials exhibit excellent near-infrared light absorbance, high photothermal efficiency, and photostability owing to their intrinsic optical properties. However, their non-biodegradable nature and potential long-term toxicity are issues of concern [51]. It has been reported that *NA*-PTT using gold nanoparticles has been shown to induce programmed cell death via protein Bid, which induces the oligomerization of proteins Bak and Bax that facilitate pore formation and result in the release of Cytochrome C from the intermembrane space. Cytochrome C interacts with other molecules and forms an apoptosome, which signals the activation of various caspases that lead to apoptotic cell death [52].

It has been observed that mild hyperthermia plays a beneficial role in wound repair, particularly for burn wounds [53]. As demonstrated by a study conducted by Shahabi et al. on BALB/c mice, wounds treated with mild hyperthermia exhibited significantly smaller size compared to untreated wounds evaluated on the same day [54]. Furthermore, treated wounds showed substantially reduced acute inflammation along with increased collagen formation and epithelialization compared with untreated wounds. With the progression of treatment, they also noticed a significant increase in neovascularization in the treated wounds. Studies also show that local hyperthermia can increase local perfusion and oxygenation at the wound site. Rabkin et al. observed increased subcutaneous tissue oxygen tension on the application of heat and a threefold increase in local perfusion, highlighting the role of hyperthermia in treating contaminated wounds and mitigating infections [55]. They found a linear relation between change in oxygen tension and reducing microbial burden.

Besides promoting cell proliferation by mild hyperthermia to accelerate wound healing and tissue regeneration, hydrogels with photothermal properties have been implicated in remotely controlled drug release. Hydrogels can absorb inflammation exudate and serve as a physical barrier by protecting the wound from bacteria. These hydrogels are formulated to resemble natural tissues and extracellular matrix, which helps them integrate with the wound and stimulate tissue regeneration [56]. Indocyanine green is an FDA-approved photothermal therapeutic agent with exceptional photothermal conversion efficacy [57]. Li et al. developed a hydrogel loaded with indocyanine green and rare-earth nanoparticles that effectively released Adriamycin upon near-infrared (NIR) activation [58].

Overall, both ablative and non-ablative PTT have significant utility in wound care that can be routinely employed in comprehensive management. To ensure appropriate biological tissue reactions and reliable therapeutic clinical outcomes, the device parameters of the device and manner of delivery must be adopted suitably.

5. Photodynamic therapy

Addressing skin wounds represents a significant global public health challenge, particularly chronic wounds, which place considerable physical and financial strain on patients and significantly diminish their quality of life [59, 60]. Photodynamic therapy (PDT) utilizes light-activated drugs called photosensitizers to achieve therapeutic effects. Initially, a photosensitizer is administered to the patient, either locally or systemically [61]. After a given period to enable optimal photosensitizer distribution, the treatment site is exposed to a specific visible or near-infrared light wavelength. The photosensitizer absorbs this light, triggering two discrete photochemical reactions, either Type I or Type II. These generate cytotoxic biochemical intermediates that ultimately lead to the desired therapeutic outcome [62]. It is worth noting that the history of PDT dates back over a 100 years and even received the 1903 Nobel Prize for Dr. Finsen Rydberg's seminal work. Dougherty and colleagues conducted the first substantial animal and human tumor studies in the late 1970s at Roswell Park, Buffalo marked the beginning of the modern PDT era [63].

PDT was originally developed for the local destruction of solid tumors and has been trialed for tumors in various sites. The first approved use was for refractory superficial bladder cancer, utilizing Photofrin as the photosensitizer and transurethral light delivery. Other approvals include the treatment of obstructive and early-stage bronchial cancers, where light is applied through a bronchoscope, and esophageal lesions for palliation or high-grade dysplasia in Barrett's Esophagus. PDT has shown high efficacy in skin cancer, particularly basal cell carcinoma, but its role compared to other treatments, such as local excision, is still being established. PDT has been less effective for squamous cell skin tumors and melanoma, where light penetration is a limitation [64]. In malignant brain tumors, PDT has been studied as an adjunctive therapy, with evidence of improved survival at high light doses. Clinical trials for prostate cancer are ongoing, using interstitial fiber-optic light delivery to treat recurrent tumors or as primary therapy for focal tumors [63, 65, 66]. PDT has also been trialed for intraperitoneal disseminated ovarian cancer and mesothelioma, with partial success. Head and neck cancer trials have targeted widespread, unresectable, or recurrent tumors, early-stage oral cancers, and nasopharyngeal tumors using a specialized trans-nasal light delivery system. PDT has been used in different stages of cancer patient management, including palliation, surgical adjuvant, stand-alone modality for primary lesion cure, and prophylactic treatment of dysplasia. Other challenging tumors under investigation include biliary tree tumors, pancreatic cancer treated laparoscopically, and spinal metastases to debulk tumor mass before vertebroplasty. PDT has also been explored for purging tumors and stem cells in bone marrow transplantation. However, this is not yet approved, as maintaining a high anti-tumor effect while preserving normal cell survival remains challenging [63, 66, 67].

5.1 Biological targets in PDT

In PDT targeting mammalian tissues, the clinical effect can result from direct target cell death (e.g., tumor cells) through necrosis or apoptosis, vascular damage leading to tissue ischemia and subsequent cell death, immune modulation, or a combination of these mechanisms. The cytotoxic impact of PDT is primarily attributed to three distinct mechanisms: Firstly, PDT exerts direct cytotoxicity toward tumor cells, precipitating their necrosis. Secondly, the generation of reactive oxygen species (ROS) during PDT provokes apoptosis by instigating alterations in oxygen free radicals, resulting in irreversible cellular and microvascular damage (**Figure 2**). Thirdly, the apoptotic or necrotic cells induced by PDT elicit immunogenic cell death, thereby instigating a cascade of immune responses and subsequent implications in the latter stages of therapy [69]. One of the potential advantages of PDT is the ability to adjust the photosensitizer choice and treatment parameters, such as the drug-light time interval, total PDT "dose," and light fluence rate, to selectively target primary biological processes and resulting responses (**Table 1**) [70–72]. For example, PDT for AMD exploits the vascular response, while bone marrow purging focuses on cellular effects. Tumor treatments often involve a combination of these biological targets and responses. Unlike radiation therapy, where DNA is the primary target, in PDT, photosensitizers typically localize in or on cell membranes, often mitochondrial membranes, resulting in somatic cell death rather than anti-proliferative effects [73]. This leads to very rapid tissue responses, sometimes detectable before treatment completion. Since PDT is usually delivered as a single, high dose rather than fractionated over many sessions, there is limited opportunity to adjust treatment parameters. Pre-treatment optimization is crucial given the potential heterogeneity of tissue responses within and between targets or patients.

The light must be efficiently delivered to the PS molecules to make PDT the most effective. Lasers and light-emitting diodes (LEDs) are currently the most common light sources used in PDT, though in some cases filtered white light can

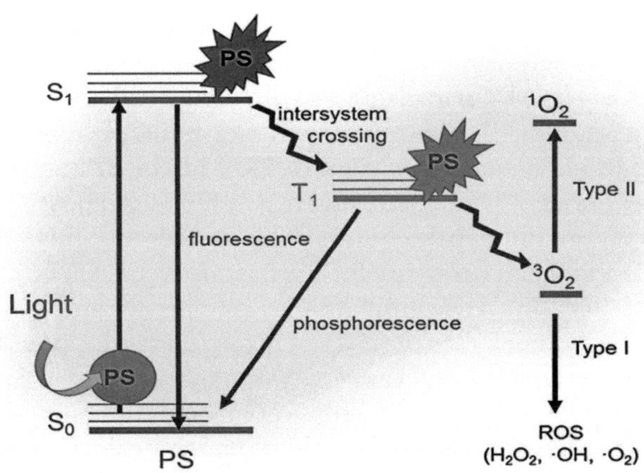

Figure 2.
The photosensitizer's (PS) electrons from the ground state (So) will absorb energy and move to singlet-excited states (S1). Some of the absorbed energy will be released via intersystem crossing, and the promoted electron will more to a triplet-excited state (T1). This triplet state has a relatively long half-life, allowing energy to be transferred to nearby oxygen molecules. This generates $^1O_2$ *in most cases via the type II pathway, which can damage the cells in the surrounding area. Adapted from Hu et al. [68].*

Photosensitizer characteristics	
Toxicity	The metabolic processes involving the photosensitizer should be structured in a manner that prevents the generation of additional harmful byproducts.
Mutagenicity and carcinogenicity	The photosensitizer's therapeutic action aimed at alleviating a particular ailment should not inadvertently lead to the onset or exacerbation of another health condition.
Biodistribution	A photosensitizer possessing the ability to specifically reach and gather in desired tissues holds potential advantages. This assumption relies on the accurate identification of the appropriate target for light exposure and activation. If the target includes intracellular sites, such as mitochondrial membranes, it can result in programmed cell death through apoptosis. On the other hand, targeting the cell membrane or extracellular regions may cause cell death via vessel collapse, resulting in necrosis. Necrosis triggers a systemic response through the cytokine family, leading to widespread effects throughout the body.

Table 1.
Guidelines for selection of photosensitizers to be used in photodynamic therapy (adapted from Refs. [70–72]).

also be used. However, most PS classes absorb ultraviolet or visible regions of the electromagnetic spectrum that overlap with the absorption of the main tissue chromophores (e.g., melanin, hemoglobin, bilirubin) [74]. The short penetration depth of visible light into tissues (<5 mm) is very effective for superficial lesions and limits the damage from reaching adjacent healthy tissues but also makes it harder to bring PDT into clinical applications that require illumination of deep tissues or large tumors [75]. Current commercial alternatives require the use of endoscopes and/or multiple optical fibers that are highly expensive and require rather specialized training for clinicians. However, because of the rapid and noticeable tissue responses, real-time monitoring of tissue response (e.g., changes in blood flow, presence of a necrotic treatment boundary) can help adjust dosing to avoid under-treating the target or over-treating adjacent normal tissues [76]. Additionally, PDT can be repeated multiple times, as seen in skin tumor treatments, without apparent induction of resistance or exceeding tissue tolerance, likely due to the preservation of collagen and tissue architecture [77–79]. Following the selection of a photosensitizer (**Table 2**), additional considerations must be addressed for its application such as targeting specific cells, the depth within the tissue where the target cell is situated, the extent of PS absorption by the target cell, as well as the prescribed protocol, including the wavelength employed in PDT to optimize the maximal convergence of PS illumination.

5.2 Photodynamic therapy in wound care

A study has demonstrated that low-dose ALA-induced PDT stimulates cell proliferation, angiogenesis, and skin homeostasis regulation, thereby enhancing wound healing through the activation of localized ROS production in an acute mouse skin excision model [80]. Studies using animal models have reported an accelerated initiation of wound re-epithelialization following PDT, characterized by the presence of active fibroblasts, fibrin, and granulation tissue [81]. Evidence suggests a robust cellular infiltrate response in the treated chronic wound as one of the various properties of PDT. Findings from a study indicate that chronic wounds subjected to ALA-PDT exhibit heightened populations of neurons containing mediators implicated in wound healing, along with an increase in the proportion of mast cells containing nerve growth factor (NGF) and vasoactive intestinal peptide (VIP).

Photosensitizers	Activation wavelength	Type of tumor
HPD (hematoporphyrin) derived	625–630 nm	Mesothelioma, high grade glioma, advanced gastrointestinal tumors, sub-foveal choroidal neovascularization
BPD (benzoporphyrin) derived	689 nm	Non-/facia port-wine stains
5-ALA (5-aminolevulinic acid)	635 nm	Malignant gliomas
5-ALA methyl ester	635 nm	Basal cell carcinoma
5-ALA benzyl ester	635 nm	Gastrointestinal tumors
HPPH (hexylether derivative of pyropheophorbide-A)	665 nm	Several Barrett's esophagus, endobronchial recurrence from lung cancer
Phthalocyanines or naphthalocyanines	650–770 nm	Cutaneous tumors, endobronchial lesions, head and neck tumors
Lutetium texaphyrin	732 nm	Cervical, prostate and brain tumors
SNET2 (tin etiopurpurin dichloride)	664 nm	Cutaneous metastatic breast cancer, basal-cell carcinoma, Kaposis's sarcoma, prostate cancer
Boronated protoporphyrin	630 nm	Brain tumors
M-THPC (meta-tetra (hydroxyphenyl) chlorin)	652 nm	Head and neck tumors

Table 2.
Types of photosensitizers used in photodynamic therapy for malignant diseases.

5.2.1 PDT for disinfections

PDT has emerged as a treatment option for localized bacterial infections, driven by the increasing problem of antibiotic resistance. Various photosensitizers have been found effective against multi-drug-resistant bacterial strains. For instance, methylene blue PDT has been approved in Canada for treating periodontitis, where a gel formulation of the drug is applied to infected gum pockets, followed by light delivery through an optical fiber placed in each pocket [82–84]. Ongoing trials explore using PDT for sterilizing chronically infected wounds, such as diabetic ulcers, and the nares to eliminate bacteria that can cause peri-operative self-infection of surgical wounds [85]. PDT has also been tested as an anti-fungal agent, including against Candida, and off-label for acne treatment, targeting the bacterium *Acne vulgaris*. These applications involve direct application of the photosensitizer and light to the infected tissue [86]. Other potential uses of PDT include sterilizing in situ implanted devices like in-dwelling catheters and field sterilization, such as in operating rooms, to prevent bacterial growth. In the 1980s, there was interest in using PDT to purge blood of viral agents pre-transfusion, particularly for HIV and hepatitis. Although technically successful, concerns about the economics of the technique and re-injection of blood-containing photosensitizer led to its limited adoption. However, with the development of photosensitizers that can be used at lower concentrations and demonstrate high anti-viral activity, this technique may regain interest in the future [87].

While bacteria colonize all chronic wounds, infected wounds hinder effective wound healing. Antibiotics provide limited respite, especially against multidrug-resistant bacteria that undergo rapid mutation to adapt to extreme environmental conditions. Additionally, bacteria can exist in colonies that form aggregates on a surface, known as biofilm, which show increased antibacterial resistance and affect antibacterial efficacy. These factors make developing strategies to combat bacterial infection an urgent necessity. Recent years have seen a positive outlook toward using nanotechnology in PTT, owing to its broad-spectrum antibacterial activity, prevention of drug resistance, and reliable controllability. However, PTT alone is often insufficient to completely eliminate bacteria due to uneven heat distribution in bacterial biofilms. To counter this, numerous recent studies have used PTT in conjugation with other therapeutic methods, such as PDT, antimicrobial peptides, or antibiotics, for better reparative outcomes [88, 89].

5.2.2 PDT for anti-angiogenesis

Photodynamic therapy has emerged as a highly effective treatment for age-related macular degeneration (AMD), the leading cause of blindness in the elderly in the Western world. The "wet" form of AMD, characterized by abnormal blood vessel growth in the choriocapillaris, can lead to central vision loss. PDT has been used in over 2 million cases to date, significantly impacting treatment outcomes. Before PDT, thermal laser coagulation was the only available treatment, but its effectiveness was limited. In PDT for AMD, a diode laser delivers light through a fundus camera to irradiate a 3 mm diameter spot shortly after intravenous injection of the photosensitizer VisudyneR while the drug is still in the vascular compartment [90]. This process targets and kills vascular endothelial cells, leading to thrombosis and vessel closure. While PDT does not restore lost vision, it can slow or halt further vision loss with several rounds of treatment over several months. Visudyne-PDT has become the standard treatment for AMD, although trials combining PDT with anti-VEGF therapy are currently underway [91]. The use of PDT in modulating angiogenesis in chronic wounds may be useful in accelerating the resolution of granulation tissue and promoting remodeling.

5.2.3 PDT for anti-inflammatory, immunomodulation, and skin remodeling

PDT has been extensively studied in dermatology, particularly for skin tumors. It has shown high efficacy in basal cell carcinoma, especially for basal cell nevus syndrome and difficult-to-treat sites like the eyelids. However, PDT has not been approved for basal cell carcinoma due to the high success rates of established alternatives like excision and cryosurgery [92, 93]. In dermatological PDT, 5-aminolevulinic acid (ALA) is used to synthesize protoporphyrin IX (PpIX) endogenously in target cells, making it effective for conditions like actinic keratosis or sun-damaged skin. ALA-PDT is approved for these indications and has led to off-label use in cosmetic dermatology for acne, hair removal, and skin remodeling [94–96]. PDT has also been studied for psoriasis, a condition characterized by uncontrolled keratinocyte proliferation leading to plaques, particularly on joints like the elbows and knees. While other forms of phototherapy, like UV-B treatment or PUVA, are options for psoriasis, they carry a risk of UV-induced skin cancer. PDT using visible light-activated photosensitizers presents a promising alternative, but its efficacy for psoriasis is still under investigation [97–99]. PDT has effectively treated specific skin conditions such as acne vulgaris, rosacea, genital warts, and superficial tumors [100]. PDT has been employed for the treatment of diverse conditions such as malignancies, microbial infections, and esthetic concerns such as actinic keratoses, squamous cell carcinoma, basal cell carcinoma, Bowen's disease, mycosis fungoid, warts, acne, rejuvenation, and necrobiosis lipoidica besides other conditions [61, 101–108]. These PDT applications suggest its immunomodulatory and anti-inflammatory responses could be utilized in chronic wound scenarios effectively, but require a more thorough investigation.

6. Photobiomodulation

The scientific study of the interaction of light in the form of non-ionizing radiation and living organisms is known as Photobiology. This includes phenomena such as photosynthesis and bioluminescence. An innovative approach to utilizing low-dose light treatments to modulate host biological responses is termed Photobiomodulation (PBM) therapy, which evokes potent therapeutic biological response [20]. PBM has gained widespread popularity and is commonly employed in clinical medicine due to its non-invasive nature and cost-effectiveness. PBM, also known as low-level laser therapy (LLLT) or light therapy, involves using low-level lasers or light-emitting diodes (LEDs) to stimulate cellular processes, promote tissue repair of skin injuries, reduce inflammation, and produce analgesia. Research with respect to PBM for wound healing has explored its effects on several types of wounds, including chronic wounds and surgical incisions. The therapeutic approaches include the PBM-induced effect in mobilizing immune cells into the bloodstream and the recruitment and modulation of their pro-regenerative activity into the wound site. PBM is performed with various wavelengths spanning visible to near-infrared and is increasingly appreciated as an energy transfer phenomenon based on absorption and inelastic scattering [20]. PBM is one of the most popular forms of light-based therapies currently due to significant recent advances in its demonstrated therapeutic benefits in supportive cancer care, where it has been noted to enhance resilience and minimize adverse side-effects of cancer treatments [109, 110].

6.1 Mechanism of action of photobiomodulation

There are over 300 terms for using this treatment such as low-level light/laser therapy, cold laser therapy, infrared or red-light therapy. This non-invasive technique utilizes low doses of light to stimulate cellular function and promote tissue repair [111]. Efficacy of PBM is dependent on several factors that include positioning of cells within the proximity of light exposure, cell type, molecular composition, cellular redox state, tissue microenvironment conditions, and various parameters related to the PBM technique itself, including wavelength, power density, delivery method (pulsed or continuous), size and shape of the light beam or spot are being used for irradiation purposes along with duration/frequency of exposure [109]. Extensive studies have been conducted to understand the mechanisms of action of PBM on biological tissues [111]. Various molecular targets and signaling pathways have been identified. These can be broadly categorized into three main compartments: the intracellular mitochondria (Cytochrome C Oxidase), the cell membrane (photosensitive transporters and receptors like TRPV-1, Opsin 2–4), and the extracellular milieu (Latent TGF-β1 activation) (**Figure 3**). Therapeutic benefits of PBM are observed owing to the direct biological effect of these discrete components. Cytochrome C Oxidase (CCO), the intracellular mitochondrial enzyme, demonstrates distinctive absorption characteristics within the non-ionizing, visible spectrum (blue and red) and near-infrared (NIR) wavelength, which is the most popular cited PBM

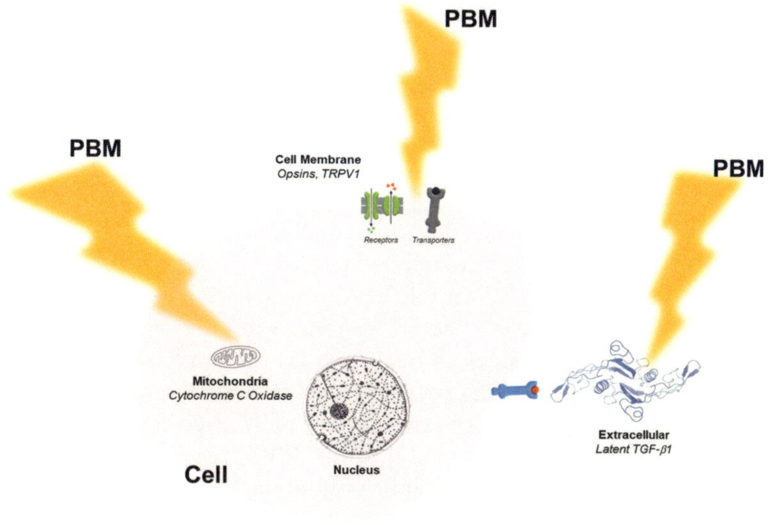

Figure 3.
Currently outlines mechanism of photobiomodulation (PBM) therapy. Broadly there are three categories: intracellular involving cytochrome C oxidase, cell membrane receptors and transporters, and extracellular latent TGF-β1. It is being increasingly appreciated that multiple pathways and synergy among them integrate into biological responses that are ultimately responsible for the therapeutic clinical outcomes.

mechanism. Direct absorption of light at specific wavelengths by CCO leads to the enhancement of mitochondrial activity, which eventually leads to an increase in ATP production, along with the generation of mild, transient reactive oxygen species (ROS) [112–115]. Studies have demonstrated that the absorption spectrum of CCO spans from 580 to 850 nm, specifically with absorption bands present at the red region (660 nm) and the near-infrared region (810 nm) [116, 117]. The enhanced mitochondrial activity directly activates several signaling pathways, leading to higher ATP/ADP ratios and transitory reactive oxygen species. Both effects can mediate the activation of signaling pathways that further induce transcription factors associated with cell migration, proliferation, protein and nucleic acid synthesis, and apoptosis inhibition [115]. Such effects allow for accelerated tissue repair, modulated inflammatory processes, and pain signaling to enhance angiogenesis, collagen synthesis, and re-epithelization [114, 117].

Improved wound healing was among the very first clinical observations with PBM treatments [118]. A key PBM mechanism mediating this response is its ability to directly activate a potent pro-healing latent growth factor complex, TGF-β1 [119, 120]. The role of TGF-β1 spans a broad range of health and wellness, including processes such as development, immune responses, wound healing, and malignancies. These growth factors have been shown to act on several cell types in a context-dependent manner and appear to play a crucial role in the healing milieu [116, 119]. Our prior work with an *in vivo* human oral tooth extraction model and PBM treatments noted increased TGF-β1 expression immediately post-injury [120]. Additionally, immunohistochemistry analysis revealed an elevated expression of TGF-β3 14 days post-treatment. Further *in vitro* and *in vivo* studies using biochemical and molecular assays, transgenic mice, and chemical inhibitors have outlined the PBM-induced redox-activated mechanism for latent TGF-β1 activation that involved a single amino acid, a methionine at position 253 on its latency-associated peptide [119, 121]. In a more recent study, Khan et al. observed the effects of PBM therapy on a modified burn wound model for third-degree burns in C57BL/6 mice [122]. Using a dynamic treatment protocol consisting of an 810 nm laser at 70 mW/cm^2 for 5 minutes, or a total dose of 21 J/cm^2 PBM-treated wounds were observed to have significantly improved closure and healing responses 9 days post-treatment when compared to controls. In wounds subjected to PBM, activation of TGF-β1 signaling was evidenced through increased nuclear localization of phospho-Smad2/3 complexes [122]. Further, to examine the mechanism of PBM-promoted wound healing, a chimeric knock-in mice model with the β1 dimer in the TGF-β1 latency-associated peptide was substituted with β3 (TGF-$\beta^{L1\beta3/L1\beta3}$). In wild type TGF-$\beta^{L1\beta1/L1\beta1}$ mice, PBM was observed to expedite the burn wound healing response, whereas a partial response was observed in the heterozygous chimeric TGF-$\beta^{L1\beta1/L1\beta3}$ mice while poor healing was noted in the homozygous chimeric TGF-$\beta^{L1\beta1/L1\beta3}$ mice. Immunostaining revealed no significant changes in the inflammatory response, further implying the central role of TGF-β1 signaling in the healing process of PBM-treated burn wounds [122]. Thus, PBM treatments via TGF-β1 activation is the primary mechanism mediating its wound healing therapeutic responses.

6.2 Cell-type responses to photobiomodulation treatments

Recent studies have observed distinct impacts of PBM on diverse types of cells during the wound healing process. Studies have highlighted PBM treatments to promote the functions of keratinocytes, fibroblasts, macrophages, neutrophils, and endothelial cells [114, 116, 117, 123]. These functions include migration and proliferation of these cells, promoting inflammatory infiltration, macrophage phagocytoses, wound contraction, angiogenesis, fibroblast matrix synthesis, and keratinocyte maturation [111]. Furthermore, a study conducted by Otterço et al. examined the effects of PBM in the kinetics of wound healing responses [114]. The experiment involved 20 male Wistar rats, with 10 rats undergoing treatment utilizing a GaAlAs laser emitting at 670 nm with a continuous pulse and an energy density of 14.28 J/cm^2 for a consecutive period of 15 days. Histopathological and immunohistochemistry analyses were conducted on the 4th, 11th, and 16th days, whereas the histopathological results revealed significantly lower values of inflammatory infiltrate on the 16th day in the laser group compared to the control. The immunochemistry analysis revealed several mechanistic effects, including reduced levels of tumor necrosis factor TNF-α, increased expression of vascular endothelial growth factor, and higher levels of collagen type 1 fiber with improved organization and arrangement, all of which promoted wound healing in the PBM-treated Wistar rats [114, 124]. Similarly, PBM treatments have recorded modulation of platelet biology within a mouse model of hemophilia, including heightened mechanical rigidity and enhanced activity of clots via improved adhesion of coagulation factors [125]. Although there is a posed risk for thrombosis, the treatments promoted wound healing and presented no signs of disruption to protective coagulation responses [111, 114]. Additionally, it was observed that the combined application of red and infrared (650 nm and 830 nm, respectively) lasers had the most pronounced systemic impact on the healing of skin wounds in athymic mice [126]. Moreover, in cultured human fibroblasts, PBM using a diode laser (red light, 660 nm) was found to stimulate gene expression in various cell adhesion molecules (CAMs) and extracellular proteins in an in vitro wound model and reduced matrix degradation and positively regulated its synthesis [127, 128].

6.3 PBM for oral wounds

Outlined in the mechanism of action, PBM treatments have been documented to directly induce reactive oxygen species that further activate latent transforming growth factors, namely TFG-β1 and TFG-β3. These growth factors have been shown to act on several cell types in a context-dependent manner and appear to play a crucial role in the healing milieu [116, 119]. With an *in vivo* model of human tooth extraction and socket healing (**Figure 4**), Arany et al. [120], showcased an augmented expression of TGF-β1 immediately following irradiation with a Gallium Arsenide far-infrared laser at 904 nm, administered at an energy dosage of 3 J/cm^2. Additionally, immunohistochemistry analysis revealed an elevated expression of TGF-β3 14 days post-treatment. This observation implies that photobiomodulation therapy has the potential to activate latent transforming growth factors, thereby playing a pivotal role in facilitating a quicker healing response [120, 122].

6.4 PBM for venous ulcers

In a recent double-blind, randomized, placebo-controlled human clinical study, Vitse et al. worked to analyze the efficacy of PBM treatments on chronic venous leg ulcers [129]. The study was designed with 24 test subjects randomized to treatments of PBM or placebo over a period of 12 weeks. The study aimed to compare ulcer size, pain reduction, and the incidence of complete wound closure between the placebo and PBM treatments. All subjects underwent standard wound healing care, encompassing necrotic tissue debridement, application of hydrating wound dressings, daily compression therapy, support stockings, and nutritional guidance. PBM treatments utilized a red laser at a wavelength of 635 nm, comprising three diodes, each with an output power of 17.5 mW. This irradiance was 2.46 mW/cm^2 during 20-minute

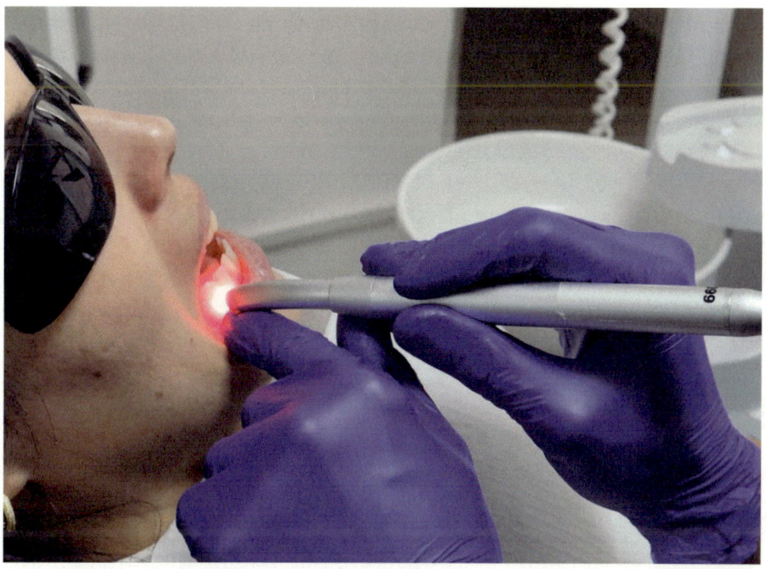

Figure 4.
Clinical PBM treatment being performed with a dental laser on a patient for mucositis.

sessions, resulting in a total fluence of 2.95 J/cm^2. Chronic leg ulcers were evaluated at 4 and 12 weeks via digital photography (laser planimetry), arterial blood flow measurements (laser Doppler), a record of pain medications, and an analog pain score (0–100) provided by the subjects [116]. The results revealed a significant reduction in mean ulcer size of 0.46 cm^2 and mean pain score of 43.54 points between the test and placebo groups [129]. Furthermore, the results indicated a significant reduction in ulcer pain at both 4 and 12 weeks after PBM treatment [116]. These positive outcomes suggest that photobiomodulation holds promise as a viable approach for the long-term treatment of chronic leg ulcers. It is imperative to explore the effects of dosage and wavelength in the modulated healing response to optimize PBM as a robust modality for venous ulcer care.

6.5 PBM for burn wounds

Khan et al. observed the effects of PBM therapy on a modified burn wound model for third-degree burns in C57BL/6 mice [122]. Using a dynamic treatment protocol consisting of an 810 nm laser at 70 mW/cm^2 for 5 minutes, or a total dose of 21 J/cm^2, PBM-treated wounds had significantly improved closure and healing responses 9 days post-treatment compared to controls. In wounds subjected to PBM, evident activation of TGF-β1 signaling was indicated through an augmented nuclear localization of phosphor-Smad2/3. This observation implies that the PBM-induced activation of TGF-β signaling may contribute to enhancing the healing and management of burn wounds. Further, they also examined the effects of PBM treatment on wild type TGF-$\beta^{L1\beta1/L1\beta1}$ mice and a chimeric knock-in mice model, featuring the replacement of the β1 dimer in the TGF-β1 latency-associated peptide with β3 (TGF-$\beta^{L1\beta1/L1\beta3}$). In wild type TGF-$\beta^{L1\beta1/L1\beta1}$ mice, PBM was observed to expedite the burn wound healing response, whereas a partial response was observed in the heterozygous chimeric TGF-$\beta^{L1\beta1/L1\beta3}$ mice. PBM treatments did not yield significant outcomes in the healing process in the heterozygous chimeric TGF-$\beta^{L1\beta1/L1\beta3}$ mice, and immunostaining revealed no significant changes in the inflammatory response, further implying the central role of TGF-β1 signaling in the healing process of PBM treated burn wounds. In summary, near-infrared and red-light treatments have been shown to be prominent biophysical therapeutic modalities. In another double-blind, placebo-controlled trial, Oliveira et al. used low-dose LED therapy (658 nm) was administered to address second and third-degree burn injuries [116]. Following treatment, all participants noted diminished pain and itching, along with reduced inflammatory exudate and fibrin, enhanced re-epithelialization, and well-organized granulation tissue at sites treated with photobiomodulation (PBM) therapy (peak power of 40 mW, beam size of 0.13 cm^2, and irradiance of 0.31 W/cm^2), as compared to control sites on the opposite side.

6.6 PBM for pressure ulcers

Pressure ulcers, often arising from reduced blood flow due to applied pressure on the skin, are characterized by a localized injury to the skin and soft tissue. Quick and effective treatment is crucial to avert potential life-threatening complications, leading to the growing popularity of PBM therapy in managing these injuries. In a randomized, single-blind clinical study, Taradaj et al. worked to evaluate the effects of three common PBM wavelengths on the healing response of pressure ulcers [116]. Their study utilized a total of 71 subjects with stage II and III pressure ulcers

(EPUAP scale), categorizing them into four groups: (1) 658 nm (red) laser, (2) 808 nm (NIR) laser, (3) 940 nm (NIR) laser, and (4) placebo. All patients underwent routine wound healing care, comprising daily wound irrigations using a 0.9% physiologic saline solution and application of 1% hydrophilic sulfadiazine cream. Furthermore, participants received adapted footwear, engaged in self-care practices, and preventive measures were implemented to mitigate the risk of disabilities. PBM treatments were performed daily, five times a week over a month, using a GaAlAs diode laser with an average dosage of 4 J/cm^2, spot size of 0.1 cm^2, maximum output power of 50 mW, and continuous radiation emission [130]. Ulcers were evaluated using planimetry with an infrared camera to obtain thermographic images and temperature profiles. At 3 months post-treatment, their findings indicated a notable increase in healing rates within the 658 nm treated group, showing a heightened rate of approximately 59%, compared to the 940, 808 nm, and placebo, exhibiting an estimated healing rate of 17% [130]. Furthermore, the 658 nm treated group demonstrated significant efficacy in facilitating wound closure, showcasing a 71% decrease in ulcer size 1-month post-treatment. On the other hand, the 808 nm and 940 nm treated groups did not exhibit a significant improvement in healing rates compared to the placebo (31%, 30%, and 28%, respectively) [116]. These findings suggest that PBM treatments within the red, visible spectrum contribute significantly to the healing process of pressure ulcers.

6.7 PBM in diabetes

Diabetes mellitus (DM) is a complex metabolic disease that compromises the metabolism of carbohydrates and lipids via an inadequate production or sensitivity to insulin [131–133]. Over the past 50 years, the prevalence of DM has risen at an unsettling rate, increasing from 108 million in 1980 to nearly 422 million in 2014 [133]. DM is associated with chronic hyperglycemia and leads to prolonged complications such as cardiovascular disease, kidney disease, peripheral and autonomic neuropathy, diabetic foot ulcers, and impaired white blood cell activity [131–135]. Among the complications outlined above, an estimated 25% of individuals with DM face the possibility of developing a diabetic foot ulcer (DFU), carrying an elevated risk for chronic wounds that may lead to infection or gangrene [135, 136]. Hyperglycemia plays a role in the impairment of white blood cells, affecting their ability to migrate and clot, ultimately leading to a delayed wound-healing process [132]. The prolonged healing process and a reoccurrence rate ranging from 40% to 65% have led to approximately 3% of DM patients requiring amputation of the lower limb, as well as a high mortality rate of 75.9% within 3 years [133, 137, 138].

Current approaches to treat and manage diabetic foot ulcers include patient education and prevention, systemic glycemic control, negative pressure therapy, topical growth factors, and local wound care [132, 133, 135]. Conventional wound care of DFUs involves a multidisciplinary team of healthcare professionals that work through a process of debridement, cleaning, antibiotic treatment, and dressing of the ulcer. Methods for debridement include autolytic, biochemical, osmotic, biological, and surgical removal of necrotic or infected tissue [135]. Nevertheless, all the aforementioned treatment methods are ineffective in delivering sufficient care as only a 50% healing rate is attained [135]. These individual treatments are focused on basic wound care and are empirical in nature.

Photobiomodulation has exhibited beneficial outcomes in treating chronic wounds and diabetic foot ulcers. In studies involving wound healing models, PBM (laser—InGaAlP) at 660 nm demonstrated the ability to expedite collagen production and increase the overall percentage of type III collagen in diabetic animals [139]. Numerous *in vivo* and *in vitro* studies have substantiated the promising effects of PBM, such as Maiya et al., who examined the impacts of PBM at a 632.8 nm visible wavelength with a fluence of 4.8 J/cm^2 administered 5 days per week on the healing of diabetic wounds in alloxan-induced diabetic animals [140]. Examination of the histopathological and biochemical characteristics of the wounds exhibited an accelerated and improved healing process from PBM treatments. On average, laser-treated groups were healed within 3 weeks, while the control groups required over 8 weeks to heal [140]. In a literature review of 13 studies conducted over the last 20 years, the most effective PBM features for healing DFUs include red light with wavelengths ranging from 630 to 660 nm, or infrared light at 850 to 890 nm, and an irradiance between 3 and 7 J/cm^2 [134]. In a challenging recent case of Fournier's syndrome that involves necrotizing gangrene of perineum and external genitalia, adjunctive use of 660 and 810 nm laser PBM treatment was noted to be extremely effective in managing these severe wounds (**Figure 5**). It should be emphasized that in this particular case of necrotizing fasciitis, infection control is of paramount importance and the use of PBM not only improves host immune defenses (via Human βDefensin-2 secretion), but also promotes the surrounding epithelium and underlying connective tissue to be effectively stimulated to heal these wounds [141–143].

Several studies have elucidated the mechanistic pathways and reactions associated with photobiomodulation in diabetic wounds. In an investigation involving a 660 nm laser at treatments of 5 J/cm^2 in diabetic wounded cells, a notable elevation in epidermal growth factor (EGF) and activation of its phosphorylated EGF receptor was observed. This activation was mediated through the Janus kinase (JAK)/Signal transducer and activators of the transcription (STAT) pathway. The activation of this pathway was identified to modulate cell migration and proliferation, indicating that PBM treatments directly affect cellular autocrine signaling [133]. Diabetic wounded fibroblast cells irradiated with a Helium-Neon laser at a wavelength of 632.8 nm with an energy density of 5 J/cm^2 corresponded to a rise in the levels of IL-6, an anti-inflammatory cytokine, and contributed to increased cellular proliferation and migration. In a follow-up study conducted by Houreld et al. diabetic wounded fibroblasts subjected to photobiomodulation irradiation at a dosage of 5 J/cm^2 and a wavelength of 830 nm exhibited a favorable impact on wound healing [144]. This effect was characterized by the reduced expression of pro-inflammatory cytokines IL-1β and TNF-α, as well as the stimulation of nitric oxide and reactive oxygen species [131, 133].

Among clinical trials conducted utilizing lasers within the red and near infrared wavelength range, Minatel et al. investigated the effects of 660 and 890 nm laser treatment in a double-blind randomized study with diabetic patients suffering from chronic leg ulcers [145]. PBM treatments were administered to the wounds twice a week, for a length of 90 days. The results have demonstrated that combined 660 and 890 nm light accelerated tissue granulation, improving the healing rate of diabetic foot ulcers that did not show improvement with other forms of intervention. A subsequent clinical trial conducted by Kaviani et al. involved 23 patients diagnosed with stages I and II chronic diabetic ulcers [146]. The ulcers were subjected to laser treatment at a wavelength of 685 nm with a dose of 10 J/cm^2. The findings indicated a notable reduction in ulcer size in 4 weeks post-treatment, with a substantial proportion of patients exhibiting complete wound healing. As already mentioned by this group, the initial benefits of PBM (low-dose light treatments), were primary

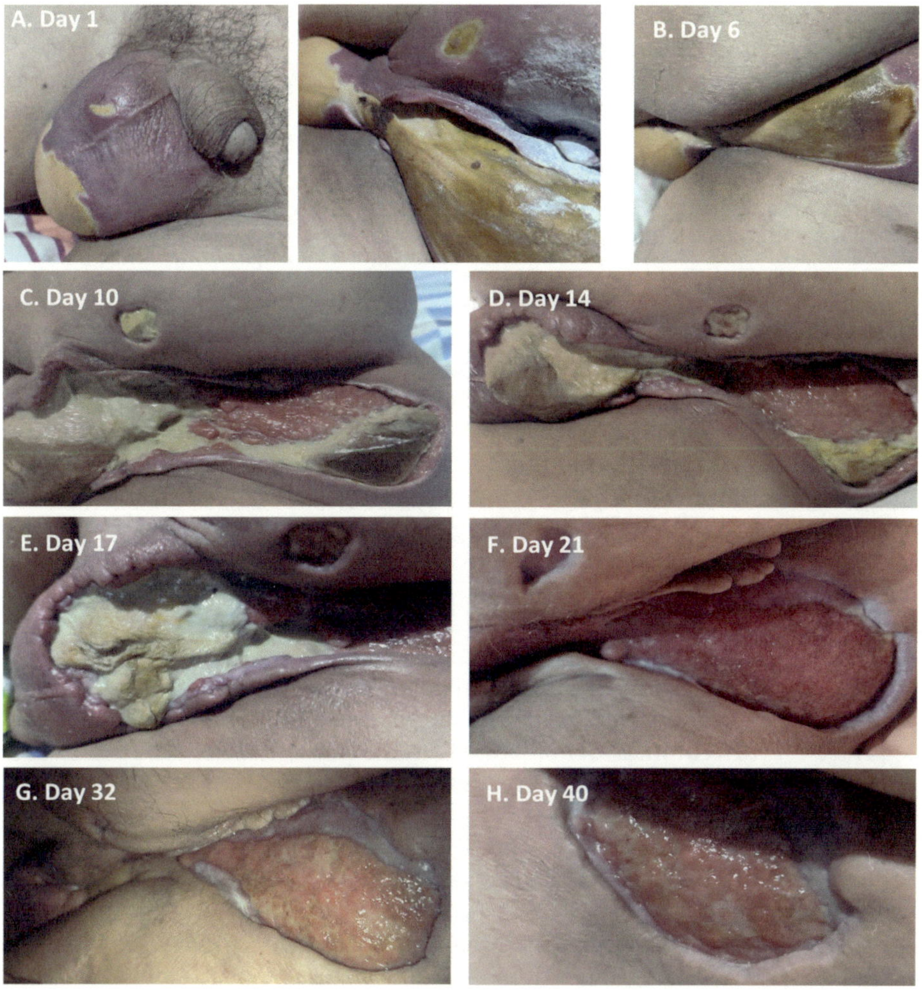

Figure 5.
Clinical progression of an ulcer caused by Fournier's syndrome treated with photobiomodulation therapy. The images chronologically depict the improvement in the ulcerated lesion over the course of 40 days of treatment, starting from day 1. Laser diodes at wavelengths of 660 and 880 nm were used to perform PBM three times per week at a fluence of 20 J/cm^2. A. Shows the initial presentation of the ulcer (yellow-brown) on day 1, prior to treatment initiation. B. to H. Demonstrate the gradual healing process, with a reduction in inflammation, wound size, and tissue damage observed over time with continued lase therapy sessions. The final image at day 40 exhibits significant healing and re-epithelialization of the affected areas, indicating the efficacy of the PBM in managing this case of Fournier's syndrome, treatments are currently continuing.

noted in the promotion of wound healing. Subsequently, well-designed controlled human studies have provided increasing evidence supporting the effectiveness of this specific application [116], for example the use of PBM in the management of chronic diabetic foot ulcers (DFUs), which diminishes the inflammatory phase, enhances angiogenesis, boosts blood circulation, refines the synthesis and organization of the extracellular matrix, and alleviates pain and infection [147]. Furthermore, a study carried out with 68 patients with chronic diabetic foot ulcers (DFU) showed a significant reduction in the area (mm^2) of ulcers in the treated group compared to the control, after 15 days of daily therapy [148]. Also, a meta-analysis which evaluated 13 randomized controlled trials (RCTs) and a total of 413 patients. In comparison with the control group, PBM significantly increased the complete healing rate, reduced the ulcer area, and shortened the mean healing time of patients with DFUs [149]. Nevertheless, although PBM shows promise as an effective adjuvant treatment for expediting diabetic wound healing, additional evidence from larger sample sizes and higher-quality RCTs is essential to establish the efficacy of PBM and determine the appropriate parameters for optimal wound healing.

Wounds arising from diabetes mellitus impose considerable socioeconomic burdens on affected individuals, contributing to heightened amputations, mortality rates and financial expenditures. Wound healing is a complex pathophysiological process that involves a variety of biological and chemical pathways. Conventional treatments adjoined with the use of low-level light therapy have shown promising efficacy in the therapeutic intervention of diabetic wounds. Photobiomodulation appears to be a viable, non-invasive, and safe alternative method for treating chronic diabetic foot ulcers. Several studies have illustrated evidence behind PBM and the effects it has on diabetic wounds. Continued exploration into the biochemical and cellular responses of photobiomodulation therapy can help translate this innovative technology into clinical applications for the effective management of diabetic lesions.

7. Conclusions

Non-healing wounds impose a substantial burden on both the healthcare system and the quality of life for affected patients. The pathogenesis of these wounds involves various factors, yet a common denominator is the consistent lack of adequate vascularization, leading to insufficient delivery of oxygen, nutrients, and growth factors to the site of the injury [150].

7.1 Sequence of different laser-based treatment modalities: PTT vs. PDT vs. PBM

A novel approach stemming from the confluence of several light-based treatment modalities termed as photoimmunotherapy is one of the recent advances focused on wound healing through the modulation of immune responses [19]. Utilizing near-infrared-induced hyperthermia to enhance the efficacy of antitumor treatments has been recognized for its ability to boost local perfusion and enhance immune reactivity, a concept also referred to as photoimmunotherapy. These approaches seem to leverage both photothermal effects and potentially photobiomodulation (nitric oxide generation), alongside non-thermal vasodilation at the tissue level, in order to alleviate hypoxia. This, in turn, improves ionizing radiation-induced tumor cytotoxicity or facilitates better tumor access to chemotherapy or immunotherapy agents [151]. Photoimmunotherapy can be accomplished through different light treatment approaches, encompassing photothermal destruction, nonspecific or targeted photodynamic responses, and Photobiomodulation therapy, which directly modulate host immune mechanisms following the antigenic stimulation induced by photothermal and photodynamic approaches. The distinct biological responses induced by light provide a strong mechanistic basis for their combined use, such as the sequential process of eliminating microbial or tumor cells followed by the stimulation of host immune responses [19].

Besides technical similarities, there are several clinically relevant differences between PTT and PDT. Firstly, due to photosensitizer accumulation and light targeting, PDT is considerably more selective than PTT. Furthermore, due to its non-thermal nature, PDT is harmless to surrounding collagenous structures and nerves. Nevertheless, in certain cases, the accumulation of ocular and cutaneous photosensitizers can lead to photosensitivity, posing challenges in treatment logistics and potentially compromising safety. In contrast to PDT, the selectivity of PTT is predominantly dependent upon localized light delivery, inevitably resulting in the formation of a temperature gradient. Another essential difference between PTT and PDT is the light source used. Additionally, oxygen requirement is a crucial point of distinction between PTT and PDT. Effective PDT requires functional vasculature and a constant supply of oxygen for the generation of reactive oxygen species. Contrastingly, PTT is essentially oxygen-independent, making it an appropriate option for treating hypoxic tumors [152].

Biophotonics seamlessly combines lasers, photonics, nanotechnology, and biotechnology, offering a novel perspective for theragnostic (diagnostic and therapeutic) applications [153, 154]. The various approaches outlined in this chapter highlight the significant utility in wound management. Synergistic and complementary modalities offer novel, cost-effective, and clinically efficacious treatments that could be employed actively.

Author details

Ridham Varsani†, Victoria Oliveira†, Rodrigo Crespo Mosca†, Mahmud Amin, Moiz Khan, Nimisha Rawat, Jonathan Kaj and Praveen Arany*
Oral Biology, Surgery, and Biomedical Engineering, University at Buffalo, New York, USA

*Address all correspondence to: prarany@buffalo.edu

† These authors are equally contributed.

References

[1] Gantwerker EA, Hom DB. Skin: Histology and physiology of wound healing. Clinics in Plastic Surgery. 2012;**39**:85-97. DOI: 10.1016/j.cps.2011.09.005

[2] Wang PH, Huang BS, Horng HC, Yeh CC, Chen YJ. Wound healing. Journal of the Chinese Medical Association. 2018;**81**:94-101. DOI: 10.1016/j.jcma.2017.11.002

[3] Eming SA, Krieg T, Davidson JM. Inflammation in wound repair: Molecular and cellular mechanisms. The Journal of Investigative Dermatology. 2007;**127**:514-525. DOI: 10.1038/sj.jid.5700701

[4] Phillipson M, Kubes P. The healing power of neutrophils. Trends in Immunology. 2019;**40**:635-647. DOI: 10.1016/j.it.2019.05.001

[5] Wang J. Neutrophils in tissue injury and repair. Cell and Tissue Research. 2018;**371**:531-539. DOI: 10.1007/s00441-017-2785-7

[6] Wilgus TA, Roy S, McDaniel JC. Neutrophils and wound repair: Positive actions and negative reactions. Advances in Wound Care (New Rochelle). 2013;**2**:379-388. DOI: 10.1089/wound.2012.0383

[7] Broughton G 2nd, Janis JE, Attinger CE. The basic science of wound healing. Plastic and Reconstructive Surgery. 2006;**117**:12S-34S. DOI: 10.1097/01.prs.0000225430.42531.c2

[8] DiPietro LA, Wilgus TA, Koh TJ. Macrophages in healing wounds: Paradoxes and paradigms. International Journal of Molecular Sciences. 19 Jan 2021;**22**(2):950. DOI: 10.3390/ijms22020950

[9] Kim SY, Nair MG. Macrophages in wound healing: Activation and plasticity. Immunology and Cell Biology. 2019;**97**:258-267. DOI: 10.1111/imcb.12236

[10] Minutti CM, Knipper JA, Allen JE, Zaiss DM. Tissue-specific contribution of macrophages to wound healing. Seminars in Cell & Developmental Biology. 2017;**61**:3-11. DOI: 10.1016/j.semcdb.2016.08.006

[11] Campos A, Borges-Branco A, Groth A. Wound healing. ABCD. Arquivos Brasileiros de Cirurgia Digestiva (São Paulo). 2007;**20**:51-58. DOI: 10.1590/S0102-67202007000100010

[12] Lawrence WT, Diegelmann RF. Growth factors in wound healing. Clinics in Dermatology. 1994;**12**:157-169. DOI: 10.1016/0738-081x(94)90266-6

[13] Childs DR, Murthy AS. Overview of wound healing and management. The Surgical Clinics of North America. 2017;**97**:189-207. DOI: 10.1016/j.suc.2016.08.013

[14] Baron JM, Glatz M, Proksch E. Optimal support of wound healing: New insights. Dermatology. 2020;**236**:593-600. DOI: 10.1159/000505291

[15] Holl J, Kowalewski C, Zimek Z, Fiedor P, Kaminski A, Oldak T, et al. Chronic diabetic wounds and their treatment with skin substitutes. Cells. 15 Mar 2021;**10**(3):655. DOI: 10.3390/cells10030655

[16] Velnar T, Bailey T, Smrkolj V. The wound healing process: An overview of the cellular and molecular mechanisms. The Journal of International Medical Research. 2009;**37**:1528-1542. DOI: 10.1177/147323000903700531

[17] Laureano A, Rodrigues A. Cicatrização de Feridas. Journal of the Portuguese Society of Dermatology and Venereology. 2011;**69**:355. DOI: 10.29021/spdv.69.3.71

[18] Parker S. Lasers in dentistry-current concepts. In: Coluzzi DJ, Parker SPA, editors. CH. 3: Laser-Tissue Interaction. Cham, Switzerland: Springer Nature; 2017. pp. 29-53. ISBN 978-3-319-51943-2

[19] Arany PR. Photoimmunotherapy: A novel field with overlapping light treatment approaches. Photobiomodulation, Photomedicine, and Laser Surgery. 29 Jun 2020. DOI: 10.1089/photob.2020.4877

[20] Parker S, Cronshaw M, Anagnostaki E, Mylona V, Lynch E, Grootveld M. Current concepts of laser-oral tissue interaction. Dentistry Journal (Basel). 28 Jun 2020;**8**(3):61. DOI: 10.3390/dj8030061

[21] Mo O et al. Periodic trends in bond dissociation energies. A theoretical study. The Journal of Physical Chemistry. A. 2005;**109**:4359-4365. DOI: 10.1021/jp050857o

[22] Anderson RR, Parrish JA. Selective photothermolysis: Precise microsurgery by selective absorption of pulsed radiation. Science. 1983;**220**:524-527. DOI: 10.1126/science.6836297

[23] Fisher JC. Photons, physiatrics, and physicians: A practical guide to understanding laser light interaction with living tissue, part I. Journal of Clinical Laser Medicine & Surgery. 1992;**10**:419-426. DOI: 10.1089/clm.1992.10.419

[24] Brandi C et al. The role of carbon dioxide therapy in the treatment of chronic wounds. In Vivo. 2010;**24**:223-226

[25] Caliskan E, Botsali A. Combination of full-field and fractional erbium: YAG laser for nonhealing wounds. Dermatologic Surgery. 2022;**48**:114-119. DOI: 10.1097/DSS.0000000000003292

[26] Guan H et al. Efficacy and safety of CO(2) laser in the treatment of chronic wounds: A Retrospective Matched Cohort Trial. Lasers in Surgery and Medicine. 2022;**54**:490-501. DOI: 10.1002/lsm.23490

[27] Hajhosseini B et al. Er:YAG laser vs. sharp debridement in management of chronic wounds: Effects on pain and bacterial load. Wound Repair and Regeneration. 2020;**28**:118-125. DOI: 10.1111/wrr.12764

[28] Jiang B et al. Clinical effectiveness of super pulsed carbon dioxide fractional laser debridement surgery in treating chronic wounds. Zhonghua Shao Shang Za Zhi. 2020;**36**:273-279. DOI: 10.3760/cma.j.cn501120-20190415-00186

[29] Mezzana P, Onesti MG, Ciotti M, Malzone G Jr, Scuderi N. Erbium:yttrium-aluminum-garnet laser debridement of chronic wounds. Plastic and Reconstructive Surgery. 2008;**122**:164e-165e. DOI: 10.1097/PRS.0b013e318186ccf2

[30] Cardinal M et al. Serial surgical debridement: A retrospective study on clinical outcomes in chronic lower extremity wounds. Wound Repair and Regeneration. 2009;**17**:306-311. DOI: 10.1111/j.1524-475X.2009.00485.x

[31] Graham JS et al. Efficacy of laser debridement with autologous split-thickness skin grafting in promoting improved healing of deep cutaneous sulfur mustard burns. Burns. 2002;**28**:719-730. DOI: 10.1016/s0305-4179(02)00198-5

[32] Lam DG, Rice P, Brown RF. The treatment of Lewisite burns with laser debridement—'lasablation'. Burns. 2002;**28**:19-25. DOI: 10.1016/s0305-4179(01)00078-x

[33] Reynolds N, Cawrse N, Burge T, Kenealy J. Debridement of a mixed partial and full thickness burn with an erbium:YAG laser. Burns. 2003;**29**:183-188. DOI: 10.1016/s0305-4179(02)00247-4

[34] Aoki A et al. Periodontal and peri-implant wound healing following laser therapy. Periodontology 2000. 2000, 2015;**68**:217-269. DOI: 10.1111/prd.12080

[35] Gaur A et al. Efficacy of diode laser ablation and low level laser therapy on healing and bacterial load reduction at intraoral biopsy site. Journal of Dentistry (Shiraz). 2022;**23**:121-128. DOI: 10.30476/DENTJODS.2021.88696.1354

[36] Jiang B et al. Impact of ultra-pulse carbon dioxide laser on the treatment of chronic refractory ulcer with bone exposure. Surgery. 2024;**175**:1184-1188. DOI: 10.1016/j.surg.2023.12.007

[37] Jiang B et al. Evaluation of the efficacy of ultrapulsed CO(2) laser in chronic wounds. Lasers in Surgery and Medicine. 2021;**53**:443-449. DOI: 10.1002/lsm.23283

[38] Lu Q et al. Clinical effects of high-intensity laser therapy on patients with chronic refractory wounds: A randomised controlled trial. BMJ Open. 2021;**11**:e045866. DOI: 10.1136/bmjopen-2020-045866

[39] Mehrabi JN, Kelly KM. Ablative fractional resurfacing for chronic wounds from traumatic scarring: A case report and literature review. Journal of Drugs in Dermatology. 2020;**19**:1112-1115. DOI: 10.36849/JDD.2020.5444

[40] Yao W et al. Laser-generated shockwaves enhance antibacterial activity against biofilms in vitro. Lasers in Surgery and Medicine. 2017;**49**:539-547. DOI: 10.1002/lsm.22627

[41] Yao W, Kuan EC, Grundfest WS, St John MA. Safety of laser-generated shockwave treatment for bacterial biofilms in a cutaneous rodent model. Lasers in Medical Science. 2021;**36**:1403-1410. DOI: 10.1007/s10103-020-03171-3

[42] Vaupel P, editor. Water-Filtered Infrared A (wIRA) Irradiation: From Research to Clinical Settings [Internet]. Cham (CH): Springer; 2022. ISBN-13: 978-3-030-92879-7. PMID: 37494506

[43] Becker A et al. Receptor-targeted optical imaging of tumors with near-infrared fluorescent ligands. Nature Biotechnology. 2001;**19**:327-331. DOI: 10.1038/86707

[44] Zhang X et al. Near-infrared light-triggered porous AuPd alloy nanoparticles to produce mild localized heat to accelerate bone regeneration. Journal of Physical Chemistry Letters. 2019;**10**:4185-4191. DOI: 10.1021/acs.jpclett.9b01735

[45] Yi X, Duan QY, Wu FG. Low-temperature photothermal therapy: Strategies and applications. Research (Washington, D.C.). 2021;**2021**:9816594. DOI: 10.34133/2021/9816594

[46] Melamed JR, Edelstein RS, Day ES. Elucidating the fundamental mechanisms of cell death triggered by photothermal therapy. ACS Nano. 2015;**9**:6-11. DOI: 10.1021/acsnano.5b00021

[47] Zhang Y et al. Temperature-dependent cell death patterns induced by functionalized gold nanoparticle photothermal therapy in melanoma

cells. Scientific Reports. 2018;**8**:8720. DOI: 10.1038/s41598-018-26978-1

[48] Knavel EM, Brace CL. Tumor ablation: Common modalities and general practices. Techniques in Vascular and Interventional Radiology. 2013;**16**: 192-200. DOI: 10.1053/j.tvir.2013.08.002

[49] Jolly C, Morimoto RI. Role of the heat shock response and molecular chaperones in oncogenesis and cell death. Journal of the National Cancer Institute. 2000;**92**:1564-1572. DOI: 10.1093/jnci/92.19.1564

[50] Han HS, Choi KY. Advances in nanomaterial-mediated photothermal cancer therapies: Toward clinical applications. Biomedicines. 16 Mar 2021;**9**(3):305. DOI: 10.3390/biomedicines9030305

[51] Bao Z, Liu X, Liu Y, Liu H, Zhao K. Near-infrared light-responsive inorganic nanomaterials for photothermal therapy. Asian Journal of Pharmaceutical Sciences. 2016;**11**:349-364. DOI: 10.1016/j.ajps.2015.11.123

[52] Pérez-Hernández M et al. Dissecting the molecular mechanism of apoptosis during photothermal therapy using gold nanoprisms. ACS Nano. 2015;**9**:52-61. DOI: 10.1021/nn505468v

[53] Shahabi S et al. Hyperthermia can accelerate the healing process of 2nd degree burn wounds. Journal of Kerman University of Medical Sciences. 2005;**12**:110-118

[54] Shahabi S et al. The effect of post-burn local hyperthermia on the reducing burn injury: The possible role of opioids. International Journal of Hyperthermia. 2006;**22**:421-431. DOI: 10.1080/02656730600841857

[55] Rabkin JM, Hunt TK. Local heat increases blood flow and oxygen tension in wounds. Archives of Surgery. 1987;**122**:221-225. DOI: 10.1001/archsurg.1987.01400140103014

[56] Li J et al. Moist-retaining, self-recoverable, bioadhesive, and transparent in situ forming hydrogels to accelerate wound healing. ACS Applied Materials & Interfaces. 2020;**12**:2023-2038. DOI: 10.1021/acsami.9b17180

[57] Huang L, Zhou J, Chen Y, Li W, Han X, Wang L. Engineering microcapsules for simultaneous delivery of combinational therapeutics. Advanced Materials Technologies. 2020;**5**(11). Article 2000623. DOI: 10.1002/admt.202000623

[58] Li L et al. Microenvironment-triggered degradable hydrogel for imaging diagnosis and combined treatment of intraocular choroidal melanoma. ACS Nano. 2020;**14**:15403-15416. DOI: 10.1021/acsnano.0c06000

[59] Garraud O, Hozzein WN, Badr G. Wound healing: Time to look for intelligent, 'natural' immunological approaches? BMC Immunology. 2017;**18**:23. DOI: 10.1186/s12865-017-0207-y

[60] Sen CK. Human wound and its burden: Updated 2020 compendium of estimates. Advances in Wound Care (New Rochelle). 2021;**10**:281-292. DOI: 10.1089/wound.2021.0026

[61] Plaetzer K, Krammer B, Berlanda J, Berr F, Kiesslich T. Photophysics and photochemistry of photodynamic therapy: Fundamental aspects. Lasers in Medical Science. 2009;**24**:259-268. DOI: 10.1007/s10103-008-0539-1

[62] Seraj H et al. The uses of photodynamic therapy versus anti-vascular endothelial growth factor in the management of acute central serous chorioretinopathy: A systematic review and meta-analysis.

Cureus. 2023;**15**:e46100. DOI: 10.7759/cureus.46100

[63] Kessel D. Photodynamic therapy: A brief history. Journal of Clinical Medicine. 2 Oct 2019;**8**(10):1581. DOI: 10.3390/jcm8101581

[64] Adnane F, El-Zayat E, Fahmy HM. The combinational application of photodynamic therapy and nanotechnology in skin cancer treatment: A review. Tissue & Cell. 2022;**77**:101856. DOI: 10.1016/j.tice.2022.101856

[65] Crous A, Abrahamse H. Photodynamic therapy of lung cancer, where are we? Frontiers in Pharmacology. 2022;**13**:932098. DOI: 10.3389/fphar.2022.932098

[66] Osuchowski M, Aebisher D, Bartusik-Aebisher D, Krupka-Olek M, Dynarowicz K, Przygoda M, et al. Photodynamic therapy-adjunctive therapy in the treatment of prostate cancer. Diagnostics (Basel). 28 Apr 2022;**12**(5):1113. DOI: 10.3390/diagnostics12051113

[67] Miyake M et al. Fluorescent cystoscopy-assisted en bloc transurethral resection versus conventional transurethral resection in patients with non-muscle invasive bladder cancer: Study protocol of a prospective, open-label, randomized control trial (the FLEBER study). Trials. 2021;**22**:136. DOI: 10.1186/s13063-021-05094-y

[68] Hu J et al. Nanocomposite-based photodynamic therapy strategies for deep tumor treatment. Small. 2015;**22**:5860-5887

[69] Hou YJ et al. Pathological mechanism of photodynamic therapy and photothermal therapy based on nanoparticles. International Journal of Nanomedicine. 2020;**15**:6827-6838. DOI: 10.2147/IJN.S269321

[70] Gulzar MA et al. Comparison of photodynamic therapy and corticosteroid therapy in management of oral lichen planus: A systematic review of randomized controlled trials. Photodiagnosis and Photodynamic Therapy. 2023;**44**:103747. DOI: 10.1016/j.pdpdt.2023.103747

[71] Hsia T, Small JL, Yekula A, Batool SM, Escobedo AK, Ekanayake E, et al. Systematic review of photodynamic therapy in gliomas. Cancers (Basel). 1 Aug 2023;**15**(15):3918. DOI: 10.3390/cancers15153918

[72] Zhang R, Gao T, Wang D. Photodynamic therapy (PDT) for oral leukoplakia: A systematic review and meta-analysis of single-arm studies examining efficacy and subgroup analyses. BMC Oral Health. 2023;**23**:568. DOI: 10.1186/s12903-023-03294-3

[73] Burloiu AM, Manda G, Lupuliasa D, Socoteanu RP, Mihai DP, Neagoe IV, et al. Assessment of some unsymmetrical porphyrins as promising molecules for photodynamic therapy of cutaneous disorders. Pharmaceuticals (Basel). 29 Dec 2023;**17**(1):62. DOI: 10.3390/ph17010062

[74] Cheon YK et al. Outcome of photodynamic therapy for early esophageal cancer. Gut and Liver. 2007;**1**:126-131. DOI: 10.5009/gnl.2007.1.2.126

[75] Sabino CP et al. The optical properties of mouse skin in the visible and near infrared spectral regions. Journal of Photochemistry and Photobiology. B. 2016;**160**:72-78. DOI: 10.1016/j.jphotobiol.2016.03.047

[76] Soto-Moreno A, Montero-Vilchez T, Diaz-Calvillo P, Molina-Leyva A, Arias-Santiago S. The impact of photodynamic therapy on skin

homeostasis in patients with actinic keratosis: A prospective observational study. Skin Research and Technology. 2023;**29**:e13493. DOI: 10.1111/srt.13493

[77] Dragicevic N, Predic-Atkinson J, Nikolic B, Pajovic SB, Ivkovic S, Adzic M. Nanocarriers in topical photodynamic therapy. Expert Opinion on Drug Delivery. Feb 2024;**21**(2):279-307. DOI: 10.1080/17425247.2024.2318460

[78] Kaneko K, Nagata H, Yang XY, Ginzel J, Hartman Z, Everitt J, et al. A non-invasive deep photoablation technique to inhibit DCIS progression and induce antitumor immunity. Cancers (Basel). 23 Nov 2022;**14**(23):5762. DOI: 10.3390/cancers14235762

[79] Zhao Y et al. Preparation and evaluation of oxidized-dextran based on antibacterial hydrogel for synergistic photodynamic therapy. International Journal of Biological Macromolecules. 2023;**253**:127648. DOI: 10.1016/j.ijbiomac.2023.127648

[80] Ning X, He G, Zeng W, Xia Y. The photosensitizer-based therapies enhance the repairing of skin wounds. Frontiers in Medicine (Lausanne). 2022;**9**:915548. DOI: 10.3389/fmed.2022.915548

[81] Yang Z et al. Photodynamic therapy accelerates skin wound healing through promoting re-epithelialization. Burns & Trauma. 2021;**9**:tkab008. DOI: 10.1093/burnst/tkab008

[82] Bourbour S, Darbandi A, Bostanghadiri N, Ghanavati R, Taheri B, Bahador A. Effects of antimicrobial photosensitizers of photodynamic therapy (PDT) to treat periodontitis. Current Pharmaceutical Biotechnology. 2024;**25**(10):1209-1229. DOI: 10.2174/138920102466623 0720104516

[83] Dunegan KA et al. Subgingival scaling and root planing during minimally invasive periodontal surgery: A randomized controlled split-mouth trial. Journal of Periodontology. 2024;**95**:9-16. DOI: 10.1002/JPER.23-0198

[84] Nie M, Yang J, Rastelli ANS, Shen Y, Deng D. Oxygen availability on the application of antimicrobial photodynamic therapy against multi-species biofilms. Pathogens. 3 Jul 2023;**12**(7):904. DOI: 10.3390/pathogens12070904

[85] Amini A et al. Photobiomodulation therapy improves inflammatory responses by modifying stereological parameters, microRNA-21 and FGF2 expression. Journal of Lasers in Medical Sciences. 2023;**14**:e16. DOI: 10.34172/jlms.2023.16

[86] Paasch U et al. Antifungal efficacy of lasers against dermatophytes and yeasts in vitro. International Journal of Hyperthermia. 2013;**29**:544-550. DOI: 10.3109/02656736.2013.823672

[87] Park JH, Yun JH, Shi Y, Han J, Li X, Jin Z, et al. Non-cryogenic structure and dynamics of HIV-1 integrase catalytic core domain by X-ray free-electron lasers. International Journal of Molecular Sciences. 20 Apr 2019;**20**(8):1943. DOI: 10.3390/ijms20081943

[88] Fan XL et al. Magainin-modified polydopamine nanoparticles for photothermal killing of bacteria at low temperature. Colloids and Surfaces. B, Biointerfaces. 2019;**183**:110423. DOI: 10.1016/j.colsurfb.2019.110423

[89] Tan L et al. Overcoming multidrug-resistant MRSA using conventional aminoglycoside antibiotics. Advanced Science (Weinh). 2020;**7**:1902070. DOI: 10.1002/advs.201902070

[90] Wang H et al. Research trends of worldwide ophthalmologic randomized controlled trials in the 21st century: A bibliometric study. Advances in Ophthalmology Practice and Research. 2023;**3**:159-170. DOI: 10.1016/j.aopr.2023.07.003

[91] Xu D, Zhu T, Huang L, Wang X, Chen M. Clinical efficacy of subthreshold micropulse laser combined with anti-VEGF drugs in the treatment of diabetic macular edema: A meta-analysis. Medicine (Baltimore). 2024;**103**:e34583. DOI: 10.1097/MD.0000000000034583

[92] Narala S, Cohen PR. Basal cell carcinoma of the umbilicus: A comprehensive literature review. Cureus. 2016;**8**:e770. DOI: 10.7759/cureus.770

[93] van der Geer S, Ostertag JU, Krekels GA. Treatment of basal cell carcinomas in patients with nevoid basal cell carcinoma syndrome. Journal of the European Academy of Dermatology and Venereology. 2009;**23**:308-313. DOI: 10.1111/j.1468-3083.2008.03040.x

[94] Pacioni S, D'Alessandris QG, Giannetti S, Della Pepa GM, Offi M, Giordano M, et al. 5-Aminolevulinic acid (5-ALA)-induced protoporphyrin IX fluorescence by glioma cells—A fluorescence microscopy clinical study. Cancers (Basel). 8 Jun 2022;**14**(12):2844. DOI: 10.3390/cancers14122844

[95] Shinoda Y, Kato D, Ando R, Endo H, Takahashi T, Tsuneoka Y, et al. Systematic review and meta-analysis of in vitro anti-human cancer experiments investigating the use of 5-aminolevulinic acid (5-ALA) for photodynamic therapy. Pharmaceuticals (Basel). 7 Mar 2021;**14**(3):229. DOI: 10.3390/ph14030229

[96] Su Y et al. Effect and rational application of topical photodynamic therapy (PDT) with 5-aminolevulinic acid (5-ALA) for treatment of cervical intraepithelial neoplasia with vaginal intraepithelial neoplasia. Photodiagnosis and Photodynamic Therapy. 2022;**37**:102634. DOI: 10.1016/j.pdpdt.2021.102634

[97] Racz E, Prens EP. Phototherapy and photochemotherapy for psoriasis. Dermatologic Clinics. 2015;**33**:79-89. DOI: 10.1016/j.det.2014.09.007

[98] Stege H, Ghoreschi K, Hunefeld C. UV phototherapy: UV phototherapy and photodiagnostics-a practical overview. Hautarzt. 2021;**72**:14-26. DOI: 10.1007/s00105-020-04744-7

[99] Totonchy MB, Chiu MW. UV-based therapy. Dermatologic Clinics. 2014;**32**:399-413, ix-x. DOI: 10.1016/j.det.2014.03.003

[100] Celli JP et al. Imaging and photodynamic therapy: Mechanisms, monitoring, and optimization. Chemical Reviews. 2010;**110**:2795-2838. DOI: 10.1021/cr900300p

[101] Almeida Issa MC et al. Immunohistochemical expression of matrix metalloproteinases in photodamaged skin by photodynamic therapy. The British Journal of Dermatology. 2009;**161**:647-653. DOI: 10.1111/j.1365-2133.2009.09326.x

[102] Berking C, Hegyi J, Arenberger P, Ruzicka T, Jemec GB. Photodynamic therapy of necrobiosis lipoidica—A multicenter study of 18 patients. Dermatology. 2009;**218**:136-139. DOI: 10.1159/000182259

[103] Morton CA et al. Guidelines for topical photodynamic therapy: Report of a workshop of the British Photodermatology Group. The British Journal of

Dermatology. 2002;**146**:552-567. DOI: 10.1046/j.1365-2133.2002.04719.x

[104] Morton CA et al. Guidelines for topical photodynamic therapy: Update. The British Journal of Dermatology. 2008;**159**:1245-1266. DOI: 10.1111/j.1365-2133.2008.08882.x

[105] Rhodes LE et al. Five-year follow-up of a randomized, prospective trial of topical methyl aminolevulinate photodynamic therapy vs surgery for nodular basal cell carcinoma. Archives of Dermatology. 2007;**143**:1131-1136. DOI: 10.1001/archderm.143.9.1131

[106] Wan MT, Lin JY. Current evidence and applications of photodynamic therapy in dermatology. Clinical, Cosmetic and Investigational Dermatology. 2014;**7**:145-163. DOI: 10.2147/CCID.S35334

[107] Szeimies RM et al. Clinical, histopathological and immuno-histochemical assessment of human skin field cancerization before and after photodynamic therapy. The British Journal of Dermatology. 2012;**167**:150-159. DOI: 10.1111/j.1365-2133.2012.10887.x

[108] Peng Q et al. 5-Aminolevulinic acid-based photodynamic therapy. Clinical research and future challenges. Cancer. 1997;**79**:2282-2308. DOI: 10.1002/(sici)1097-0142(19970615)79:12<2282::aid-cncr2>3.0.co;2-o

[109] Robijns J et al. Photobiomodulation therapy in management of cancer therapy-induced side effects: WALT position paper 2022. Frontiers in Oncology. 2022;**12**:927685. DOI: 10.3389/fonc.2022.927685

[110] Zadik Y et al. Systematic review of photobiomodulation for the management of oral mucositis in cancer patients and clinical practice guidelines. Support Care Cancer. 2019;**27**:3969-3983. DOI: 10.1007/s00520-019-04890-2

[111] Arany PR. Craniofacial wound healing with photobiomodulation therapy: New insights and current challenges. Journal of Dental Research. 2016;**95**:977-984. DOI: 10.1177/0022034516648939

[112] Karu TI, Pyatibrat LV, Kolyakov SF, Afanasyeva NI. Absorption measurements of a cell monolayer relevant to phototherapy: Reduction of cytochrome c oxidase under near IR radiation. Journal of Photochemistry and Photobiology. B. 2005;**81**:98-106. DOI: S1011-1344(05)00130-2 [pii]10.1016/j.jphotobiol.2005.07.002

[113] Wong-Riley MT et al. Photobiomodulation directly benefits primary neurons functionally inactivated by toxins: Role of cytochrome c oxidase. The Journal of Biological Chemistry. 2005;**280**:4761-4771. DOI: 10.1074/jbc.M409650200

[114] Otterço AN et al. Photobiomodulation mechanisms in the kinetics of the wound healing process in rats. Journal of Photochemistry and Photobiology B: Biology. 2018;**183**:22-29. DOI: 10.1016/j.jphotobiol.2018.04.010

[115] Mosca RC et al. The efficacy of photobiomodulation therapy in improving tissue resilience and healing of radiation skin damage. Photonics. 2022;**9**:10

[116] Mosca RC, Ong AA, Albasha O, Bass K, Arany P. Photobiomodulation therapy for wound care: A potent, noninvasive, photoceutical approach. Advances in Skin & Wound Care. 2019;**32**:157-167. DOI: 10.1097/01.ASW.0000553600.97572.d2

[117] Mathioudaki E, Rallis M, Politopoulos K, Alexandratou E. Photobiomodulation and wound healing: Low-level laser therapy at 661 nm in a scratch assay keratinocyte model. Annals of Biomedical Engineering. Feb 2024;**52**(2):376-385. DOI: 10.1007/s10439-023-03384-x

[118] Mester E, Korenyi-Both A, Spiry T, Scher A, Tisza S. Stimulation of wound healing by means of laser rays. (Clinical and electron microscopical study). Acta Chirurgica Academiae Scientiarum Hungaricae. 1973;**14**:347-356

[119] Arany PR et al. Photoactivation of endogenous latent transforming growth factor-beta1 directs dental stem cell differentiation for regeneration. Science Translational Medicine. 2014;**6**:238ra269. DOI: 10.1126/scitranslmed.3008234

[120] Arany PR et al. Activation of latent TGF-beta1 by low-power laser in vitro correlates with increased TGF-beta1 levels in laser-enhanced oral wound healing. Wound Repair and Regeneration. 2007;**15**:866-874. DOI: 10.1111/j.1524-475X.2007.00306.x

[121] Arany PR. Photobiomodulation-activated latent transforming growth factor-beta1: A critical clinical therapeutic pathway and an endogenous optogenetic tool for discovery. Photobiomodulation, Photomedicine, and Laser Surgery. 2022;**40**:136-147. DOI: 10.1089/photob.2021.0109

[122] Khan I et al. Accelerated burn wound healing with photobiomodulation therapy involves activation of endogenous latent TGF-β1. Scientific Reports. 2021;**11**:13371. DOI: 10.1038/s41598-021-92650-w

[123] Rohringer S et al. The impact of wavelengths of LED light-therapy on endothelial cells. Scientific Reports. 2017;**7**:10700. DOI: 10.1038/s41598-017-11061-y

[124] Rezende SB, Ribeiro MS, Nunez SC, Garcia VG, Maldonado EP. Effects of a single near-infrared laser treatment on cutaneous wound healing: Biometrical and histological study in rats. Journal of Photochemistry and Photobiology. B. 2007;**87**:145-153. DOI: 10.1016/j.jphotobiol.2007.02.005

[125] Hoffman M, Monroe DM. Low intensity laser therapy speeds wound healing in hemophilia by enhancing platelet procoagulant activity. Wound Repair and Regeneration. 2012;**20**:770-777. DOI: 10.1111/j.1524-475X.2012.00828.x

[126] Rodrigo SM et al. Analysis of the systemic effect of red and infrared laser therapy on wound repair. Photomedicine and Laser Surgery. 2009;**27**:929-935. DOI: 10.1089/pho.2008.2306

[127] Ayuk SM, Houreld NN, Abrahamse H. Effect of 660 nm visible red light on cell proliferation and viability in diabetic models in vitro under stressed conditions. Lasers in Medical Science. 2018;**33**:1085-1093. DOI: 10.1007/s10103-017-2432-2

[128] Ayuk SM, Houreld NN, Abrahamse H. Laser irradiation alters the expression profile of genes involved in the extracellular matrix. International Journal of Photoenergy in vitro. 2014;**2014**:17. Article ID 604518. DOI: 10.1155/2014/604518

[129] Vitse J, Bekara F, Byun S, Herlin C, Teot L. A double-blind, placebo-controlled randomized evaluation of the effect of low-level laser therapy on venous leg ulcers. The International Journal of Lower Extremity Wounds. 2017;**16**:29-35. DOI: 10.1177/1534734617690948

[130] Taradaj J et al. Effect of laser irradiation at different wavelengths (940, 808, and 658 nm) on pressure ulcer healing: Results from a clinical study. Evidence-Based Complementary and Alternative Medicine. 2013;**2013**:960240. DOI: 10.1155/2013/960240

[131] Karkada G et al. Effect of photobiomodulation therapy on inflammatory cytokines in healing dynamics of diabetic wounds: A systematic review of preclinical studies. Archives of Physiology and Biochemistry. 2023;**129**:663-670. DOI: 10.1080/13813455.2020.1861025

[132] Oyebode O, Houreld NN, Abrahamse H. Photobiomodulation in diabetic wound healing: A review of red and near-infrared wavelength applications. Cell Biochemistry and Function. 2021;**39**:596-612. DOI: 10.1002/cbf.3629

[133] Ponnusamy S, Mosca R, Desai K, Arany P. Photobiomodulation therapy in diabetic wound healing. In: Bagchi D, Das A, Roy S, editors. Wound Healing, Tissue Repair, and Regeneration in Diabetes. San Diego, CA, USA: Academic Press; 2020. pp. 305-321

[134] Sutton E, Ganie S, Chan C, Kaur A, Nussbaum E. Photobiomodulation and diabetic foot and lower leg ulcer healing: A narrative synthesis. The Foot. 2021;**48**:101847. DOI: 10.1016/j.foot.2021.101847

[135] Dhlamini T, Houreld NN. Clinical effect of photobiomodulation on wound healing of diabetic foot ulcers: Does skin color needs to be considered? Journal of Diabetes Research. 2022;**2022**:3312840. DOI: 10.1155/2022/3312840

[136] Dungel P et al. Wavelength-dependent effects of photobiomodulation for wound care in diabetic wounds. International Journal of Molecular Sciences. 2023;**24**:5895

[137] Reardon R et al. The diabetic foot ulcer. Australian Journal of General Practice. 2020;**49**:250-255. DOI: 10.31128/ajgp-11-19-5161

[138] Houreld N. Healing effects of photobiomodulation on diabetic wounds. Applied Sciences. 2019;**9**:5114

[139] Silva DCGGE et al. Low level laser therapy (AlGaInP) applied at 5J/cm2 reduces the proliferation of MRSA in infected wounds and intact skin of rats. Anais Brasileiros de Dermatologia. 2013;**88**:50-55. DOI: 10.1590/S0365-05962013000100005

[140] Maiya GA, Kumar P, Rao L. Effect of low intensity helium-neon (He-Ne) laser irradiation on diabetic wound healing dynamics. Photomedicine and Laser Surgery. 2005;**23**:187-190. DOI: 10.1089/pho.2005.23.187

[141] Engel KW, Khan I, Arany PR. Cell lineage responses to photobiomodulation therapy. Journal of Biophotonics. 2016;**9**:1148-1156. DOI: 10.1002/jbio.201600025

[142] Khan I, Arany PR. Photobiomodulation therapy promotes expansion of epithelial colony forming units. Photomedicine and Laser Surgery. 2016;**34**:550-555. DOI: 10.1089/pho.2015.4054

[143] Tang E, Khan I, Andreana S, Arany PR. Laser-activated transforming growth factor-beta1 induces human beta-defensin 2: Implications for laser therapies for periodontitis and peri-implantitis. Journal of Periodontal Research. 2017;**52**:360-367. DOI: 10.1111/jre.12399

[144] Houreld NN, Sekhejane PR, Abrahamse H. Irradiation at 830 nm

stimulates nitric oxide production and inhibits pro-inflammatory cytokines in diabetic wounded fibroblast cells. Lasers in Surgery and Medicine. 2010;**42**:494-502. DOI: 10.1002/lsm.20812

[145] Minatel DG, Frade MA, Franca SC, Enwemeka CS. Phototherapy promotes healing of chronic diabetic leg ulcers that failed to respond to other therapies. Lasers in Surgery and Medicine. 2009;**41**:433-441. DOI: 10.1002/lsm.20789

[146] Kaviani A et al. A randomized clinical trial on the effect of low-level laser therapy on chronic diabetic foot wound healing: A preliminary report. Photomedicine and Laser Surgery. 2011;**29**:109-114. DOI: 10.1089/pho.2009.2680

[147] Oyebode OA, Jere SW, Houreld NN. Current therapeutic modalities for the management of chronic diabetic wounds of the foot. Journal Diabetes Research. 2023;**2023**:1359537. DOI: 10.1155/2023/1359537

[148] Kajagar BM, Godhi AS, Pandit A, Khatri S. Efficacy of low level laser therapy on wound healing in patients with chronic diabetic foot ulcers—A randomised control trial. The Indian Journal of Surgery. 2012;**74**:359-363. DOI: 10.1007/s12262-011-0393-4

[149] Huang J, Chen J, Xiong S, Huang J, Liu Z. The effect of low-level laser therapy on diabetic foot ulcers: A meta-analysis of randomised controlled trials. International Wound Journal. 2021;**18**:763-776. DOI: 10.1111/iwj.13577

[150] Groppa E, Colliva A, Vuerich R, Kocijan T, Zacchigna S. Immune cell therapies to improve regeneration and revascularization of non-healing wounds. International Journal of Molecular Sciences. 23 Jul 2020;**21**(15):5235. DOI: 10.3390/ijms21155235

[151] Skitzki JJ, Repasky EA, Evans SS. Hyperthermia as an immunotherapy strategy for cancer. Current Opinion in Investigational Drugs. 2009;**10**:550-558

[152] Overchuk M, Weersink RA, Wilson BC, Zheng G. Photodynamic and photothermal therapies: Synergy opportunities for nanomedicine. ACS Nano. 9 May 2023;**17**(9):7979-8003. DOI: 10.1021/acsnano.3c00891

[153] Rahman SU et al. Learning from clinical phenotypes: Low-dose biophotonics therapies in oral diseases. Oral Diseases. 2018;**24**:261-276. DOI: 10.1111/odi.12796

[154] Besegato JF, de Melo PBG, Tamae PE, Alves APAR, Rondón LF, Leanse LG, et al. How can biophotonics help dentistry to avoid or minimize cross infection by SARS-CoV-2? Photodiagnosis and Photodynamic Therapy. Mar 2022;**37**:102682. DOI: 10.1016/j.pdpdt.2021.102682

Chapter 7

The Evolving Role of Dermal Matrices in Reconstructive Surgery

Rohan Rajaram, Min Zhang, Smitha Segu and Sally Kiu-Huen Ng

Abstract

Dermal matrices are an integral part of the reconstructive ladder. Their introduction has significantly changed the way burns and soft tissue infection such as necrotising fasciitis are managed and offer new options for aesthetic and reconstructive breast surgery. They have also allowed surgeons to reconstruct complex wounds without the need for challenging microsurgical techniques, especially for the elderly or patients who have multiple co-morbidities. The current suite of biological and synthetic dermal matrices has evolved over time to facilitate optimal wound healing and reconstruction of various soft tissue defects. The current suite of biological and synthetic dermal matrices has evolved over time to facilitate optimal wound healing and reconstruction of various soft tissue defects. This book chapter presents a comprehensive review of the concept and development of dermal matrices in reconstructive surgery. The most popular dermal matrices available in clinical use will be explored and their biology, immunology, and clinical applications in reconstructive surgery will be examined. Finally, the frontiers and future of dermal matrix technology will be discussed.

Keywords: dermal matrix, reconstructive surgery, plastic surgery, skin substitutes, skin

1. Introduction

The necessity to cover a wound vastly predates the intricate understanding of wound healing we have today. Thousands of years before Koch and Pasteur's germ theory and much before the advanced biological understanding of cellular wound healing, the ancient Sumerians believed in a triad of wound care revolving around 'washing the wound, preparing a plaster and plastering the wound' [1]. From these foundations, the Ebers Papyrus—an ancient Egyptian manuscript on medicine and surgery from the fifteenth century BC described the first attempt at dermal substitution in burn wound care—the use of frog skin xenografting [2]. Since then, scientific understanding of wound care has advanced considerably but still adheres to similar ancient principles: prevention of infection, containment of insensible water loss, encouragement of healing and restoration of form and function. Following these principles, advances in dressing technologies have resulted in improvements in the antimicrobial properties and selective environmental permeability of dressings (**Figure 1**).

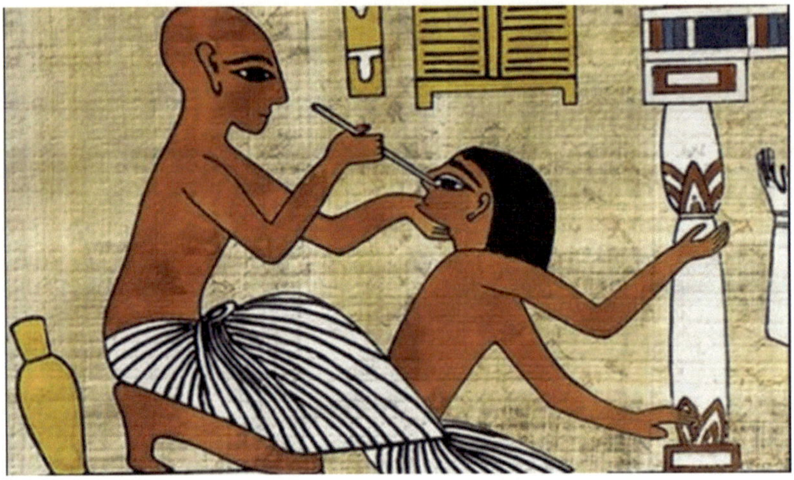

Figure 1.
An ancient Egyptian doctor painting over a wound of the eye with salve prior to xenografting. Creative Commons [3].

Comparatively, the advent of dermal matrices represents a paradigm shift from simple dressing based wound care. Dermal matrices are a product distinguishable from dressings by their innate ability to encourage and expedite the cellular factors involved in wound care while still providing coverage, protection, and infection control. This is born out of a necessity for rapid restoration of the dermis which can be extensively lost in soft tissue injury from burns, trauma or infection. In wounds that are lacking substantial dermis, normal wound healing is slow and inconsistent, leading to patients facing a protracted recovery period without protection from infection, water and heat loss which can lead to hemodynamic compromise and death. Furthermore, any wound healing achieved without considerable dermis suffers from extensive scarring, contracture and depigmentation which can be chronically painful, limit motion and be psychologically destabilising to individuals. As such, dermal matrices through a multitude of mechanisms promote the regrowth of dermis over injured areas such that effective wound healing can be achieved.

The technology utilised in dermal matrices has evolved with time and as such these products have taken on an increasingly reconstructive role through their ability to incorporate into recipient skin. Initially through xeno- and allografting, a favourable extracellular milieu was provided onto a wound bed to encourage neodermis formation, while the graft itself served as a temporary physical barrier before immunogenic rejection would cause it to be shed from the wound bed [4].

As scientific technology evolved, the ability to decellularize the graft was discovered. This left behind a scaffold rich with extracellular matrix proteins which would integrate into the recipient wound bed. The development of semisynthetic dermal matrices in the late twentieth century reduced the need to source and decellularize the graft. These products were largely comprised of biological extracellular matrix (ECM) proteins held together by linking molecules a synthetic dermal frame (e.g. nylon or polyurethane) into which biological ECM (bovine/porcine collagen) were added. While these products significantly improved healing in extensive cutaneous injury, their main fallbacks were allergy, immunogenicity and infection owing to their partial biological composition [5]. Patients, due to religious or personal preference for animal free products may also hold reservations against xenogenic products.

Dermal Matrices					
Biological		Bio- Synthetic		Synthetic	
Xenogeneic	Allogeneic	Artificial	Cellularly Enhanced	Wound Healing	Structural Support
Examples: • **Preserved Animal Skin Grafting** (e.g. Porcine, Tilapia, Bull Frog) • **Xenogeneic Acellular Dermal Matrix** (e.g. Dispase II, Triton X-100, TS-ADM)	Examples: • **Preserved Cadaver Skin** (e.g. Cryopreserved, Glycerol Preserved) • **Allogeneic Acellular Dermal Matrix** (e.g. Alloderm®, Flex HD ®)	Examples: • **Integra ®** • **Matriderm ®** • Oasis ®	Examples: • **Apligraft®** • Dermagraft® • Transcyte® • Orcel®	Example: • **NovoSorb BTM®**	Example: • **Galaflex®** • **TIGR Matrix®**
Clinical Application: • External Cutaneous Reconstruction: Most use seen in **burns.** Rarely other injuries such as necrotising infection, cancer reconstruction	Clinical Application: • External Cutaneous Reconstruction: Burns, necrotising infection, cancer reconstruction • Internal support and reconstruction: **implant-based breast surgery, abdominal hernia repair, gingival recession**	Clinical Application: • External Cutaneous Reconstruction: Burns, necrotising infection, cancer reconstruction, scalp reconstruction, single stage wound reconstruction • Not generally used internally	Clinical Application: • External Cutaneous Reconstruction: As previous but **especially used in chronic wound settings such as diabetic foot ulcer due to cellular components**	Clinical Application: • External Cutaneous Reconstruction: As previously, with an advantage in **infectious settings** due **to lack of biological components**	Clinical Application: • Volumizing and scaffolding agent for aesthetic breast and facial surgery • Abdominal wall reconstruction

Figure 2.
Overview of classifications of dermal matrices.

Considering this, the next logical step in dermal matrix technology was the development of a fully synthetic dermal matrix that is biodegradable. To date there is only one widely available synthetic dermal matrix product. Developed by Polynovo®, the Novosorb® Biodegradable Temporising Matrix (BTM) follows similar principles to existing dermal matrices, with both a dermal template layer and silicon epidermal layer, with the key difference of containing no biological products [6]. BTM provides an environment for rapid neodermis formation without any of the immunogenic, infectious, or ethical qualms faced by other products.

However, the advancement of these technologies does not necessarily result in the obsolescence of previous dermal matrices. This is due to innovations in using historical acellular dermal matrices, once used only in external skin cover, for the reconstruction of various internal defects. For example, AlloDerm® is now widely used as a mucosal graft for gingival recession [7] in dentistry and as an implant covering in breast reconstruction to prevent capsular contraction.

This chapter will cover the main classes of dermal matrices: biological, semi-synthetic and completely synthetic. It will discuss the detailed biology of products that fall into each of these categories and how they influence dermal genesis. Finally, it will cover clinical applications and present clinical cases for completeness (**Figure 2**).

2. Autologous reconstruction

2.1 Autologous skin grafting

The mainstay of cutaneous reconstruction is the autologous skin graft [8]. Compared to some biological methods, the skin graft as we know it today is a relatively contemporary technique. The technique utilises the ability for immunologically identical autologous skin to re-establish a vascular supply within a recipient wound bed. It is important to note that a graft may only be placed over clean, well vascularised tissue such as: fascia, epitenon, periosteum or perineurium in order to diffuse oxygen in the early stages of graft take. As such, bare tendon, muscle or bone are unsuitable for grafting and require another form of reconstruction. Understanding the way in which skin grafts take can help to provide a basis of understanding for new innovative biological, bio-synthetic, and fully synthetic dermal matrices.

There are two broad varieties of skin grafting based on the degree of donor dermis harvested, and each variety brings with it advantages and disadvantages:

1. The most substantial, 'full thickness' skin graft (FTSG), takes the epidermis and entire dermis from a donor site. Therefore, it necessitates reconstruction of the donor site, whether this be from primary closure, local flap coverage or through its own split thickness grafting. Generally, primary closure of the donor site is preferred and as such the potential donor locations (only those with enough laxity to close primarily can be utilised) and graft size are limited. The FTSG is preferred over the split thickness skin graft (STSG) for smaller wound defects due to its ability to heal with limited scarring and depigmentation, often yielding cosmetically identical results. This is due to the greater level of dermis providing an extracellular environment that is supportive of wound healing. Furthermore, when applied, the increased thickness of the graft allows for more robust and durable coverage.

2. When only a part of the entire thickness of the dermis is harvested, the skin graft is deemed 'split thickness' (STSG). As part of the donor dermis is left behind, the donor site is expected to heal on its own with dressing based wound care. This qualifies any site in the body to be utilised for harvest, increasing availability of donor skin. In these instances, the size of reconstruction is limited only by available undamaged skin and other operative considerations (e.g. in burns generally up to 20% total body surface area can be reconstructed in a single operation due to blood loss incurred from excising burn wounds). Size maybe further augmented by meshing or pie crusting. However, the resultant reconstruction with a thin STSG is often prone to contracture formation, scarring and discolouration and depigmentation. Furthermore, the interim wound is often fragile and prone to sheering forces which may damage the graft.

Healing in skin grafting happens in four main steps:

1. Imbibition: as the graft is applied to a vascularised wound bed, oxygen and nutrients are diffused into the graft. Lacking a blood supply, the graft appears pale and can tolerate this state for up to 4 days.

2. Inosculation: Relative hypoxia signals for the ingrowth and anastomoses between donor and recipient capillary beds, restoring blood supply, nutrition, immunological function and proliferative function to the graft. The graft now appears pink.

3. Revascularisation: The release of VEGF factors from fibroblasts now able to travel to the graft cause the ingrowth of vascular endothelial cells into the graft. This establishes a bolstered vascular network through which further wound remodelling and maturation can occur.

4. Remodelling: This step is similar to primary and secondary intention wound healing where fibroblasts convert to myofibroblasts and type III collagen is replaced with type I collagen, though this happens at a lower scale due to the existing anatomical organisation provided by a graft. The graft has now fully taken (**Figure 3**).

2.2 The cutting edge of autologous reconstruction: cultured epithelial autograft

Much of the cutaneous reconstructive effort is focused on restoring lost dermis with epithelial reconstruction usually being achieved with a thin split thickness skin graft. As such, skin availability as well as donor side pain and morbidity still remain important considerations in the ultimate reconstructive effort. The frontier of epithelial reconstruction is the concept of the cultured epithelial autograft (CEA). This technology uses donor epithelial cells which are expanded and structured in vitro to create an epithelial replacement for a defect [10]. Currently the two main brands offering CEAs are Re-Cell®, which offers an epithelial cell spray [10] and Epicel®, which offers a sheet like cultured epithelial layer [8].

While culturing and preparation differ between providers, the essential steps are similar. A biopsy is taken from the patient, sterilised with antibiotics, and sectioned in vitro. Dermis is separated from epidermis using thermolysin and heat. Remaining epidermal cells are then separated from one another within a trypsin bath and are cultured within a culture medium. These expanded colonies of epidermal keratinocytes can either be organised into a sheet or manufactured into a suspension for spray onto wounds [8].

Currently CEAs have shown promise as a standalone cover for extensive superficial thickness wounds or to be used in conjunction with dermal substitutes for full thickness wounds.

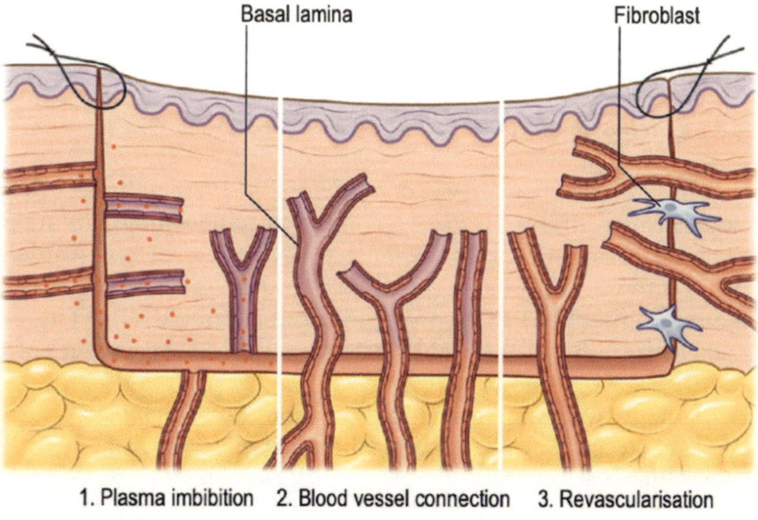

Figure 3.
Graphical representation of stages of skin graft take. Courtesy: Capla et al. [9].

3. Biological dermal matrices

The earliest attempts at wound reconstruction were done by entirely biological means [2]. This was due to the instinctive reasoning that covering a wound with a substance that was similar in composition to the lost tissue would encourage healing. To an extent, these concepts still hold true. The provision of a wound covering rich in extracellular matrix elements and skin cells does promote the chemical signalling implicated in wound healing. However, this modern understanding also helps to explain many of the pitfalls experienced by those who attempted to close a wound by entirely biological means. Our interaction with biological dermal matrices underpinned our understanding of their shortcomings of infection and immunogenicity and drove us to develop the complex dermal matrices we readily use today. This section will discuss the biology and contemporary uses for xenogenic and allogeneic dermal matrices.

3.1 Xenografting

As previously mentioned, the genesis of biological wound healing was founded in the Ancient Egyptian Ebers Papyrus, with the use of frog xenografting. Since then, skin from sheep, cats, dogs, and pigs have also been used both historically and in modern clinical settings to provide a wound coverage option that is also biologically active [4]. Pedantic adherence to nomenclature would dictate that naming the use of animal skin as xenografting is actually incorrect. This is due to the necessity for a graft to be completely incorporated into the skin. The understanding that immunological rejection of non-native skin results in the xenograft being shed from the wound bed is sound [11]. Therefore, current uses for xenografting are as a temporary wound coverage that can encourage the rapid formation of granulation tissue and expedite the preparation of a wound bed for skin grafting. The bulk of modern uses of xenografting occur in burns, where rapid and large-scale wound coverage to prevent insensible water losses and hypothermia while also encouraging healing is necessary. Currently, porcine skin is the most widely used xenografting modality with emerging evidence demonstrating the efficacy of Bullfrog (*Rana catesbeiana*) and Tilapia skin in promoting re-epithelialization and preventing moisture loss [12].

3.1.1 The efficacy of xenografts explained through the porcine xenograft

The modern use of porcine skin was documented in 1983 by Robert Ersek as a temporary wound cover for burns [13]. Currently, porcine xenografts are prepared in one of three preparation methods: 'fresh', 'cryopreserved', or 'glutaraldehyde preserved' [13]. Of these, the most common preparation method is glutaraldehyde preservation, which cross links ECM proteins found in animal skin. This cross-linking increases shelf life and has germicidal effects, reducing the chances of infection further [14].

In addition to their roles as a physical barrier, xenografts, rich in extracellular matrix proteins, encourage vascularisation, fibroblast migration and organisation of a neodermis. This increase growth of dermis as well as protection from infection and desiccation allows for rapid re-epithelialisation and wound healing. It is important to note that the cells in the xenograft are non-viable and do not contribute to wound healing.

3.1.2 Mechanisms of immunogenicity and future directions for xenografting

The largest shortcoming of porcine xenografts is their high degree of immunogenicity, which results in rapid rejection and shedding. The main antigen found on porcine xenografts that initiates cellular mediated immunity is known as 'gal'. Gal, an endothelial protein, is not found in human tissue and as a result is recognised by T cells resulting in both a CD4 and CD8 mediated immune response which results in sensitisation and cytotoxic rejection [15]. Two other antigens 'Neu5Gc' and 'Sda' have also been found to confer immunogenic properties to porcine xenografts. Beyond this porcine xenografts are also susceptible to other mechanisms of immunogenicity such as presentation of xenogenic intracellular compounds on major histocompatibility complexes (MHC) by native cells, and macrophage mediated antigen presentation as well as systemic inflammatory pathways due to their lack of human anti-inflammatory proteins such as human Heme Oxygenase-1. Finally, some reports claim that the application of porcine xenograft can sensitise patients to cadaveric skin based allografting, reducing the efficacy of cadaver skin [16].

In response to this, experimental studies that explore using CRISPR Cas 9 gene editing technology to engineer pigs with the genes controlling the production of the above [17]. These efforts endeavour to increase immune tolerance towards porcine xenografts and increase the time that they can spend on the wound bed.

Despite this, xenografting remains a temporary wound cover measure until there is further development in immune tolerance that will allow the incorporation of porcine dermis into the human wound bed.

3.1.3 Clinical applications: porcine xenografting in burns

Clinical outcomes for the use of xenografts in burns have largely reflected the pedagogy elucidated in experimental testing. Large systematic reviews and meta-analyses of xenograft use in the management of burns have demonstrated superior barrier protection, neoepithelialisation, infection control and water and heat insulation as compared to regular synthetic dressings [18]. Within these, individual studies have demonstrated that re-epithelialisation in burns treated with porcine skin grafts can occur up to 1 week ahead of silver sulfadiazine dressings. Furthermore, both porcine and fish-based skin grafts demonstrate a significant reduction in scar index of approximately five points across all studies (**Figure 4**) [20].

3.1.4 Decellularised xenografting: Veritas

Veritas Collagen Matrix is a non-fenestrated xenograft developed by Synovis Surgical Innovations in the United States in 2007 that is derived from non-cross linked bovine pericardium and FDA approved in 2019 [21]. The manufacturing process involves treating the decellularized pericardium with propylene oxide to reduce immunogenicity [22]. Once implanted, Veritas rapidly degrades and stimulates host tissue cell infiltration and neovascularization, in order to promote remodelling of the scaffold with collagen almost entirely by 3 months [22, 23]. Veritas is associated with reduced antigenicity by nature of being a non-cross-linked mesh, and therefore has a reduced foreign body reaction and inflammatory response, facilitating earlier integration into native tissue [24].

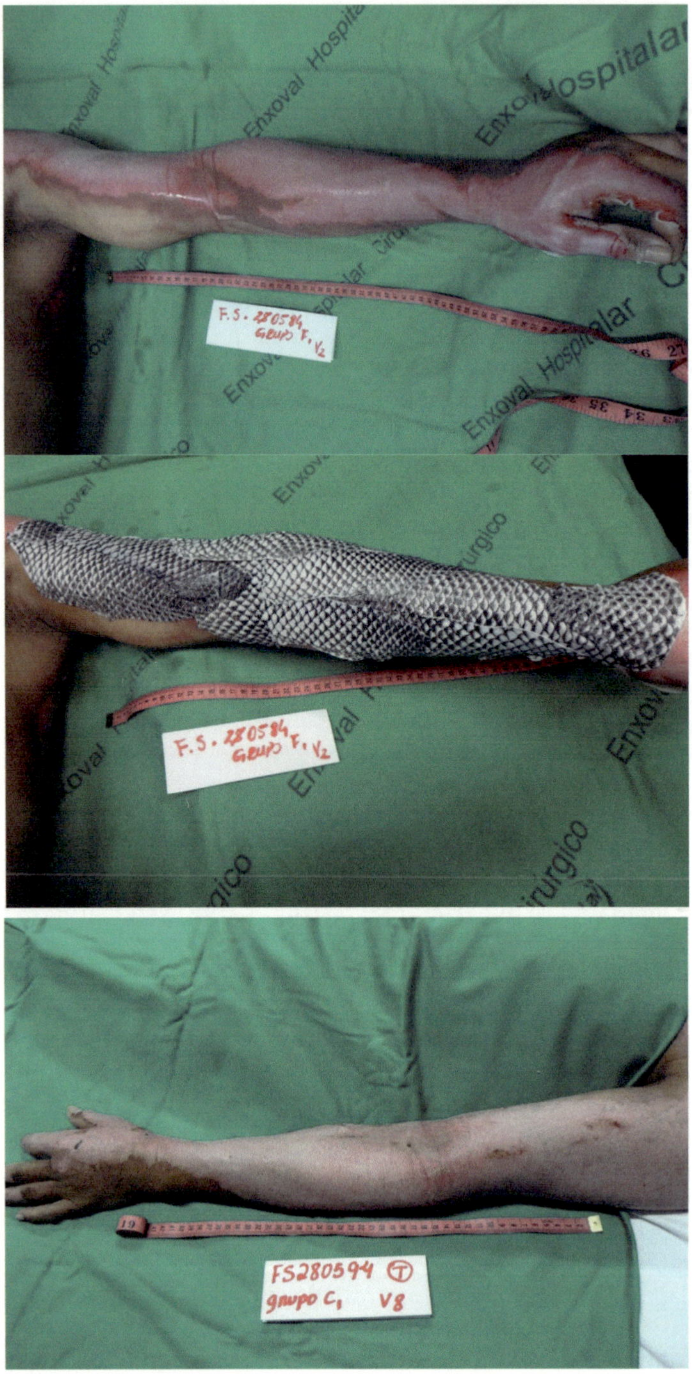

Figure 4.
Tilapia based dressing used to encourage early epithelialisation in 23M suffering partial thickness burns. Courtesy: Lima-Junior et al. [19].

3.1.4.1 Clinical applications: Veritas in abdominal wall hernia repair

The use of Veritas in ventral hernia repairs, even those complex defects such as patients with severe obesity, diabetes, and exposed synthetic mesh, is well documented [21, 24, 25] due to its minimal infection rate, low rates of adhesions, and cost effectiveness [25]. Veritas is easy to handle and does not require product-specific preparation or reconstitution with saline prior to use [24]. However, Veritas has reduced long-term tensile strength compared to its cross-linked counterparts, resulting in increased risk of hernia recurrence [23, 25].

3.2 Allografting

Allografting refers to a broad range of techniques that are united by their basis in cadaveric human origin. As with most innovations in wound cover, early attempts at using cadaver skin were born out of burn injury where large surface areas of skin required temporary cover and protection. While historically there have been accounts of ancient civilisations using cadaver skin for wound reconstruction, robust allografting techniques did not exist until the days of John Girdner in 1891, where for the first time allografting from the thigh of a deceased 6-year-old boy was performed onto a lightning strike victim [26]. Contextually, the first documented successful skin autografts, described by Reverdin, had only recently been developed. While initially ground-breaking, they suffered from inefficiencies of infection, inability to produce a split thickness graft and donor site morbidity. As such the use of cadaver skin was intended to support donor site pressures on autologous skin grafting and actually be used as a permanent wound cover technique. Initial techniques were rudimentary and involved the direct application of fresh, untreated cadaver skin onto wounds and applying dressings [26]. This method had significant drawbacks which included the necessity to use fresh cadavers at the time of injury and infection risk. Whist the development of the skin bank in the 1930s resolved some of these drawbacks through the sterilisation and cryopreservation of harvested skin, the main issue with allogeneic skin was its immunogenicity [27]. As such, much like a xenograft, most allografts would shed from the wound bed and could only be used as a temporary wound cover (**Figure 5**).

Modern cadaver skin can be classified into the following categories: 1. viable: where cells are still alive and able to function to increase re-epithelialisation but also contribute further to immunogenicity. These include fresh and cryopreserved grafts. 2. non-viable: where processing inactivates skin cells, therefore converting the graft into a biological dressing that also takes longer to be rejected. Glycerol preserved and irradiated skin grafts fall under the non-viable category [28]. It is globally understood that cadaver allografts are a method of temporary wound cover which increase keratinocyte proliferation and vascularisation of the wound bed to encourage epithelialisation. Immunogenicity results in rejection 2–4 weeks after placement of the allograft [29]. Thus, to overcome this issue and introduce an allogeneic product that permanently integrates into the wound bed, the acellular allogeneic dermal matrix was developed. The pioneering product, AlloDerm®, was developed in 1994 based on the success of its semi synthetic counterpart in

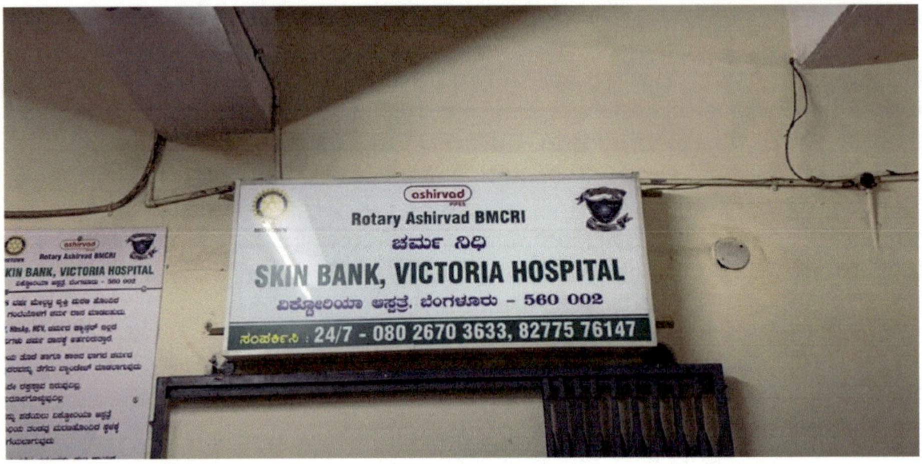

Figure 5.
The popularisation of the concept of a skin bank which now provides valuable temporary wound cover especially in middle- and lower-income countries such as India. Credit: AO.

Integra® [30]. Initially intended for burn reconstruction, it has been superseded by more contemporary products in burn care and is now used in contexts such as implant-based breast reconstruction. This section will discuss the mechanisms behind the immunogenicity of allografting as well as the specifics of AlloDerm® and similar products.

3.2.1 Immunogenicity of allografting

Immune rejection of allografts is mostly a T cell determined process with contributions for B and natural killer (NK) cells.

Within 3–4 days of placement, dendritic cells from cadaver skin travel to recipient lymph nodes and present cadaveric antigens on MHC molecules. These cause activation of T cells which then act in two major ways to cause rejection. Firstly, CD8 (Killer) T cells migrate to the wound bed and begin directly inducing apoptosis in the donor cells. Secondary CD4 (Helper) T cells are activated and secrete cytokines that prime CD8 T cells to target donor cells and instruct B cells to secrete antibodies against donor skin cells. This forms humoral immunity against cadaver skin grafts. B cell mediated antibody production works to destroy donor skin cells through complement mediated cellular lysis as well as resulting in immunological memory, whereby an additional cadaver graft is rejected at a faster rate than initial placement. Finally, NK cells recognise that the donor skin cells do not present native 'self' antigens and therefore also contribute to the destruction of the allograft [29].

As such, there exists a necessity for reducing immunogenicity. Many techniques such as reducing cellular viability, human leukocyte antigen (HLA) type matching grafts and immunosuppression had variable success in increasing graft survival [31]. However, the most successful technique to date is the decellularisation of cadaver skin to develop an immunologically inert dermal matrix that will permanently integrate into skin as a new dermis. Through this technique, products such as AlloDerm® and Flex HD® have become popular clinical products (**Figure 6**).

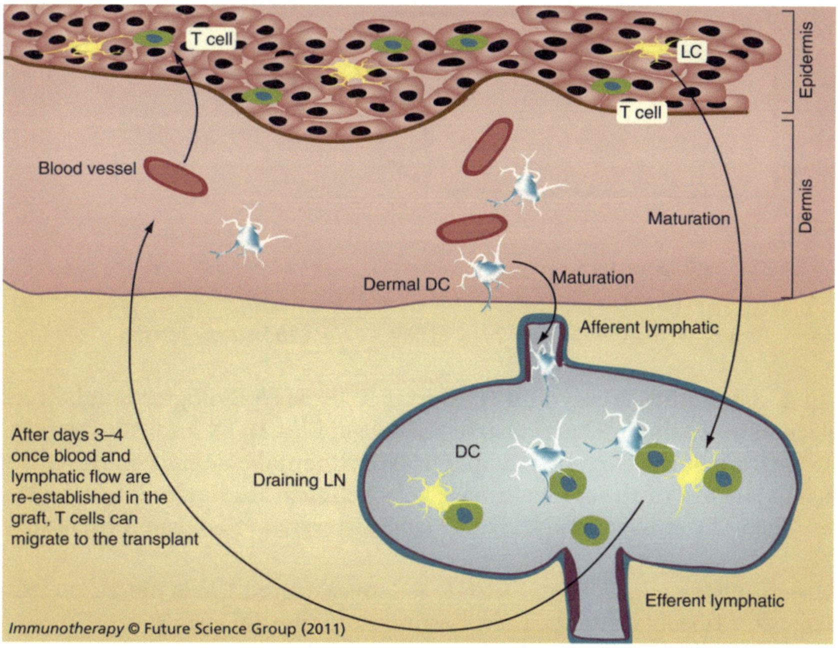

Figure 6.
Schematic demonstrating cellular immunity against allogenic skin transplantation. Rejection is largely T cell mediated with a delayed B cell response. Courtesy: Benichou et al. [29].

3.2.2 Developments in allografting technology

3.2.2.1 AlloDerm® and Flex HD®

AlloDerm® (Lifecell, Branchburg NJ) was the result of decellularisation of cadaver skin and was first described for full thickness burns in 1996 [30] and received FDA approval for this indication in 1998. Since then, novel uses for the acellular dermal matrix (ADM) have been described in breast, hernia, and gingival surgery to provide strength and substance to these various defects. The process of converting donated human skin into AlloDerm® involves separating the epidermis through using a buffered saline solution. Subsequently dermal cells such as fibroblasts are dissolved in a detergent solution, ECM proteins are not denatured in this process. Finally, the remaining acellular matrix is cryopreserved for later use. The resultant product contains a mesh made up of type 1 collagen, elastin, proteoglycans and glycosaminoglycans. It forms a mesh with pore size of 40–200 micrometres in size. The combined effect of having a porous matrix rich in ECM proteins is that vascularisation and fibroblast migration is expedited. The cost of AlloDerm® is USD 30/cm^2 [32].

Flex HD® (MTF Biologics, NJ) was developed in 2010 for the purposes of returning allogeneic acellular dermal matrices to the frontier of cutaneous wound healing. In particular, it derived its dermal source from only the reticular layer of the human dermis, which has been shown to be more loosely packed with extracellular matrix. Furthermore, the product is glycerol preserved rather than cryopreserved which obviates any need for rehydration prior to application. Ultimately the aim of this is to produce an ADM like AlloDerm® that integrated faster into a cutaneous wound and conformed more easily to the topography of different wounds [33]. Flex HD is similarly priced to AlloDerm® at USD 27/cm^2 (**Figure 7**) [34].

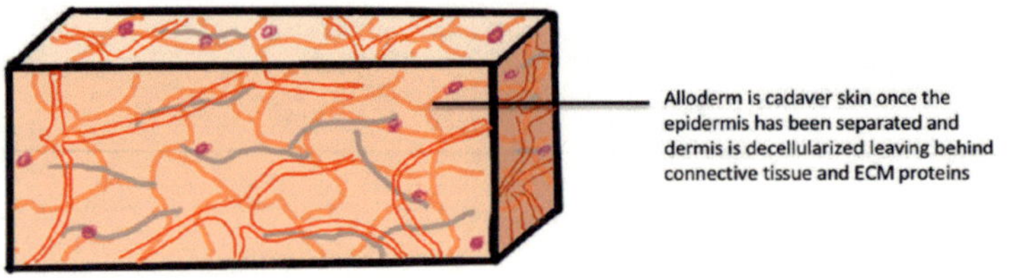

Figure 7.
Schematic of AlloDerm®. Credit: AO.

3.2.3 Comparison of AlloDerm® and Flex HD® in the laboratory setting

A singular laboratory-based study undertaken by MTF Biologics sought to compare molecular and cellular characteristics between Flex HD® and AlloDerm®. This forms the entirety of the currently available experimental evidence on the two ADMs, with much of the rest of the evidence base being clinical studies looking at patient outcomes. The MTF study found the following differences between AlloDerm® and Flex HD®:

Increased fibroblast attachment: FlexHD® demonstrated 100% increased fibroblast attachment after fibroblast application as compared to AlloDerm®.

Comparable tensile strength: Both FlexHD® products and AlloDerm® were able to similarly resist tensile strength and elongate to similar lengths before breaking.

Comparable suture retention: Both Flex HD® and AlloDerm® were able to retain a similar length of suture being pulled through before cheese-wiring occurred [35].

3.2.3.1 Pitfalls of AlloDerm® and Flex HD

AlloDerm® and Flex HD® have routine concerns of infection and immunogenicity despite measures taken to minimise these described above. Furthermore, being a biologically derived product, increased costs as well as careful consideration for donor, storage and expiry are needed.

Unique to AlloDerm® are documented cases of poor take when cutaneous reconstruction is attempted. Additionally, there have been some reports of hypertrophic scarring despite using AlloDerm® for burn reconstruction. As such, in the presence of superior contemporary products, AlloDerm® has been transitioned to be used as a scaffolding for implant-based breast reconstruction, hernia repair and gingival surgeries [36].

Both AlloDerm® and FlexHD® have been implicated in the development of 'red breast syndrome' (RBS), an inflammatory reaction exclusive to ADM used in breast reconstruction [37]. Currently there are fewer than 10 reported cases of RBS, as such the exact mechanism for its development is not yet established. It is likely an immunologic inflammatory reaction to the ADM and may be more prevalent in cases where the ADM is inserted incorrectly, or rigorous sterilisation is not performed [38]. The clinical presentation is that of localised erythema over the inferior part of the breast with variable ulceration and pustule formation. Investigation findings are similarly variable with some cases reporting leukocytosis and fever and others simply demonstrating a rise in C-reactive protein levels [39]. Histology of removed ADM show sterile abscess formation [37]. Finally, treatment is eminence based involving the use of corticosteroids to dampen immune response and broad-spectrum antibiotics to control superimposed infection. Failing this, surgery to remove and exchange the ADM is considered [37, 38].

3.2.4 Clinical applications: the breadth of uses for AlloDerm®

Since being transitioned away from cutaneous reconstruction, AlloDerm® is widely used in implant-based breast reconstruction and gingival grafting.

Within the realm of tissue expander and implant-based breast reconstruction, a multistage process is often necessitated due to a lack of sufficient soft tissue for creating a tension-free closure and preventing implant herniation. An ADM like AlloDerm® can be used to address these issues, if sculpted into a lower pole hammock, for two-stage tissue expander or by enveloping the entire implant for single-stage direct-to-implant reconstruction [36]. The AlloDerm® helps to stabilise the implant by providing internal soft tissue support, facilitates greater control on implant projection and lower pole fullness [40]. Moreover, AlloDerm® covered breast implants not only induce less post-operative pain from pectoralis muscle mobilisation but also reduces scarring and capsular contracture by forming a fibrous capsule around the implant, thereby dampening potential immunological rejection [41]. AlloDerm® is also a valuable recourse for weakened or thin skin flaps after a mastectomy at risk of wound spread or necrosis, with documented cases also demonstrating improved performance in tissue following radiotherapy. Importantly, implant-based reconstruction with AlloDerm® has been shown to be more cost-effective for patients than its absence.

AlloDerm® also has a role in aesthetic breast surgery and the treatment of implant-associated breast deformities, with applications that include the correction of symmastia or malposition by buttressing the implant into position, or the correction of surface irregularities by overlaying the AlloDerm® over the surface of the implant (**Figure 8**).

AlloDerm® is also widely used in periodontics to provide increased gingival support to patients who receive oral implants. In clinical studies it has been shown to increase the rate of gingival regrowth by providing a template for growth of new gingiva. In comparative studies it has been shown to provide the same net benefit as a free gingival graft, with increased ease of handling while obviating the necessity for donor site morbidity [43].

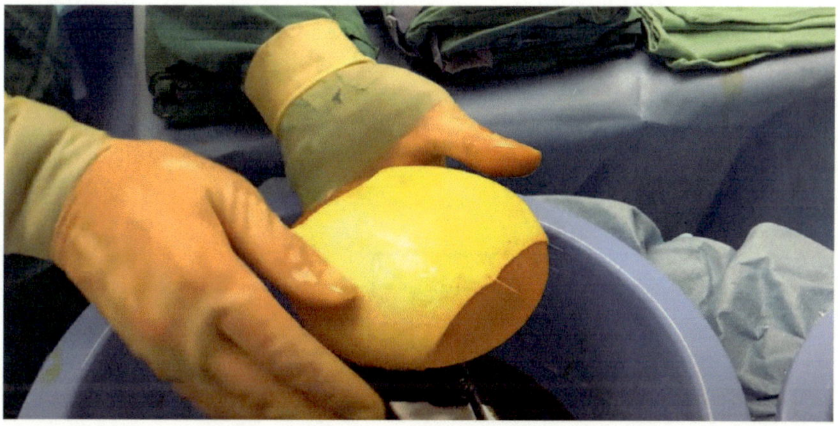

Figure 8.
Breast implant wrapped in AlloDerm® prior to insertion to prevent capsule formation and rippling. Courtesy: Changes Plastic Surgery [42].

4. Bio-synthetic dermal matrices

As technology continues to evolve, newer options in the form of hybrid biological/synthetic products are developed to overcome some of the detriments associated with decellularized biological dermal substitutes.

Biosynthetic products may be divided into the following subcategories: artificial biological matrices, such as Integra® and Matriderm®, and cellularly enhanced synthetic matrices such as Apligraf®. The main advantage of bio-synthetic substitutes is that they are not limited by donor site availability.

4.1 Artificial biological matrices

4.1.1 Integra

Integra® (Integra LifeSciences, Plainsboro, New Jersey) began development in the late 1970s as a combined endeavour between Boston Shriners burns centre, Massachusetts Institute of Technology and Massachusetts General Hospital in order to provide temporary wound coverage for large surface area full thickness burns [5]. It was first approved by the FDA for use in full thickness burns in 1996. It is a bilayered product that contains a neodermis manufactured with bovine derived collagen linked together with shark glycosaminoglycan, and a silicone sealing membrane that can be peeled when the neodermis becomes integrated to the wound bed. While it was initially designed for use in burns, the breadth of clinical applications of Integra® extends to traumatic wounds, diabetic ulcers, cancer reconstruction and even as a focused antibiotic delivery device [44]. The cost of Integra® appears to be much cheaper than other dermal matrices at USD 14/cm^2 (**Figure 9**) [45].

4.1.2 Biology of Integra®

Type I collagen from adult bovine calcaneal tendons is cross linked by glutaraldehyde to provide a controlled rate of biodegradation as the dermal substitute integrates into the wound. Type I collagen is the main form of collagen secreted by fibroblasts towards the end of wound healing. It is tougher and less elastic than type III collagen and provides a strong framework for the neodermis to develop. The orientation of the collagen fibres is maintained and stabilised by a shark derived glycosaminoglycan (GAG) known as chondroitin-6-sulphate (C-6-S), which is a long repeating polysaccharide. The thickness of this layer is approximately 1 mm with a 0.23 mm silicon sealing membrane superficial to it. The dermal matrix structure is porous with a random arrangement of pores of size 30–120 microns in size [46].

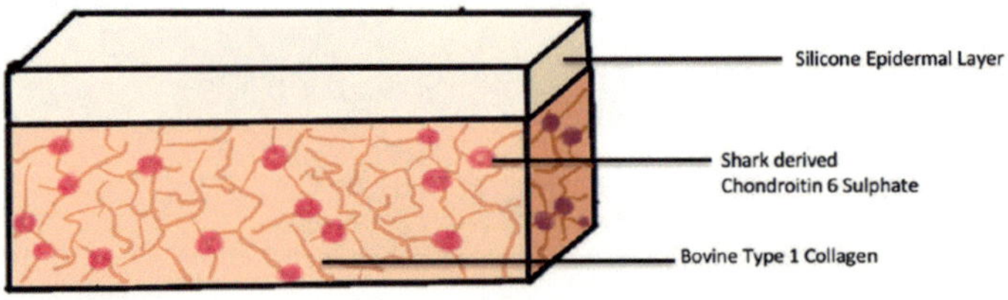

Figure 9.
Schematic of Integra®. Credit: AO.

Both the bovine type I collagen and shark C-6-S have limited immunogenicity. Alone, the type I collagen fibrils induce a negligible immune response. However, cross linked type I collagen has been shown to induce an immune response via promoting platelet aggregation. This is where the included shark GAGs play an important role in blocking thrombin induced platelet aggregation. Reducing immunogenicity and resultant inflammation is an important step in ensuring that the dermal matrix is not rejected by the host. On a more cellular level, the tempering of inflammation in wound healing settings also reduces myofibroblast induced wound contraction and scar formation [47].

4.1.3 Mechanism of action in wound healing

Wound healing in Integra® can be conceptualised as a hybrid between native wound healing and skin graft take. It occurs through four processes: imbibition, fibroblast migration, neovascularization, and remodelling.

Imbibition: As Integra® is applied, exudate from the wound, which contains fibrin, holds the matrix to the wound bed. The level of proinflammatory cytokines such as tumour growth factor (TGF)-beta begin to rise but are limited by the anti-immunogenic properties of the GAGs. This process begins as soon as the product is applied and continues for approximately 7–10 days.

Fibroblast Migration: At day 7, fibroblasts migrate into the porous neodermis. Due to both the random pattern pore structure and the dampening of immunogenicity, fibroblast to myofibroblast differentiation is inhibited. This leads to reduced wound contracture and scarring. This process continues until day 14.

Neovascularization: From day 14 to day 21 endothelial cells migrate to the wound bed and vascularize the forming neodermis to support an influx of fibroblasts. At the end of 21 days, the silicone epidermal layer can be removed, and a thin split thickness skin autograft can be applied.

Remodelling: From the third week of Integra® application, the bovine collagen is replaced with native collagen. This collagen is identical to dermal collagen and does not resemble keloid or hypertrophic scar. This near native neodermis also encourages the take of the split thickness skin graft thereby completely reconstructing the wound [46].

4.1.4 Main pitfalls

Infection: This is the main complication encountered in biological and biosynthetic dermal matrices. Integra® itself has an estimated infection rate of 16.9% [47]. Bacteria from contaminated wounds may feed on the biological components of Integra and similar matrices and cause infection. This can be limited by ensuring that the wound bed is thoroughly washed and debrided before the application of Integra. Appropriate systemic antibiotic therapy can also be used depending on the aetiology of the wound [48].

Hematoma/Seroma Formation: This occurs for similar reasons to hematoma and seroma formation in skin grafts and should be managed as such. Either by evacuating the blood/fluid with a 20G needle or by incising the Integra to evacuate the clot [48].

Two Stage Procedure: While there is a single stage Integra® product available, generally it is maintained that reconstruction with Integra requires two stages [49]. Prior to split thickness autografting, a neodermis must be formed in order for the graft to take. Patients require at least two procedures [50].

4.1.5 Clinical applications: Integra in full thickness scalp defects

Reconstruction of the scalp presents unique challenges due to the cutaneous tension of the area and the necessity to reconstruct with hair bearing skin. In full thickness scalp defects, reconstruction with a skin graft often results in patchy and scarred healing resulting in a poor aesthetic and functional outcome. Integra® has been reported in numerous studies to provide effective, aesthetic, and functional reconstruction of full thickness defects of the scalp. Systematic reviews of these studies found effective and robust wound coverage, even in patients who underwent radiotherapy prior to reconstruction [51]. Additionally, radiotherapy post reconstruction with Integra® was shown to be well tolerated. Finally, adjuvant techniques such as skull bone burring to encourage take as well as intraoperative fenestration of Integra® were shown to be effective in increasing reconstruction (**Figure 10**) [51].

4.1.6 Matriderm®

Matriderm® (Dr. Suwelack Skin and Health Care AG, Billerbeck, Germany) is a porous matrix made up of non cross-linked bovine collagen and elastin hydrolysate. It was developed in the late 1990s and made commercially available in 2004 for the cover of a variety of soft tissue wounds [52]. It is a single layer matrix and does not include an epidermal silicon layer. Matriderm costs USD 4.50/cm^2 [53].

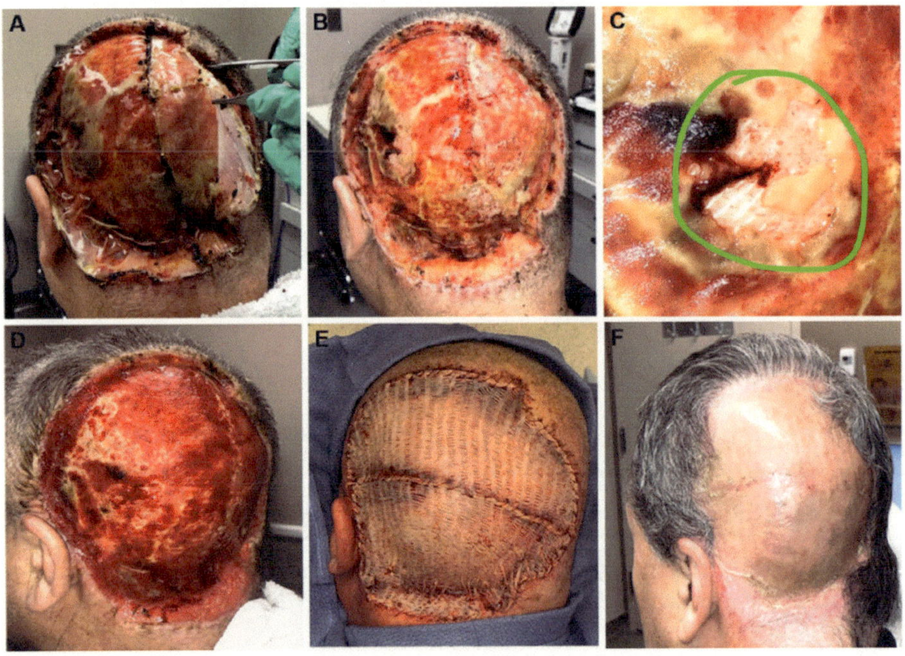

Figure 10.
Dermatofibrosarcoma excision and reconstruction with Integra® and SSG. (A) Large full-thickness scalp defect after dermatofibrosarcoma excision reconstructed with Integra. Silicone sheet removal 3 weeks after Integra placement. (B) Area of exposed bone with incomplete coverage with granulation tissue. (C) Close examination of the area reveals neovascularization of the bone. (D) The second layer of Integra placed. (E) Three weeks after second Integra placement, wound bed covered with a meshed skin graft. (F) Four months post-reconstruction. © {2021} {Yang S, Wu MS, Pittman AL}. Originally published in Plast Aesthet Res 2021 under CC BY 4.0 license. Available from: 10.20517/2347-9264.2021.40.

4.1.7 Biology

Matriderm® contains type I, III and IV collagen also derived from adult bovine calcaneal tendons as well as elastin hydrolysate. In addition to collagen, the elastin has been shown to improve wound healing by promoting early vascularisation. This encourages the migration of macrophages and fibroblasts involved in the process of wound healing, and also combats subclinical infection by the increased transportation of leukocytes to the wound bed [54].

A key difference between Matriderm® and other artificial biological matrices is that it contains collagen that is not cross linked, thereby increasing the absorption rate of the matrix into the native wound bed. This has three key benefits to wound reconstruction. Firstly, it reduces the time that a foreign matrix spends in the wound bed which provides less time for platelet aggregation, and therefore further reduces immunogenicity. Secondly, it allows for rapid formation of a neodermis through the absorption of collagen. Finally, and most distinctly, it allows for single stage wound healing (i.e. where the dermal matrix and a split thickness skin graft are applied in the one operation). Matriderm® is available in dermal matrix thicknesses of 1 and 2 mm with pore sizes between 18 and 34 microns, smaller on average than those of Integra® (**Figure 11**) [55].

4.1.8 Mechanism of action in single stage wound healing

Matriderm® may be used in a two-stage fashion in poorly vascularised wound beds or over exposed bare tendon or bone. In these instances, the mechanism of wound healing is similar to that of Integra®. The current concept on how Matriderm® works in a single staged fashion is as follows:

Imbibition: When a combination of Matriderm® and a skin graft are applied to the wound bed, diffusion provides the graft with oxygen. In the case of other dermal matrices such as Integra®, this process is not feasible as the graft cannot survive the usual 14 days for neovascularization to begin. This time constraint does not exist with Matriderm® [55].

Neovascularization: Due to the presence of elastin hydrolysate within Matriderm®, vascularisation can be seen as soon as 5 days post application. This promotes the rapid regeneration of dermis to support the skin graft and confers immunological defence to the wound. Rapid neovascularization of the wound bed is thought to be the key process underpinning the ability to perform single stage reconstruction with Matriderm® [55].

Remodelling: Matriderm® begins degrading by day 16 and is rapidly replaced by native dermis and extracellular matrix proteins [55].

The convenience and reduction in operative burden that single stage split skin grafting with Matriderm® offers in full thickness defects has been reported

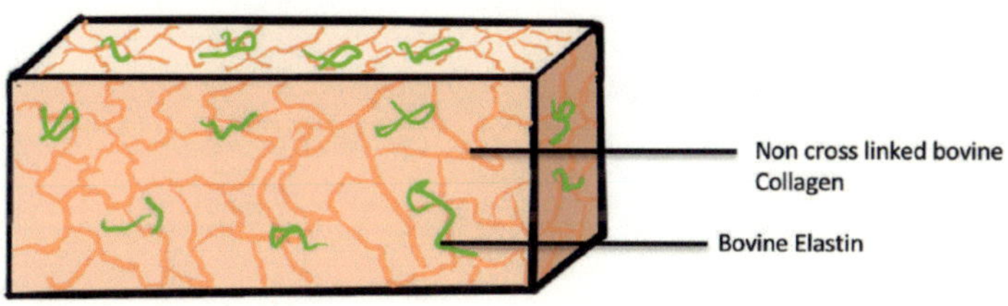

Figure 11.
Schematic of Matriderm®. Credit: AO.

numerous times. Cohort studies have demonstrated that single stage wound reconstruction is viable, effective and provides a cosmetic effect that is appreciated by patients [53]. Furthermore, in surgeons' experience, using Matriderm® with immediate skin grafting produces wound coverage with comparable robustness to delayed phase skin grafting [53].

More objectively, cohort studies in post-traumatic reconstruction have shown that Matriderm® provides re-epithelialisation 20% faster than skin grafting alone and a scar that is perceived to be better to statistical significance in: colour, contour, texture, appearance, and margins according to the Manchester Scar Scale [56].

4.1.9 Pitfalls

Outside of the regular complications of infection, haematoma, seroma, and immunogenicity, it must be noted that some studies suggest Matriderm® may be less robust compared to Integra® with regards to discoloration and wound contracture (**Figure 12**) [57].

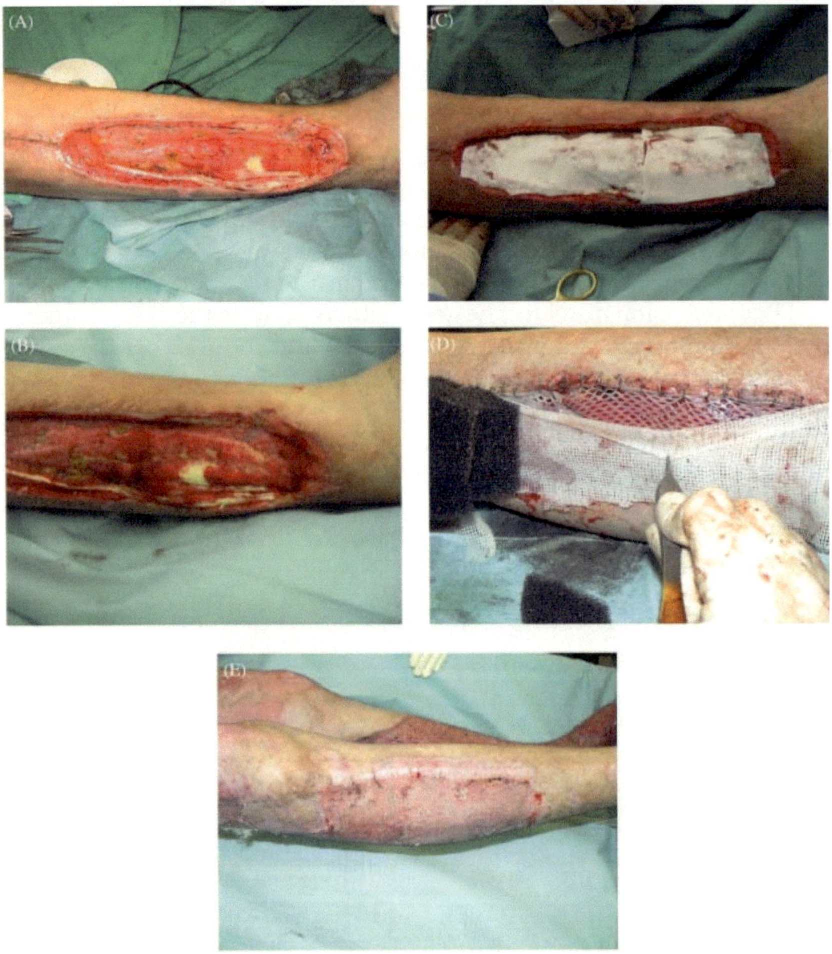

Figure 12.
34M with electrical burn to lateral lower leg has wounds successfully closed with single stage Matriderm + SSG. Courtesy: Ryssel et al. [53].

4.2 Cellularly enhanced synthetic matrix

4.2.1 Apligraf®

The cellular and immunological environment of the chronic wound (such as in venous and diabetic ulcers) differs considerably from those of acute wounds (such as burns, cancer excision and trauma). As such a skin substitute that behaves in a different way from those thus far examined may be necessary to heal the chronic non-healing wound. Departing from the paradigm of decellularized dermal substitutes is Apligraf® which is a bovine type I collagen-based skin substitute containing both human neonatal fibroblasts and keratinocytes (FDA approval 1998) [58]. It has been shown in multiple clinical trials to create low immunogenicity and be efficacious in the healing of chronic wounds. Beyond this, Apligraf® has a broad application in paediatric populations and in some acute wounds (**Figure 13**).

4.2.2 Biology

Apligraf® has the most intricate composition of the dermal matrices thus far discussed. The superficial epidermal layer contains living keratinocytes and epidermal stem cells. These are derived from neonatal foreskin and are able to actively signal to the native wound bed in order to encourage neovascularisation, proliferation, and wound healing. Furthermore, until a neo-epidermis is established, Apligraf® provides a near native temporary wound coverage. The deeper, dermal layer is similarly structured to resemble the native skin on which it is applied. It contains a template of type I bovine collagen with human fibroblasts which further encourages vascularisation and expedites the regeneration of the extracellular matrix in the dermis. Intuitive concerns with using cellular allogenic material in wound reconstruction surround immunogenicity which is antithetical to wound healing. To this end, Apligraf® has demonstrated low immunogenicity across multiple studies. There are two proposed reasons for this. Firstly, the use of neonatal cells which are often more immunologically naive as compared to adult cells minimises the risk of antigen recognition. Secondly, Apligraf® does not contain any immune cells such as Langerhans cells, dendritic cells, or monocytes, further reducing the possibility for antigen presentation and the mounting of an innate immune response [59]. As such the biologically intricate yet immunologically inert composition of Apligraf® allows for powerful cell signalling and fast wound healing without running a significant risk of rejection.

4.2.3 Mechanism of action in chronic wound healing

The cellular environment of the chronic wound is altered compared to the acute wound, with chronic inflammation creating resistance to wound healing.

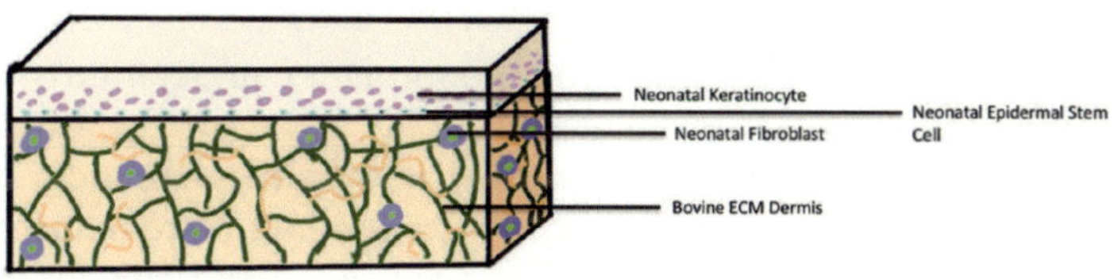

Figure 13.
Schematic of Apligraf®. Credit: AO.

This occurs due to a multitude of factors dependent on the aetiology of the chronic wound e.g. arterial vs. venous vs. diabetic ulcers. Nonetheless, failure of wound healing in chronic wounds can be generally conceptualised as four main processes of dysfunction.

1. Keratinocyte dysfunction: Keratinocytes found within venous ulcers and diabetic ulcers have been shown to have decreased rates of proliferation, increased senescence and reduced production of cytokines. This further hampers wound healing [60]

2. Imbalance of matrix metalloproteinases (MMP) to MMP inhibitor ratio: While MMPs are integral to wound healing, overproduction of these as seen in diabetic and venous ulcers leads to an inappropriate activation of inflammatory chemokines which halt the wound in the inflammatory stage and do not allow it to progress into proliferation [60].

3. General growth factor dysfunction: Chronic inflammation halts the production of TGF-beta and VEGF-alpha while also resulting in the receptors for growth factors becoming increasingly desensitised [60].

4. Increased fibrosis: Uncontrolled extracellular matrix deposition due to the unopposed action of myofibroblasts leads to fibrosis and inhibits proper wound healing [60].

Apligraf® targets these deficits in the following ways:

1. Dermal level: The addition of new fibroblasts found in Apligraf® begin to down-regulate cellular signalling pathways that cause fibrosis. This has been shown to reverse the level of fibrosis within a chronic wound and encourage the formation of new granulation tissue. Granulation tissue is a hallmark of acute wound healing. As such the fibroblast component acts to transform the chronic wound into an acute wound [60].

2. Epidermal level: Keratinocytes found in Apligraf® also signal to surrounding dysfunctional keratinocytes to proliferate and migrate. This results in the size of the wound edge decreasing until eventual closure [60].

As the wound heals, foreign cells found in Apligraf® are gradually replaced by native cells, having gained the ability for migration and revascularisation to the wound.

4.2.4 Pitfalls

Being a highly biological product with a predominant composition of cellular matter, Apligraf® is expensive to produce (USD \$28/cm^2) with a significantly short shelf life of 5 days after delivery. This necessitates a 'made to order' methodology and therefore limits the possibility of mass production to reduce the cost. Furthermore, Apligraf® is incredibly volatile once opened and must be used within 15 minutes of opening to prevent cell death, once again adding a time pressure to the reconstruction [61].

4.2.5 Clinical applications: Apligraf® in diabetic foot ulcer management

In addition to underlying chronic vascular, neuropathic and biochemical impairments caused by diabetes, the cellular environment of the chronic wound hampers the healing of a diabetic foot ulcer. Apligraf® claims to reduce the burden of the dysregulated cellular environment to wound healing. Comparative studies have demonstrated that the use of Apligraf® doubled the proportion of patients who achieved complete re-epithelialisation while also expediting the time taken for wound healing by 20% [62]. Another large scale multi-centre study confirmed these findings while also demonstrating that the difference between Apligraf® and traditional diabetic foot ulcer management is especially profound in the first 4 weeks of wound healing, with almost 10 times as many patients demonstrating effective wound healing within 4 weeks of Apligraf® application as compared to a control (**Figure 14**) [64].

5. Fully synthetic dermal matrices

Thus far, the suite of dermal matrices available to the reconstructive surgeon are vast. Xenografts provide extensive wound cover and protection from infection and desiccation but require definitive wound closure. Allografts have facilitated the advent of acellular dermal matrices which integrate into the wound and provide increased structure to the wound healing process yet still have issues of poor take and residual infection, immunogenicity and complex storage and handling requirements. Finally, semi synthetic matrices are effective and wide spanning in their use cases, representing the frontier of dermal substitution yet are hindered by cost and availability. Additionally, the use of animal products, whether bovine, porcine or human may spark religious or ethical concerns amongst patients, reducing overall acceptance of dermal matrices.

In these cases, a dermal matrix containing no biological products may prove advantageous. Currently three main products exist in this space: Novosorb® BTM (Polynovo®, Melbourne), Galaflex® (Galatea Surgical, MA) and TIGR Matrix® (Novus Scientific, Uppsala). This section will discuss the composition and mechanism of action of Novosorb® BTM, Galaflex® and TIGR Matrix®.

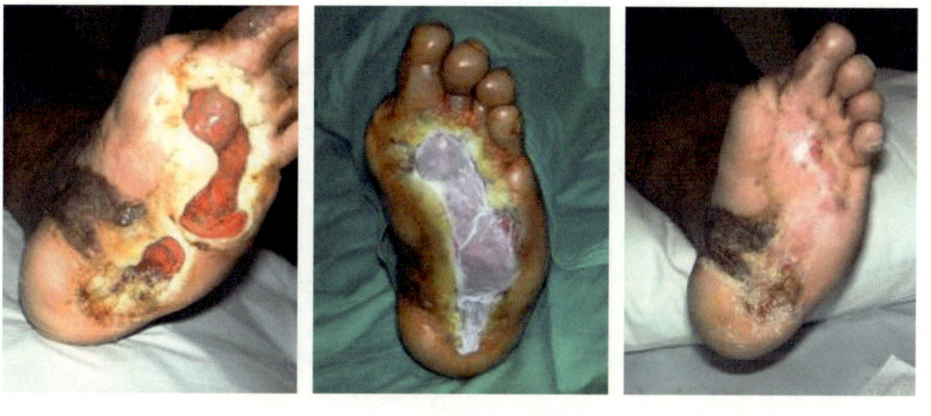

Figure 14.
Diabetic foot ulcer prior to Apligraf® application, upon Apligraf® application and after wound healing. Courtesy: Vowden et al. [63].

5.1 Novosorb® BTM

Novosorb® BTM (henceforth, BTM) was released by Polynovo® in 2018 (after receiving FDA approval in 2015) as a fully synthetic bi-layered dermal matrix for the management of full thickness burns. Since then, it has seen high volume widespread use in free flap donor site reconstruction, trauma, chronic ulcer as well as its original use case in burns [65]. Like many of the dermal matrices already discussed, its porous structure and epidermal layer allows for vascularisation and ingrowth of a neodermis to be contained within the dermal matrix area [6]. Being of completely synthetic origin, it has a high shelf life of at least 3 years and can be stored in temperatures of up to 25°C. Furthermore, it has been shown to display virtually no immunogenicity and when applied to a clean wound demonstrates low infection rates [65]. Cost per cm^2 of BTM is USD 10.50 (**Figure 15**) [66].

5.1.1 Composition and mechanism of action of BTM

Macroscopically, BTM consists of two layers to mimic the dermis and epidermis of native skin. The epidermal layer is made up of non-porous silicone which is non-biodegradable and is intended to be delaminated and grafted over once the neodermis is ready. The dermal layer is a porous foam made up of a biodegradable polymer known as polycaprolactone. Pore sizes are between 20 and 150 microns, dermal thickness options of 1 and 2 mm and a variety of sheet sizes are available [67].

Wound healing in BTM is similar to that of Integra with the key steps of fibroblast migration, revascularisation, extracellular matrix proliferation and delamination and skin grafting being retained. From a timeline perspective: within 2 weeks neovascularisation should be established and extracellular matrix proliferation should begin. The porous structure of BTM also prevents long contiguous strands of collagen being deposited, thereby limiting wound contracture and scarring. At 4–6 weeks, notwithstanding infection or other complications, the neodermis is ready. BTM may be delaminated and grafted [6].

A key advantage of the synthetic nature of BTM is its resistance to infection. While the exact underlying mechanism is thus far not identified, BTM has been shown to be used in cases of necrotising fasciitis and where the wound bed has not achieved culture proven sterility post infection to good effect. Clinicians often report BTM being 'undisturbed' by infection, facilitating the drainage of an infective collection while still encouraging wound healing [68].

5.1.2 Clinical application: Novosorb® BTM in challenging wounds

BTM has shown promise in complex and variable wound healing situations. Early reports have shown that BTM can be used over exposed tendon and bone where

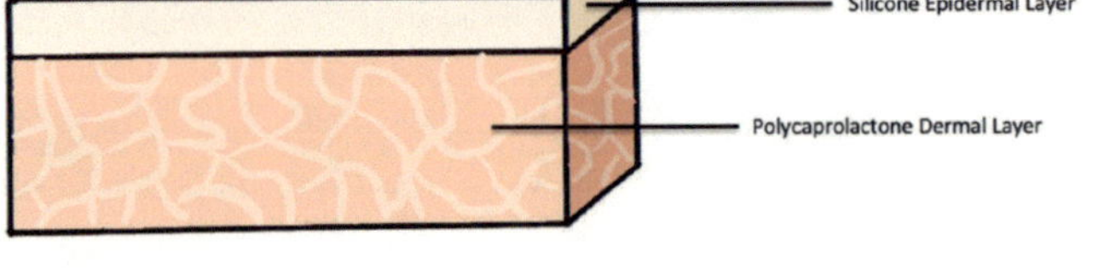

Figure 15.
Schematic of BTM. Credit: AO.

conventional split skin grafting has failed. This has positioned BTM as a staple matrix in the closure of wounds with exposed bone and tendon found in joint replacement and free flap donor sites such as the free fibular flap. In addition to its extensive use in orthopaedic surgeries and free flap donor site reconstruction, the entirely synthetic nature of BTM has been demonstrated in early case series to be unaffected by the presence of infection [69]. This resistance to infection is especially encouraging in cases of necrotising fasciitis, where a significant concern held by the reconstructive surgeon is the potential for recurrence of infection despite appropriate debridement. Emerging research shows that the use of BTM for dermal regeneration in necrotising fasciitis yields almost no skin graft loss once reconstruction is complete [68].

Aesthetic outcomes are also excellent with no range of motion deficit due to scarring reported (**Figure 16**) [68].

5.1.3 Galaflex®

Galaflex® (Galatea Surgical) is a similarly designed completely synthetic dermal matrix designed primarily for soft tissue support in reconstructive and aesthetic

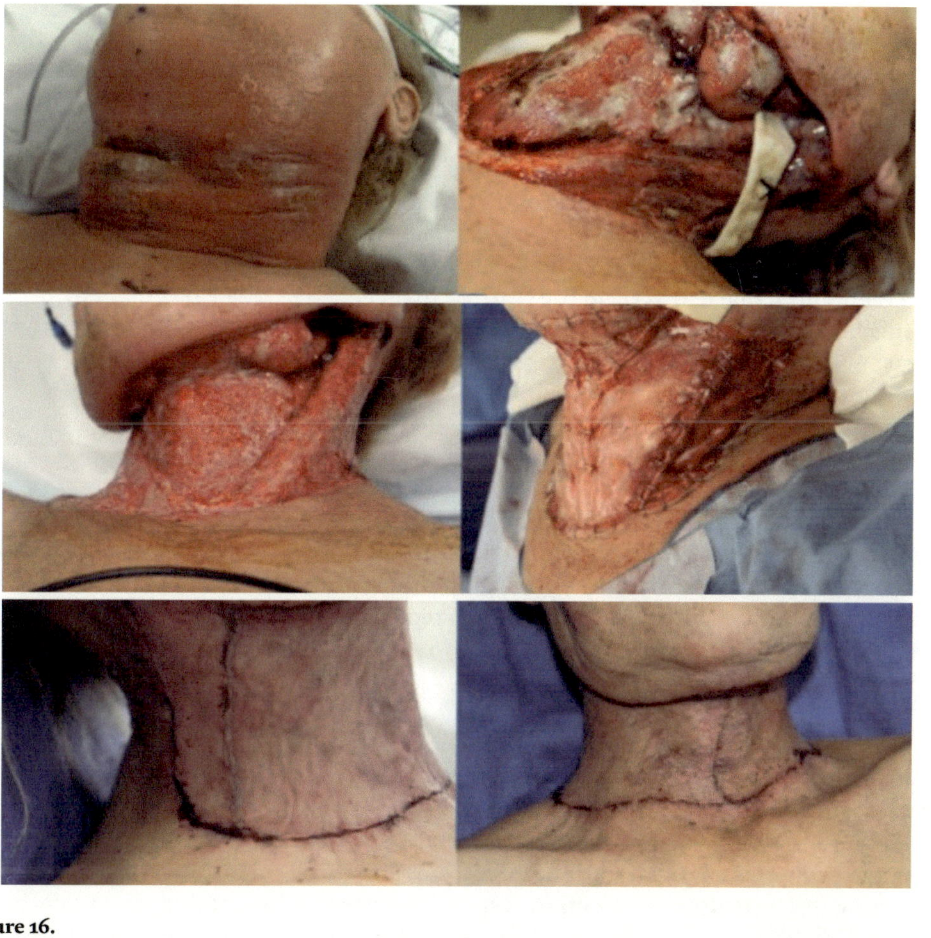

Figure 16.
Novosorb® BTM in the reconstruction of necrotising fasciitis of the neck. Courtesy: © 2017. Wagstaff MJ, Caplash Y, Greenwood JE. Originally published in Eplasty under the CC BY 3.0 license. Available from: PMID 28197297 [68].

surgeries. As such it is intended for internal use and does not have an epidermal layer and is completely biodegradable. It received FDA approval as a surgical mesh in 2014. It is comprised of a slightly different polymer, poly-4-hydroxybutyrate which has a half-life greater than that of polycaprolactone, consistent with its use as a soft tissue support [70]. It is an example of how dermal matrix technology, while initially designed for wound healing, can provide usefulness in a breadth of surgical applications.

5.1.4 TIGR® Matrix

TIGR® Matrix Surgical Mesh is a fully synthetic dermal matrix launched in 2010, after receiving FDA approval that year, by Novus Scientific in the Uppsala, Sweden [71]. The intent was to create a biocompatible polymer material that could stimulate functional connective tissue regeneration whilst avoiding a chronic inflammatory response [71]. Several indications have since been described, such as in abdominal wall repair and prosthetic breast reconstruction [71–74] as it is associated with low complication rates and cost [73–75].

TIGR® Matrix is a macroporous absorbable mesh constructed using a warp knitting technique from two different synthetic resorbable fibres [71]. These fibres are designed to degrade by bulk hydrolysis at different time frames to promote functional soft tissue remodelling via a process known as mechanotransduction [71]—a physiological process by which cells sense and respond to mechanical loads. Firstly, a fast-degrading fibre composed from a co-polymer of glycolide, lactide and trimethylene carbonate [71] provides a stable healing environment and reinforces the wound defect before losing its strength after 2 weeks [76]. Secondly, a slower-degrading fibre composed from a co-polymer lactide and trimethylene carbonate which has greater elastic properties promotes scar tissue remodelling and functional collagen regeneration through a transfer of mechanical load from the scaffold to regenerated tissue by gradually increasing mechanical compliance [71]. This mesh can maintain half of its initial strength for at least 6 months and is completely resorbed at approximately 3 years [71].

6. Future developments in dermal matrix technology

As the popularity of dermal matrices continues to grow and the boundaries of their potential surgical applications are explored, a critical imperative emerges. The need to further optimise dermal matrices and their properties become paramount to ascertain their definitive role within each reconstructive algorithm. Below are just some examples of the novel concepts currently being explored.

6.1 Source

Efforts to create viable alternatives to dermal matrices have been encouraging. Novel scaffolds such as decellularized adipose tissue or amniotic membrane which innately feature biological properties important for tissue engineering, such as the ability to promote cell proliferation, migration, and differentiation; whilst also inhibiting inflammatory or rejection responses, fibrosis and scarring, and microbial burden [77]. The possibility of creating an entirely synthetic composite graft generated from a fasciocutaneous flap design and dermal matrices show promise as an exciting potential substitute for human tissue.

6.2 Manufacturing process

The production of dermal matrices involves crucial modifications to its physicochemical properties, microstructure, biocompatibility, and functionality. Sterile pre-hydrated dermal matrices used for implant-based breast reconstruction improves post-operative breast texture, volume, and symmetry in comparison to freeze dried dermal matrices. Wound healing can be improved by cross-linking porcine dermal matrices with epoxidized natural polysaccharides to improve its thermal stability and hydrophilicity or with dialdehyde heparin to enhance its anticoagulant properties. Dermal matrices can also be drilled with micropore lasers to improve their permeability and promote cell adhesion and migration [78].

At a macroscopic level, one avenue under investigation is the physical form by which dermal matrices are produced. The most used is a sheet-type structure, but recently other forms are being explored. Paste-type micronised dermal matrices has been studied as an alternative material for soft tissue filler in tissue replacement and has been shown efficacy in human patients with diabetic foot ulcers to reduce the risk of recurrence and eliminate the need for skin grafts when combined with negative pressure wound therapy, demonstrating comparable or superior tissue incorporation and long-term structural integrity compared with sheet-type dermal matrices [79]. With respect to the physical properties, dermal matrices with smaller surface area have been associated with reduced risk of seroma and infection when used for direct-to-implant breast reconstruction. No difference was observed with thickness or manufacturer. Meanwhile, in rodent animal models for full thickness burn wounds, wound contracture and graft take was significantly worse when thicker ADM was applied, highlighting the importance of customisable dermal matrices.

6.3 Carrier potential

Another dynamic area of interest is the ability to impregnate the dermal matrix scaffold with endogenous or exogenous factors to promote better angiogenesis, facilitate improved tissue integration, and enhance reconstructive performance. Possibilities include the addition of autologous cells such as stem cells or dermal cells, cytokines such as IL-4, or endogenous molecules such as hyaluronic acid as well as antibiotics to reduce wound infection [80]. Furthermore, the incorporation of blood products such as platelet rich plasma (PRP) within an ADM has been shown to enhance matrix integration and dermal regeneration in a variety of settings such as, gingival recession [81] and Hidradenitis Suppurativa [82] in both animal [83] and human studies. Inorganic compounds can also be incorporated to provide beneficial properties, such as nano silver as an antibacterial agent or graphene oxide as a transplantation system for mesenchymal stem cells.

6.3.1 Intra-operative technique

The method of intra-operative use is another domain in which researchers have endeavoured to identify ways to reduce financial burdens and improve patient outcomes. Within breast reconstruction, dermal matrices can be manipulated using a kirigami strategy to ensure greater precision for moulding the sheet around the implant; or wrapped in a knitted Vicryl mesh to circumvent the need of tacking sutures. Both these methods have been identified to minimise both operative time and cost [84]. Biological barriers such as tyramine-substituted hyaluronan hydrogel coatings are also being developed to help mitigate premature graft degradation, such as the case with dermal matrix usage in ventral hernia repair [85].

7. Conclusion

The heterogeneity and variety of dermal matrices may be overwhelming to the reconstructive surgeon on first glance. However, their ontology may be explained by the diverse and ever challenging frontiers that wound healing present. Ultimately this chapter should provide both a panoramic view at the multifaceted nature of dermal matrices while also delving into the complexities of their cellular biology, immunology, and real-world applications.

Author details

Rohan Rajaram[1], Min Zhang[1], Smitha Segu[2] and Sally Kiu-Huen Ng[1*]

1 Department of Plastic and Reconstructive Surgery, Austin Health, Heidelberg, Victoria, Australia

2 Department of Plastic and Reconstructive Surgery, Bangalore Medical College and Research Institute, Bangalore, India

*Address all correspondence to: sally.ng@austin.org.au

References

[1] Shah JB. The history of wound care. The Journal of the American College of Certified Wound Specialists. 2011;**3**(3):65-66. DOI: 10.1016/j.jcws.2012.04.002

[2] Tran A, Desai S, Mraz RD. From ancient Egypt to the dermatologic office: An overview of skin substitutes and modern-day applications in dermatologic surgery. Health Science Reports. 2023;**6**(1):e1067. DOI: 10.1002/hsr2.1067

[3] Medicine in ancient Egypt: How did the pharaohs treat wounds and broken bones? EgyptToday. 2022;(January 12). Available from: https://www.egypttoday.com/Article/4/111766/Medicine-in-ancient-Egypt-How-did-the-pharaohs-treat-wounds [Accessed: January 22, 2024]

[4] Yamamoto T, Iwase H, King TW, Hara H, Cooper DKC. Skin xenotransplantation: Historical review and clinical potential. Burns. 2018;**44**(7):1738-1749. DOI: 10.1016/j.burns.2018.02.029

[5] Integra Life Sciences. Integra Overview. Integralife.com; 2020. Available from: https://www.integralife.com/integra-dermal-regeneration-template/product/wound-reconstruction-care-inpatient-acute-or-integra-dermal-regeneration-template [Accessed: January 22, 2020]

[6] Polynovo®. NovoSorb® BTM: Synthetic Polymer for Traumatic Wound Treatment. Australia: Novosorb BTM; 2022. Available from: https://polynovo.com/product-btm/ [Accessed: January 22, 2024]

[7] Shanmugam M, Sivakumar V, Anitha V, Sivakumar B. Clinical evaluation of alloderm for root coverage and colour match. Journal of Indian Society of Periodontology. 2012;**16**(2):218-223. DOI: 10.4103/0972-124X.99265

[8] Prohaska J, Cook C. Skin grafting. In: StatPearls. Treasure Island (FL): StatPearls Publishing; 2023

[9] Revised from Capla JM, Ceradini DJ, Tepper OM, et al. Skin graft vascularization involves precisely regulated regression and replacement of endothelial cells through both angiogenesis and vasculogenesis. Plastic and Reconstructive Surgery. 2006;**117**:836-844

[10] Wright KA, Nadire KB, Busto P, Tubo R, McPherson JM, Wentworth BM. Alternative delivery of keratinocytes using a polyurethane membrane and the implications for its use in the treatment of full-thickness burn injury. Burns. 1998;**24**(1):7-17. DOI: 10.1016/s0305-4179(97)00075-2

[11] Griesemer A, Yamada K, Sykes M. Xenotransplantation: Immunological hurdles and progress toward tolerance. Immunological Reviews. 2014;**258**(1):241-258. DOI: 10.1111/imr.12152

[12] Cadri S, Elrosasy A, Al Mawla AM, et al. The efficacy of Nile tilapia skin xenograft for treating superficial partial-thickness burn versus the standard of care: A meta-analysis of published trials. Archives of Dermatological Research. 2023;**316**(1):33. DOI: 10.1007/s00403-023-02755-7

[13] Deschamps JY, Roux FA, Saï P, Gouin E. History of xenotransplantation. Xenotransplantation. 2005;**12**(2):91-109. DOI: 10.1111/j.1399-3089.2004.00199.x

[14] Hermans MH. Porcine xenografts vs. (cryopreserved) allografts in the management of partial thickness burns: Is there a clinical difference? Burns. 2014;**40**(3):408-415. DOI: 10.1016/j.burns.2013.08.020

[15] Good AH, Cooper DK, Malcolm AJ, et al. Identification of carbohydrate structures that bind human antiporcine antibodies: Implications for discordant xenografting in humans. Transplantation Proceedings. 1992;**24**(2):559-562

[16] Cooper DK. Depletion of natural antibodies in non-human primates—A step towards successful discordant xenografting in humans. Clinical Transplantation. 1992;**6**(3 part 1):178-183

[17] Phelps CJ, Koike C, Vaught TD, et al. Production of alpha 1,3-galactosyltransferase-deficient pigs. Science. 2003;**299**(5605):411-414. DOI: 10.1126/science.1078942

[18] Irilouzadian R, Khalaji A, Baghsheikhi H, et al. The clinical outcomes of xenografts in the treatment of burn patients: A systematic review and meta-analysis. European Journal of Medical Research. 2023;**28**(1):524. DOI: 10.1186/s40001-023-01505-9

[19] Lima-Junior EM, de Moraes Filho MO, Costa BA, et al. Innovative treatment using tilapia skin as a xenograft for partial thickness burns after a gunpowder explosion. Journal of Surgical Case Reports. 2019;**2019**(6):rjz181. DOI: 10.1093/jscr/rjz181

[20] Salloum A, Bazzi N, Squires S, Chu T, Benedetto P, Benedetto A. Comparing the application of various engineered xenografts for skin defects: A systematic review. Journal of Cosmetic Dermatology. 2023;**22**(3):921-931. DOI: 10.1111/jocd.15517

[21] Baxter Professional. Veritas Brochure. Germany: Baxter Professional; 2017. Available from: https://www.baxterprofessional.de/system/files/2017-08/DE-Veritas_Broschuere.pdf [Accessed: February 19, 2024]

[22] Sun WQ, Xu H, Sandor M, Lombardi J. Process-induced extracellular matrix alterations affect the mechanisms of soft tissue repair and regeneration. Journal of Tissue Engineering. 2013;**4**:2041731413505305. DOI: 10.1177/2041731413505305

[23] Rastegarpour A, Cheung M, Vardhan M, Ibrahim MM, Butler CE, Levinson H. Surgical mesh for ventral incisional hernia repairs: Understanding mesh design. Plastic Surgery (Oakv). 2016;**24**(1):41-50. DOI: 10.4172/plastic-surgery.1000955

[24] Shieh MK. Use of bovine pericardium in complex hernia repair. Bariatric Times. 2011;**8**(8):14-16

[25] Gaertner WB, Bonsack ME, Delaney JP. Experimental evaluation of four biologic prostheses for ventral hernia repair. Journal of Gastrointestinal Surgery. 2007;**11**(10):1275-1285. DOI: 10.1007/s11605-007-0242-8

[26] Girnder JH. Skin grafting with grafts taken from the dead subject. Medical Record (1866-1922) New York. 1881;**20**(5):119

[27] Pianigiani E, Ierardi F, Cherubini Di Simplicio F, Andreassi A. Skin bank organization. Clinics in Dermatology. 2005;**23**(4):353-356. DOI: 10.1016/j.clindermatol.2004.07.016

[28] Kua EH, Goh CQ, Ting Y, Chua A, Song C. Comparing the use of glycerol preserved and cryopreserved allogenic skin for the treatment of severe burns: Differences in clinical outcomes and in

vitro tissue viability. Cell and Tissue Banking. 2012;**13**(2):269-279. DOI: 10.1007/s10561-011-9254-4

[29] Benichou G, Yamada Y, Yun SH, Lin C, Fray M, Tocco G. Immune recognition and rejection of allogeneic skin grafts. Immunotherapy. 2011;**3**(6):757-770. DOI: 10.2217/imt.11.2

[30] Introduction to AlloDerm Dermal Matrix. USA: AlloDerm RTM; 2019. Available from: https://hcp.alloderm.com/ [Accessed: January 22, 2024]

[31] Muratov R, Britikov D, Sachkov A, et al. New approach to reduce allograft tissue immunogenicity. Experimental data. Interactive Cardiovascular and Thoracic Surgery. 2019;**10**(3):408-412. DOI: 10.1510/icvts.2009.216549

[32] Mark Mofid M, Singh NK. Pocket conversion made easy: A simple technique using Alloderm to convert subglandular breast implants to the dual-plane position. Aesthetic Surgery Journal. 2009;**29**(1):12-18. DOI: 10.1016/j.asj.2008.12.005

[33] The Surgeon's Choice in ADMs-FlexHD. USA: FlexHD Pliable Products; 2019. Available from: https://www.mtfbiologics.org/flexhd?utm_source=Google&utm_medium=cpc&utm_campaign=mtf_google_ppc_prs_flexhd_2022247&utm_id=20556709403&utm_term=flexhd; [Accessed: January 22, 2024]

[34] Lu KW, Khachemoune A. Skin substitutes for the management of mohs micrographic surgery wounds: A systematic review. Archives of Dermatological Research. 2023;**315**:17-31. DOI: 10.1007/s00403-022-02327-1

[35] Development of a Novel Acellular Dermal Matrix (ADM) Designed Specifically for Plastic and Reconstructive Surgery. MTF Biologics Research & Development; 2019

[36] Cheng A, Saint-Cyr M. Comparison of different ADM materials in breast surgery. Clinics in Plastic Surgery. 2012;**39**(2):167-175. DOI: 10.1016/j.cps.2012.02.004

[37] Phan R, Lin F, White D. Local reaction to FlexHD® acellular dermal matrix in breast reconstruction: A case report and review of the literature. Australasian. Journal of Plastic Surgery. 2018;**1**:140-146

[38] Carminati M, Sempf D, Bonfirraro PP, Devalle L, Verga M, Righi B, et al. Immediate implant-based breast reconstruction with acellular dermal matrix compared with tissue-expander breast reconstruction: Rate of infection. Plastic and Reconstructive Surgery - Global Open;**6**(12):e1949

[39] James J, Jackson L, Saunders C. Florid pustular dermatitis of breast: A case report on a unusual complication from acellular dermal matrix use. International Journal of Surgery Case Reports. 2016;**22**:59-61. DOI: 10.1016/j.ijscr.2016.02.040

[40] Jansen LA, Macadam SA. The use of AlloDerm in postmastectomy alloplastic breast reconstruction: Part I. A systematic review. Plastic and Reconstructive Surgery. 2011;**127**(6):2232-2244. DOI: 10.1097/PRS.0b013e3182131c56

[41] Fosnot J, Kovach SJ, Scarlatti JM. Acellular dermal matrix: General principles for the plastic surgeon. Aesthetic Surgery Journal. 2011;**31**(Suppl. 7):5S-12S

[42] Breast Reconstruction with Acellular Dermal Matrix. USA: YouTube; 2018. Available from: https://www.youtube.

com/watch?v=hBN_wKswn6g [Accessed: January 22, 2024]

[43] Balaji VR, Ramakrishnan T, Manikandan D, et al. Management of gingival recession with acellular dermal matrix graft: A clinical study. Journal of Pharmacy & Bioallied Sciences. 2016;**8**(Suppl. 1):S59-S64. DOI: 10.4103/0975-7406.191970

[44] Chalmers RL, Smock E, Geh JL. Experience of Integra(®) in cancer reconstructive surgery. Journal of Plastic, Reconstructive & Aesthetic Surgery. 2010;**63**(12):2081-2090. DOI: 10.1016/j.bjps.2010.02.025

[45] Lei YH, Huang SH. Single-stage acellular dermal matrix reconstruction of defects in the nose and ears with exposed cartilage: A prospective case series. BMC Surgery. 2022;**22**:444. DOI: 10.1186/s12893-022-01859-7

[46] Taupin P, Gandhi A, Saini S. Integra® dermal regeneration template: From design to clinical use. Cureus. 2023;**15**(5):e38608. DOI: 10.7759/cureus.38608

[47] Chang DK, Louis MR, Gimenez A, Reece EM. The basics of Integra dermal regeneration template and its expanding clinical applications. Seminars in Plastic Surgery. 2019;**33**(3):185-189. DOI: 10.1055/s-0039-1693401

[48] Gonzalez SR, Wolter KG, Yuen JC. Infectious complications associated with the use of Integra: A systematic review of the literature. Plastic and Reconstructive Surgery. Global Open. 2020;**8**(7):e2869. DOI: 10.1097/GOX.0000000000002869

[49] Rudnicki PA, Purt B, True D, Siordia H, Lohmeier S, Chan RK. Single-stage composite skin reconstruction using a dermal regeneration template. Plastic and Reconstructive Surgery. Global Open. 2020;**8**(2):e2622. DOI: 10.1097/GOX.0000000000002622

[50] Nicoli F, Rampinelli I, Godwin Y. The application of Integra in a challenging context. Scars, Burns & Healing. 2016;**2**:2059513116672789. DOI: 10.1177/2059513116672789

[51] Johnson MB, Wong AK. Integra-based reconstruction of large scalp wounds: A case report and systematic review of the literature. Plastic and Reconstructive Surgery. Global Open. 2016;**4**(10):e1074. DOI: 10.1097/GOX.0000000000001074

[52] MATRIDERM® by MedSkin Solutions dr. suwelack. MatriDerm®—MedSkin Solutions Dr. Suwelack AG. 2021. Available from: https://matriderm.com/ [Accessed: January 22, 2024]

[53] Ryssel H, Radu CA, Germann G, Otte M, Gazyakan E. Single-stage Matriderm® and skin grafting as an alternative reconstruction in high-voltage injuries. International Wound Journal. 2010;**7**(5):385-392. DOI: 10.1111/j.1742-481X.2010.00703.x

[54] Min JH, Yun IS, Lew DH, Roh TS, Lee WJ. The use of matriderm and autologous skin graft in the treatment of full thickness skin defects. Archives of Plastic Surgery. 2021;**41**(4):330-336. DOI: 10.5999/aps.2014.41.4.330

[55] de Vries HJ, Middelkoop E, Mekkes JR, Dutrieux RP, Wildevuur CH, Westerhof H. Dermal regeneration in native non-cross-linked collagen sponges with different extracellular matrix molecules. Wound Repair and Regeneration. 1994;**2**(1):37-47. DOI: 10.1046/j.1524-475X.1994.20107.x

[56] Cervelli V, Brinci L, Spallone D, et al. The use of MatriDerm® and skin grafting in post-traumatic wounds. International

Wound Journal. 2011;**8**(4):400-405. DOI: 10.1111/j.1742-481X.2011.00806.x

[57] Choi JY, Kim SH, Oh GJ, Roh SG, Lee NH, Yang KM. Management of defects on lower extremities with the use of matriderm and skin graft. Archives of Plastic Surgery. 2014;**41**(4):337-343. DOI: 10.5999/aps.2014.41.4.337

[58] Apligraf. USA; 2018. Available from: https://apligraf.com/ [Accessed: January 22, 2024]

[59] Eaglstein WH, Alvarez OM, Auletta M, et al. Acute excisional wounds treated with a tissue-engineered skin (Apligraf). Dermatologic Surgery. 2018;**25**(3):195-201. DOI: 10.1046/j.1524-4725.1999.08186.x

[60] The Challenges of Healing Stalled VLUs and DFUs. USA: Apligraf; 2018. Available from: https://apligraf.com/challenges-of-healing-vlus-dfus/ [Accessed: January 22, 2024]

[61] Podiatry Today. USA: Apligraf; 2020. Available from: https://www.hmpgloballearningnetwork.com/site/podiatry/article/1771#:~:text=Apligraf%20is%20supplied%20as%20a,%241%2C000%20to%20%241%2C200%20per%20use [Accessed: January 22, 2024]

[62] Zaulyanov L, Kirsner RS. A review of a bi-layered living cell treatment (Apligraf) in the treatment of venous leg ulcers and diabetic foot ulcers. Clinical Interventions in Aging. 2020;**2**(1):93-98. DOI: 10.2147/ciia.2007.2.1.93

[63] Vowden K et al. Management of a Complex Neuropathic Foot Ulcer: A Case Report. 2002. Available from: http://www.worldwidewounds.com/2002/may/Vowden/Complex-Foot-Ulcer.html#bibliography [Accessed: January 22, 2024]

[64] Dinh TL, Veves A. The efficacy of Apligraf in the treatment of diabetic foot ulcers. Plastic and Reconstructive Surgery. 2006;**117**(Suppl. 7):152S-159S. DOI: 10.1097/01.prs.0000222534.79915.d3

[65] Li H, Lim P, Stanley E, et al. Experience with NovoSorb® Biodegradable Temporising Matrix in reconstruction of complex wounds. ANZ Journal of Surgery. 2021;**91**(9):1744-1750. DOI: 10.1111/ans.16936

[66] Patel NK, Tipps JA, Graham EM, Taylor JA, Mendenhall SD. Reconstruction of a near-total scalp avulsion with NovoSorb biodegradable temporizing matrix: Pediatric case report. Plastic and Reconstructive Surgery. Global Open. 2022;**10**(12):e4717. DOI: 10.1097/GOX.0000000000004717

[67] Li A, Dearman BL, Crompton KE, Moore TG, Greenwood JE. Evaluation of a novel biodegradable polymer for the generation of a dermal matrix. Journal of Burn Care & Research. 2009;**30**(4):717-728. DOI: 10.1097/BCR.0b013e3181abffca

[68] Wagstaff MJ, Caplash Y, Greenwood JE. Reconstruction of an anterior cervical necrotizing fasciitis defect using a biodegradable polyurethane dermal substitute. Eplasty. 2017;**17**:e3

[69] Lim P, Li H, Ng S. Novosorb® biodegradable temporising matrix (BTM) and its applications. Surgical Technology International. 2023

[70] Galaflex Surgical Scaffold: Strength from Within. Galatea Surgical; 2023. Available from: https://www.galateasurgical.com/surgical-scaffolds/galaflex-surgical-scaffold/ [Accessed: January 22, 2024]

[71] Novus Scientific. TIGR Matrix Development Story. Sweden: Novus

Scientific; 2024. Available from: https://novusscientific.com/us/tigr-matrix-product-information/tigr-matrix-development-story/ [Accessed: February 19, 2024]

[72] Hjort H, Mathisen T, Alves A, Clermont G, Boutrand JP. Three-year results from a preclinical implantation study of a long-term resorbable surgical mesh with time-dependent mechanical characteristics. Hernia. 2012;**16**(2):191-197. DOI: 10.1007/s10029-011-0885-y

[73] Hallberg H, Lewin R, Elander A, Hansson E. TIGR® matrix surgical mesh—A two-year follow-up study and complication analysis in 65 immediate breast reconstructions. Journal of Plastic Surgery and Hand Surgery. 2018;**52**(4):253-258. DOI: 10.1080/2000656X.2018.1478841

[74] Becker H, Lind JG 2nd. The use of synthetic mesh in reconstructive, revision, and cosmetic breast surgery. Aesthetic Plastic Surgery. 2013;**37**(5):914-921. DOI: 10.1007/s00266-013-0171-8

[75] Schrenk P. Immediate implant-based breast reconstruction using the TIGR® Matrix mesh. Future Medicine. 2016;**5**(2)

[76] Stephan B, Ramshaw B, Forman B. Value-based clinical quality improvement (CQI) for patients undergoing abdominal wall reconstruction. Surgical Technology International. 2015;**26**:135-142

[77] Yu C, Bianco J, Brown C, Fuetterer L, Watkins JF, Samani A, et al. Porous decellularized adipose tissue foams for soft tissue regeneration. Biomaterials. 2013;**34**(13):3290-3302

[78] Park KC. Comparative analysis of sterile freeze-dried versus sterile pre-hydration acellular dermal matrix in implant-based breast reconstruction. Aesthetic Plastic Surgery. 2023;**47**(5):1671-1677

[79] Feng R. Crosslinking of dialdehyde heparin: A new strategy for improving the anticoagulant properties of porcine acellular dermal matrix. RSC Advances. 2022;**12**(11):6811-6820

[80] Wang Z. Single-stage transplantation combined with epidermal stem cells promotes the survival of tissue-engineered skin by inducing early angiogenesis. Stem Cell Research & Therapy. 2023;**14**(1):51

[81] Çetiner D, Gökalp Kalabay P, Özdemir B, Çankaya ZT. Efficiency of platelet-rich plasma on acellular dermal matrix application with coronally advanced flap in the treatment of multiple adjacent gingival recessions: A randomized controlled clinical trial. Journal of Dental Sciences. 2018;**13**(3):198-206. DOI: 10.1016/j.jds.2017.11.002

[82] Gierek M, Klama-Baryła A, Łabuś W, Bergler-Czop B, Pietrauszka K, Niemiec P. Platelet-rich plasma and acellular dermal matrix in the surgical treatment of hidradenitis suppurativa: A comparative retrospective study. Journal of Clinical Medicine. 2023;**12**(6):2112. DOI: 10.3390/jcm12062112

[83] Araujo-Gutierrez R, Van Eps JL, Scherba JC, et al. Platelet rich plasma concentration improves biologic mesh incorporation and decreases multinucleated giant cells in a dose dependent fashion. Journal of Tissue Engineering and Regenerative Medicine. 2021;**15**(11):1037-1046. DOI: 10.1002/term.3247

[84] Lee YJ. Natural shaping of acellular dermal matrices for implant-based breast reconstruction via Expansile Kirigami. Advanced Materials. 2023;**35**(6):e2208088

[85] Mookerjee VG. Single stitch vicryl mesh wrap for prepectoral implant breast reconstruction. Plastic and Reconstructive Surgery. Global Open. 2023;**11**(6):e5058

Chapter 8

Innovative Biologic Dressings for Neonatal and Pediatric Wounds

Vita Boyar

Abstract

The landscape of neonatal and pediatric care has changed dramatically in the last decade. As more immature and critically ill neonates survive, newer treatments are offered, innovative approaches are tried and novel medications are developed. The growth and capabilities of clinical care have exploded, but with those, new complications in the care of neonatal and pediatric skin have surfaced. The intricacies of neonatal skin development are many. Birth and survival of extremely premature and critically ill infants facilitated the development of wounds of "immaturity" and wounds of "critical illness" such as extravasations, ostomies, and pressure injuries (PI) related to medical devices. Surgical wound dehiscence has become a familiar entity in neonatal units, as treatments for critical, previously incompatible-with-life conditions offer surgical hope every day. Understanding of pathophysiology of neonatal wounds, challenges in healing, nuances of treatment product compatibility, and safety can guide optimal care pathways. This chapter will offer a discussion on the common neonatal and pediatric wounds, healing stages, and approaches to safe and effective wound healing products, including amniotic membranes and umbilical cord dressings, collagen products, and fish skin grafts.

Keywords: pediatrics, neonate, wound healing, collagen products, umbilical membranes, fish skin graft

1. Introduction

We live in the era of cell therapies renaissance in neonatal and pediatric medicine. Cell therapies do not always imply multipotent "stem" cells, but any biological precursors that have the potential to repair and grow body tissues. Discoveries in the regenerative medicine field identified various components of tissues as an effective therapy to induce the generation and differentiation of cells. These cells can be sourced from many sources, including human and mammalian tissues or synthetic, laboratory-grown preparations. Amniotic membranes and umbilical cord tissues, mammalian, piscine, or synthetic collagens combinations, or fish skin grafts offer new horizons in modern wound care. Research in the regenerative and anti-inflammatory capabilities of these tissues extends into the neonatal lung, brain, and gastrointestinal injury arena. Many are promising to change the trajectory of neonatal medicine but are investigational at this point. However, cutaneous applications of these therapies have been widespread in the adult wound arena and have gained acceptance in the pediatric and neonatal wound community.

The landscape of neonatal care has changed dramatically in the last decade. As more immature and critically ill neonates survive, newer treatments are offered, innovative approaches are tried and novel medications are developed. The growth and capabilities of neonatal care have exploded, but with those, new complications and old inadequacies have come to the surface. The intricacies of neonatal skin development are many. Birth and survival of extremely premature and critically ill infants facilitated the development of wounds of "immaturity" such as medical adhesive related skin injury (MARSI), peripheral venous catheters (PIV) extravasations (PIVE), and wounds of "critical illness" such as pressure injuries (PI) related to medical devices and life-threatening conditions [1–4]. Surgical wound dehiscence has become a familiar entity in neonatal units. Conditions necessitating gastrostomy, tracheostomy, and intestinal stoma placement have propelled the enterostomal field forward, but have left the neonatal products manufacturers trailing behind. On the flip side of that, care for congenital conditions such as epidermolysis bullosa, ichthyosis, aplasia cutis congenita, and omphalocele have evolved tremendously over the last decade. Understanding of pathophysiology of neonatal wounds, challenges in healing, nuances of treatment product compatibility, and safety can guide optimal care pathways. This chapter will offer a discussion on common neonatal and pediatric wounds, healing stages, and approaches to safe and effective wound healing products, including amniotic membranes and umbilical cord grafts, collagen products, and fish skin grafts.

2. Neonatal skin

Skin is the largest organ and, in a neonate, the one injured the most frequently. Preterm neonatal skin is poorly prepared for the transition to the dry, cool, organism-rich outside environment. The stratum corneum (SC) layer is barely present, leading to increased transepidermal water loss, electrolyte and temperature fluctuations, increased transcutaneous absorption of caustic substances, decreased protection from microbes as acid mantle takes time to develop, and increased susceptibility to dermatitis [1–6]. Unlike a full-term infant's skin, preterm skin lacks vernix, important for the formation of the acid mantle, hydration via fatty acids donation, and provision of an antimicrobial barrier. SC cell cohesiveness, important for preventing mechanical trauma, is lacking. Fewer dermal/epidermal fibrils connect the layers, leading to stronger adhesion between the epidermis and an outer dressing than between the dermal/epidermal bond [1–6]. The dermis is 30% of adult thickness, with minimal subcutaneous fat support. These characteristics amplify the risks for pressure injury and extravasations. Absorption of transcutaneous substances is greater in neonates, leading to a concern of toxicity and suppression of cellular growth, often rendering topical products unsafe or simply not studied and therefore not used in the neonatal population [1–7].

Infants treated in the neonatal intensive care unit (NICU) are at increased risk of bacterial colonization [8]. Birth via cesarian section predisposes skin to colonization by pathogenic bacteria [8]. Prolonged exposure to antibiotics and invasive devices changes the microbiome milieu, supporting pathogenic microbes' growth [8–10]. Critical illness, suboptimal nutrient intake, and hypercatabolic state decrease calorie and protein available for wound healing. In addition, many neonates are deficient in vitamins and trace elements such as zinc, copper, and selenium [11–15]. Their frequent exposure to oxygen and lack of adequate oxygen radicals' scavengers leaves tissues exposed to radical damage and inflammation.

3. Neonatal skin injuries

3.1 Medical adhesive related skin injury (MARSI)

Advancements in technology and survival led to the increasing number of gadgets and monitoring devices placed on tiny neonatal bodies. Removal and attachment of adhesive products happens many times a day, leading to a prevalence of MARSI up to 40% in neonatal units [16–20]. Epidermal stripping, skin tears, and irritant contact dermatitis dominate this class of injuries, but tension blisters, allergic contact dermatitis, and maceration have been reported as well [16, 17]. In 2001 an evidence-based practice project determined that adhesive removal was the primary cause of neonatal skin breakdown, with tape removal contributing 17% of all injuries [17–20]. A consensus statement on MARSI was published in 2013, including risk factors and prevention guidance [16]. A variety of papers have addressed neonatal MARSI. Functional and structural immaturity of the skin is the most important factor predisposing to MARSI [18–20]. Yet, because adhesives are so widespread, familiar, and necessary, caregivers fail to recognize the imminent danger they represent; 10–15% of neonatal graduates leave the NICUs with a scar; approximately 15% are functionally and cosmetically significant.

Epidermal stripping is a subtype of MARSI. Studies have documented those certain dressings (films with acrylate adhesives and hydrocolloids) increase the risk of epidermal stripping [16–19]. Silicone-based is the only atraumatic dressing on the market; it should be used as much as possible in the neonatal population [16]. Few products mitigate the risk for MARSI. A nonalcoholic liquid skin barrier may provide a protective layer between epidermal and adhesives as well as minimize irritation from caustic substances, and bonding agents should not be used in the neonatal population. These agents can increase epidermal stripping, and cases of skin necrosis have been described. A silicone-based adhesive remover should be used with all adhesives; it releases the adhesive bond without leaving the residue (the downfall of oil-based solvent or the toxicity of alcohol-based one), allowing immediate dressing repositioning if desired or complete removal without pain and injury to the SC [17–19]. Techniques of dressing removal, such as stabilizing the skin and rolling tape/dressing on itself may lessen MARSI [16, 17]. Finally, awareness and understanding of the risks of MARSI, along with an emphasis on prevention reduces these injuries.

3.2 Peripheral intravenous vascular extravasation (PIVE)

Peripheral intravenous vascular catheter placement is the most common procedure performed in the neonatal intensive care unit, yet over 60% of PIV catheters are removed before their intended time due to complications such as occlusion, dislodgement, leaking, phlebitis, infiltration, or extravasation. Up to 70% are reported to be infiltrations and up to 25% are extravasations [21]. Infusion Nurses Society defines extravasation as an inadvertent administration of a vesicant solution or medication that causes the formation of blisters leading to tissue apoptosis or necrosis, whereas infiltration causes damage via hypoxia and mass effect, eventually leading to tissue necrosis [22, 23]. Neonates are at increased risk for extravasations. Immature skin, lack of robust subcutaneous tissue, small vessel diameter, disadvantaged site of IV placement (joint), and inability to verbalize pain are just a few factors [23, 24]. The nature of infuscate neonates receives places them at risk every day. Vesicants injure endothelial cells through direct medication effects, increased osmolality, poor solubility, and non-neutral pH [21–24]. Once injured, cells trigger an inflammatory cascade by releasing oxygen radicals and pro-inflammatory cytokines. Preterm neonates and sick children are not able to counterbalance this process due to ongoing hypoxemia, mitochondrial injury, lack of energy resources, and limited oxygen radicals' scavengers. A vicious cycle leads to cellular apoptosis and necrosis, skin, and soft tissue injury, leading to partial or full-thickness wounds [21–24]. Wound development following PIVE occurs in about 6% [21–23].

3.3 Pressure injury

Skin is one of the most underdeveloped organs in neonates and, therefore least prepared to withstand the effects of multiple forces exerted by devices. PI due to intrinsic factors (such as immobility, nutrition, and perfusion) are fairly uncommon in neonates. The majority of PI are device-related and non-invasive respiratory devices are most commonly involved [25–29]. These injuries are followed by injuries from the PIV hub, oxygen saturation probe, and electroencephalography lead [25, 27]. The most common areas injured in neonates as a result of a medical device are the nose and its surrounding area [28]. Transmitted pressure leads to deformation of the cellular cytoskeleton as well as obstructed blood flow, ischemia, further inflammation, and cell death [28]. The sensation can be diminished in the tiniest and sickest babies, and so is mobility as special developmental positioners limit body and head movement. National and international agencies have recommended various bundle elements to reduce PI in general and device-specific PI [29]. Literature questions the utility of available PI skin assessment scales and their ability to statistically prevent pediatric PI occurrence [30]. This translates into the importance of clinical risk understanding. National Pressure Injury Advisory Panel states that all patients with medical devices are considered at risk; certain clinical scenarios (intubation, hypotension, edema, sepsis) multiply the risk [1]. Preventative measures are at the forefront of pediatric PI eradication. Once developed, pressure wounds are treated as wounds from other etiologies.

3.4 Surgical wounds

Surgical wounds in neonates are often a consequence of immaturity, such as dehisced wounds after necrotizing enterocolitis, ostomies due to congenital and acquired conditions, and unanticipated complications following congenital defects repairs. Dehisced wounds are always concerning for developing surgical site infection and optimal wound preparation is required. Effective debridement means biofilm removal and prevention of further formation, followed by antimicrobial coverage, appropriate packing, moisture balance, and protection from the outside environment. Deeper and slow-healing wounds are not uncommon in the high acuity intensive care units. Understanding of cells important in healing stages enhances care and appropriate product selection for these patients.

4. Wound healing stages

Despite the functional and structural immaturity of neonatal skin, the physiologic principles of wound healing are similar along the age continuum. Healing wounds evolve through four distinct dynamic and intertwined stages of healing [31]. Stage 1 starts with hemostasis. Hemostasis is initiated through the activation of a coagulation cascade, attracting various cells, and releasing cytokines as chemical messengers. Platelets are paramount for the fibrin plug formation, local vasodilation, differentiation of cells, and release of chemoattractants. Chemoattractants such as epidermal growth factor, fibroblast growth factor, insulin-like growth factor, and keratinocyte growth factor are instrumental in facilitating the beginning of the inflammatory stage (stage2) and targeted cell movement within the wound in addition to the targeted cellular differentiation [31, 32]. Vasoactive substances such as bradykinin, serotonin, and prostaglandins increase endothelial permeability and cell influx [31, 32]. Cell-to-cell communication and cytokines attract neutrophils, monocytes, and lymphocytes. These cells debride the area from the bacteria, dead cells, and inflammatory milieu. In addition, monocytes differentiate into macrophages, ensuring optimal pro-inflammatory/anti-inflammatory macrophage subtypes ratio. The macrophage becomes the main cell to orchestrate the transition between inflammatory and stage 3, the proliferative stage [31, 32]. Many ancillary chemokines affect this stage. For example, omega-6 polyunsaturated fatty acids intermediates such as linoleic acid, arachidonic acid, leukotrienes, and endothelin are integral in pro-inflammatory chemokines communication. Concomitantly anti-inflammatory omega-3 pathway mediators, such as eicosapentaenoic and docosahexaenoic acids increase over time, leading the wound to the proliferative stage. As the inflammatory stage progresses macrophages signal an influx of fibroblasts and endothelial growth factors; together they facilitate collagen production, and vascular growth, mediated by the production of nitric oxide. The proliferation stage starts with the extracellular matrix deposition via granulation tissue and angiogenesis. Along with the above-mentioned cells, chemokines, growth factors, and matrix elements (such as elastin, hyaluronic acid, proteoglycans, and fibronectin) orchestrate the new tissue formation [31, 32]. Adequate energy and protein building blocks are essential in this stage, together with communication co-factors such as vitamin C, vitamin B, iron, zinc, and copper. Optimal oxygen delivery promotes angiogenesis. Antioxidants and anti-inflammatory mediators are delivered continuously to the area, removing oxygen radicals, pro-inflammatory mediators, and excessive matrix metalloproteinases. Micronutrients such as selenium and Vitamin E are integral for this and inflammatory stages, especially in patients who do not have an adequate supply of superoxide dismutase and other oxygen radical scavengers. As the proliferation stage progresses, the new epithelial tissue growth over the granulation tissue signals the beginning of the final stage- remodeling. Remodeling can last months, ensuring collagen transformation toward mostly type 1 and 3, wound contraction, and scar tissue thinning by selective apoptosis of the described cells [31, 32]. The injured area will not have the same tensile strength as once intact tissue, but the remodeling stage ensures the optimal capacity the tissue can obtain.

Clinical implications of understanding these stages are essential. It is well documented that slowly healing wounds tend to have delayed inflammatory and/or proliferative stages. Such wounds may benefit from a scaffold for the ingrowing cells, exogenous matrix components, growth factors and at times anti-inflammatory mediators as slowly healing wounds may show an overabundance of matrix proteases or may need of a proliferative boost.

4.1 Wound care management

Comprehensive and holistic approach to wound care is recommended. All wounds should be assessed for the debridement need. While sharp debridement is non-specific, painful and rarely performed in pediatrics, the mechanical, enzymatic and autolytic types are common. For wounds with minimal slough I use medical grade honey, surfactant-based gel and rarely hydrogel. I favor medical honey gel for its acidic, hyperosmolar properties, anti-bacterial action and concomitant extracellular matrix growth inducer. Enzymatic collagenase ointment is a potent and safe debrider, especially when thicker slough or eschar is encountered. Finally, mechanical debridement with a monofilament fiber pad or lolly is an effective, quick and relatively painless option when scrubbing is considered. The product needs to be copiously moistened with normal saline, although I often use stabilized hypochlorous acid as my moisture. Hypochlorous acid is non-cytotoxic, gentle and safe. All debridement products I use are safe even in the smallest preterm neonates.

Neonatal and pediatric wound care is a relatively young field. Standard-of-care is mostly established from many case series, opinion leaders and somewhat recently from the societal guidelines. Prior to cellular therapies, packing with hydrogel, hydrofiber, silver-based products and recently medical honey has been the standard. The last decade brought an increased use of NPWT both single-use and canister based. While all the products mentioned are still the standard-of-care in many pediatric practices, newer, advanced therapies are changing the landscape of what pediatric wound doctors are using as their first choice now. Atraumatic wound dressings, NPWT and other supportive measures are out of scope of this chapter.

5. Advanced wound care products

5.1 Collagen

Collagen, produced by fibroblasts, accounts for 30% of the protein in humans and 77% of the dry weight of the skin. Collagen molecules are composed of 3 polypeptide chains that are aligned in a parallel manner and coiled in a left-handed helix. Types 1, 2, 3, 5, and 11 collagens have fibrillary quaternary structures. Type 1 collagen is the most abundant type in animals and most often used in medicine [33, 34, 36].

Collagen is paramount for the healing cascade, stimulating cellular migration in inflammatory and proliferative stages, contributing to the extracellular matrix, and ensuring tissue elasticity and strength in the regenerative stage [35]. Natural collagens can be prepared in many ways, but overall belong to two categories: a decellularized matrix that maintains original tissue properties and extracellular structure or a collagen scaffold prepared by extraction, purification, or polymerization [36, 37]. Collagen dressings take form as sponges, powders, gels, films, membranes or collagen–impregnated cellulose dressings, as well as varieties of skin substitutes auto and allografts [33–37].

5.2 Use of collagen in wounds

Challenges in neonatal or pediatric wound's proliferative stage may stem from insufficient amino acids and therefore protein and collagen secondary to frequent hypercatabolic or hyperproliferative state. Most critically ill neonates have increased protein consumption due to ongoing growth, losses (renal disease, congenital heart disease and ostomy patients), cellular differentiation, pro- and anti-inflammatory mediators' formation, and at times inadequate provision. Most pediatric wounds can benefit from collagen dressing. Given the patient's small size and at times challenging location of these wounds, collagen gel or powder preparations can be advantageous in application. Wounds with larger wound beds and an easier placement benefit from classic dressing varieties. Most neonatal practitioners use pure collagen preparations, without antimicrobial additives as systemic absorption of additive substances through the immature neonatal skin can be significant.

In my neonatal practice, most wounds respond well to collagen products. Clinically, I see faster and more robust extracellular matrix deposition compared to plain packing or application of hydrogel or medical-grade honey. Appropriate gentle debridement must take place first as wound bed slough slows down ECM growth. A combination of collagen with NPWT works well with dehisced surgical wounds.

Adult and pediatric literature has reported improved outcomes with various collagen preparations, including gels, sheets, and powders. Product versatility, faster healing rates due to the immediate bioavailability and expedited cellular matrix incorporation, and robust fibroblast response are cited [33–37]. This becomes important as the recruitment of fibroblasts, the cells dominant in the proliferative phase of normal wound healing, can be retarded [35]. In addition, the expression of the collagen gene in some fibroblasts can be suppressed [36]. Collagen products diminish the inflammatory process and decrease matrix metalloprotease destruction of the native intact collagen in the ECM [36, 37].

Case 1 illustrates a dehisced thoracic wound. This patient was born with congenital heart disease and needed a repair at 1 week of age. His wound dehisced by 5 days (**Figure 1A**). After gentle debridement and decolonization with medical- grade honey for 2 days, collagen gel was applied and covered by portable NPWT. **Figure 2B** illustrates the wound after 2 applications on Day 3 and Day 9. Robust ECM is appreciated. Collagen gel was reapplied on Days 10 and 15 (**Figure 1C**). The wound was completely closed in 3 weeks.

Extravasation wounds can be deep in neonates. Collagen dressings offer scaffold to exogenous cells and afford faster healing compared to common management with hydrogel or medical grade honey and secondary dressings. Case 2 shows severe extravasation (**Figure 2A**) that was deep (once the eschar was debrided) and slow to heal. Using collagen powder allowed for easy and precise application (**Figure 2B** and **C**). This wound took 3 weeks to heal, but as you can see on the follow-up 1 month later the scar is soft, pliable, and no limitation of motion despite the location over a wrist joint (**Figure 2D**).

5.3 Amniotic membranes (AM) and umbilical cord (UC)-based dressings

The fetal membrane is the original cell-based biologic scaffold that is well suited to integrate with the host tissue and provide an optimal environment for cell growth and differentiation. The main mechanisms of action in animals seem to be immune

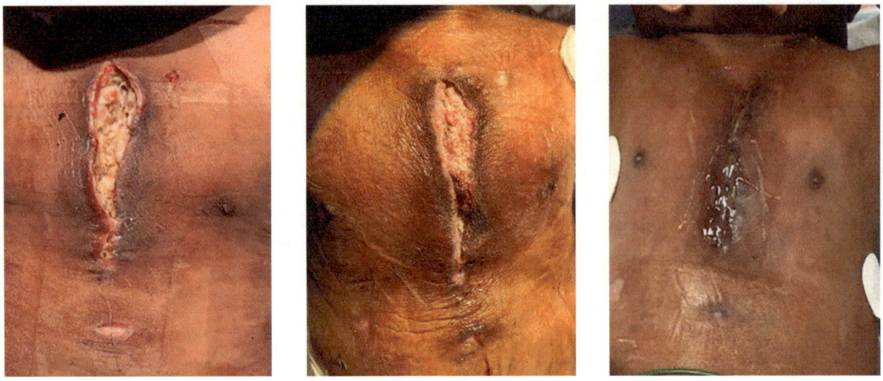

Figure 1.
A. Dehisced thoracic wound in a full term, now 2 weeks old neonate. Wound was colonized with MSSA and had slough over the wound bed. After decolonization and debridement, collagen gel was applied under NPWT. B. 11 days later wound is contracting and granulation tissue is appreciated. Wound had 2 applications of collagen gel and portable NPWT. C. Day 15. Collagen gel is applied under a secondary silicon-based dressing as wound is almost fully closed.

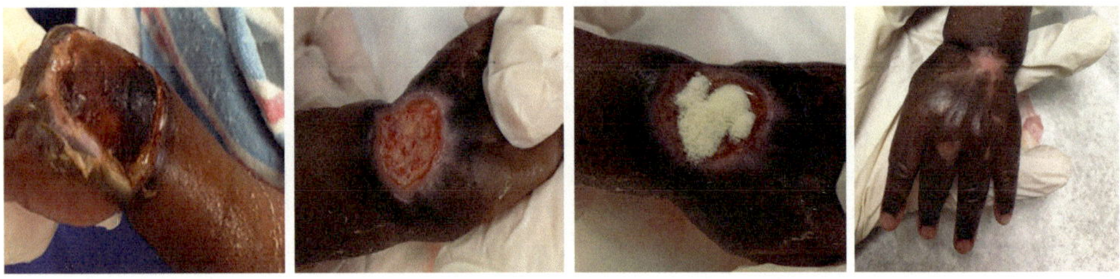

Figure 2.
A. Appearance of an eschar from severe peripheral intravenous extravasation. Once debrided, deep thickness wound through the dermis was appreciated. B and C. Collagen powder was applied every 5 days. D. Soft scar with minimal pigmentation loss. Full range-of-motion of the wrist was appreciated at 1-month follow-up clinic visit, despite location over a joint.

modulation, pro-angiogenic, anti-oxidant, anti-fibrotic, and pro-fibroblast growth. Lack of graft vs. host reaction and human leukocyte antigens immunization makes this product ideal in preterm neonates and critically ill children, where strong immune responses may cause systemic instability. First introduced in 1910 for skin transplantation, it was subsequently found to be useful in the management of burns, and diabetic ulcers, the creation of surgical dressings, and the reconstruction of various tissues [38].

The fetal membranes are composed of two layers: the outer chorion that is in contact with maternal tissue and the thin, avascular inner amniotic membrane that surrounds the embryo. Amnion has 5 layers: epithelium, basement membrane, compact layer, fibroblast layer, and spongy layer. Amniotic epithelial cells produce essential growth factors for epithelization, including epidermal growth factor (EGF), transforming growth factor-a (TGF-a), keratinocyte growth factor, hepatocyte growth factor, nerve growth factor (NGF) and brain-derived neurotrophic factor (BDNF) in addition to transforming growth factor-b (TGF-b) and basic fibroblast growth factor (bFGF), important for angiogenesis.

The epithelium sits on a basement membrane (BM), which is the most pertinent structural part of the amnion from the perspective of application in wound healing. The organizational framework of the basement membrane, provided by the ECM, contains not only an intricate network of macromolecules produced and assembled by surrounding cells but also numerous growth factors along with collagens, laminins, nidogen-1 and 2, fibronectin, fibulin-2, fibrillin-2, perlecan, and agrin. Collagen in BM decreases microbial accumulation, along with cystatin-E, an anti-infective inhibitor, and beta 3-defensin, an antimicrobial peptide [38–41]. Additionally, many growth factors are found within basal membrane ECM. ECM also contains fibroblasts and neonatal mesenchymal cells (MSCs). MSCs release soluble factors that stimulate proliferation and migration within the wound [39, 40]. MSCs also provide anti-scarring properties via stimulation of the release of vascular endothelial growth factor (VEGF) and hepatocyte growth factor (HGF). Modern evidence shows that MSC cells may exert their effects via MSC-derived extra-cellular vesicles (EV), small secreted membrane vesicles formed through the fusion of endosomes with the cell membrane. EVs are known for their cell-to-cell communication, genetic information transfer via mRNA, and guidance to macrophage differentiation from pro-inflammatory to pro-repair phenotype [38, 40]. The anti-inflammatory effect is moderated by the release of interleukin 10 and thrombospondin-1 [39].

Umbilical cord tissue contains Wharton's jelly, a rich source of proteoglycans, heavy-chain hyaluronic acid, and glycoproteins. Many dressings incorporate umbilical cord tissue to incorporate the glycoprotein complex for inhibition of pro-inflammatory cell adhesion and their apoptosis, promotion of anti-inflammatory cytokines, and increased dressing integrity.

Both AM and UC dressings have an analgesic effect by covering nerve endings and minimizing wound desiccation. Multiple studies from adult patients revealed the efficacy of AM/UC dressings, including those for chronic wounds, burns, diabetic foot ulcers, and PI. All show successful epithelization with minimum dressing manipulation, softer scars, and shortened time to closure compared to other modalities. Pediatric literature focuses on burn care, while neonatal report superior results with extravasation injuries [39–45].

In my experience, AM or UC dressings have been excellent in utilization for pressure injuries, deep extravasation wounds, dehisced surgical wounds, and complex congenital conditions. Case 4 images illustrate challenging neonatal PIVI wounds. Location over a joint was concerning for potential contractures affecting limb function, if significant scarring occurred in the healing process. Dehydrated amniotic membrane graft and NPWT were used and resulted in timely healing, with a soft scar and no contractures or limitation of walking.

Case 3 illustrates the application of AM in a stagnant deep sacral PI. This pediatric patient was in a critical state for a few weeks after his diagnosis of cancer and the transplant that followed. He was intubated, septic, immunocompromised and suffered from protein-calorie malnutrition. His repositioning and offloading were dependent on the caregivers and medical staff but were challenging due to a limited reserve and movement tolerance. The sacral pressure injury developed and continued to progress as evidenced by significant depth, tunneling, and undermining. His medical team tried packing the wound with different products but failed to stimulate tissue growth (**Figure 3A**). At this point, the wound was gently cleaned with hypochlorous acid as aggressive debridement was contraindicated in this coagulopathic patient and packed with cryopreserved umbilical cord allograft. **Figure 3B** shows tremendous progress after 2.5 weeks and 2 applications of UC products. As wound became

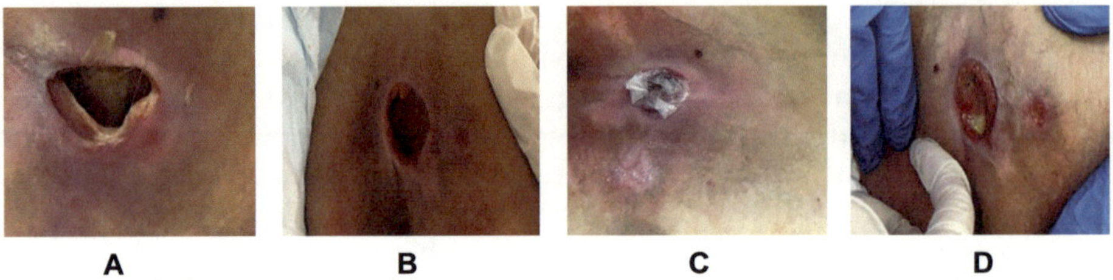

Figure 3.
A. Stage 3 sacral pressure injury. Tunneling and undermining are present. Thin slough covers wound bed and senescent edges are appreciated. B. Day 8. Wound after 1 application of cryopreserved UC. C. Day 17. As wound is smaller and shallow dehydrated amnion allograph placed. D. Day 30. Wound bed is filled-in with robust granulation tissue.

shallower, we transitioned to a dehydrated amniotic allograft membrane (**Figure 3C**). As you can see **Figure 3D** illustrates healthy, robust granulation tissue we achieved after 2 weeks of AM dressings.

5.4 Intact fish graft

The newest development in xenograft therapies is an intact acellular fish skin graft (FSG), the only non-mammalian piscine xenograft minimally processed from the skin of North Atlantic cod or Nile Tilapia. Research demonstrated that this graft is rich in fats, collagen, fibrin, proteoglycans, and glycosaminoglycans [46, 47]. Omega-3 polyunsaturated fatty acids are particularly plentiful; their anti-inflammatory messengers (resolvins and protectins) promote fibroblast proliferation, endothelial revascularization, and ECM remodeling. Its unique porosity and infrastructure mimic human three-dimensional skin, facilitating cell ingrowth [46–48]. Since no known viral or prion diseases can be transmitted via this fish to humans, mild chemical skin alteration preserves the original architecture, which seems to be homologous to the human skin [46–48].

Pediatric studies report on the theoretical advantages of using FSG in young patients, eliminating the need for donor sites and minimizing the risk of infection [49, 50]. Pediatric and especially neonatal dermis is much thinner than adult, which makes pediatric allograft suboptimal. Anti-inflammatory properties of omega-3 PUFAs decrease the propensity for hypertrophic scars, not an uncommon concern in pediatrics. Ciprandi et al. described a large series of pediatric wounds treated successfully and expeditiously with GSG, with shorter application time, faster healing time and shorter hospital stays [49]. Literature demonstrated its effectiveness across burns, surgical wounds, trauma, PI, and in adult diabetic ulcers [46–50]. Interestingly, all papers noted faster healing compared to previous standards of care(some compared to AM, dermal allogeneic grafts, or intestinal submucosa) and decreased use of antibiotics in adult studies, likely secondary to omega-3 fatty acids support of production of anti-bacterial and anti-viral messengers [47–50].

I have found success in using novel FSG in challenging wounds, such as Case 4. This neonatal wound was a result of severe necrotizing enterocolitis, requiring extensive surgical bowel resection, ostomy, and mucous fistula creation followed by two bouts of dehiscence. This infant was critically ill, edematous, and malnourished due to a limited remaining bowel. The wound proved challenging to dress due to its proximity to ostomy where an appliance hindered access to the full wound and very limited tolerance of any "hands-on" care. His first dehiscence was successfully closed

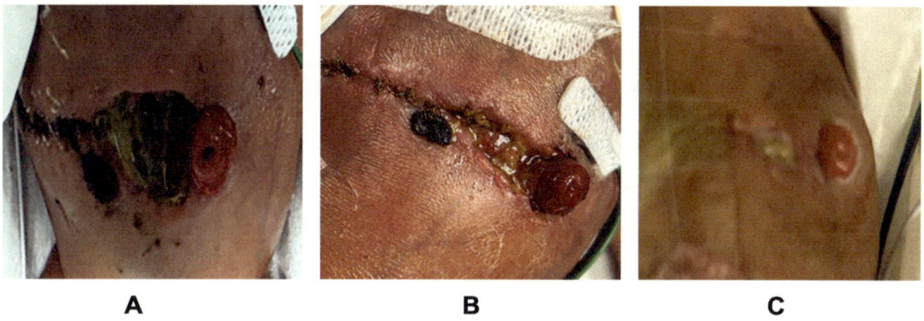

Figure 4.
A. Dehisced abdominal wound. Wound is colonized by enteric organisms as stoma opening is within the wound dehiscence. B. Day 15. S/P 2 GSG applications. Significant wound contraction. C. Follow-up visit 2 months later before ostomy reversal. Soft, pliable scar with normal pigmentation.

with collagen therapy; the second though did not respond as well. The skin was thin and ragged, and overall immune and proliferative systems were weak and deficient in nutrients and growth factors. A solid FSG sheet was cut into multiple small pieces, rehydrated with normal saline, and applied across the wound surface (**Figure 4A** shows dehiscence before FSG application), followed by hydrofiber packing and a hydrocolloid sheet to serve as a base for ostomy appliance placement. Application of FSG was repeated in 10 days for a total of 2 applications (**Figure 4B**). the wound closed completely in 4 weeks (**Figure 4C** shows the wound at 10 weeks) and importantly with minimal manipulations, which was essential given the patient's propensity to deteriorate with clinical care.

6. Discussion

While comparisons of FSG and AM/UC or collagens are scant in pediatric literature, adult -based data has been accumulating. Systematic review of literature comparing FSG and alternative wound dressings was published in 2023 [51]. Overall, literature supports superior healing with FSG in the variety of wounds, comparing to amniotic membranes, collagen-based dressing, silver sulfadiazine cream or bovine dermis. Kirshner et al. compared FSG with dehydrated human amnio-chorion membrane (dHACM) in diabetic ulcers. Fish graft afforded healing more rapidly, was 75% less expensive and had no difference between adverse outcomes in 2 groups [52]. Stone et al. compared FSG and fetal bovine dermis (FBD) as treatments for deep burns [53]. FSG integrated quicker into the wound, wounds required fewer treatments and resulted in faster re-epithelization and wound contraction. Level of blood flow and hydration was superior in FSG treated wounds compared to FBD wounds. Wallner et al. published similar results in the study of deep burns [54] as well as Lima, who compared FSG to a common standard-of-care burn dressing with silver sulfadiazine [55]. His results highlighted 3 times less dressing application and decreased analgesia requirement, decreasing cost of care overall in the group treated with FSG. Winters et al. compared cost-effectiveness of FSG to collagen dressings [55]. The cost savings with FSG was significant, about 25%, in addition to a higher number of fully healed wounds. A large trial by Lullove et al. compared collagen alginate dressings with FSG [56]. Number of required applications was 3 times higher in the collagen group and twice as many patients in the FSG had complete wound resolution.

Advanced wound therapies			
	Collagen	**AM/UC**	**FSG**
Origin	Human Bovine Porcine Equine Piscine Synthetic Plant-based	Human	Piscine
Preparation forms	Dehydrated Powder Gel	Dehydrated Cryopreserved Fresh Lyophilized	Dehydrated
Immunogenicity	Depends on preparation	Low	Low
Anti-inflammatory effect	Yes, indirectly	Yes	Yes
Anti-fibrotic effect	No	Yes	No
Anti-microbial effect	No	No	Yes
Pain relieving effect	No	Yes	Yes
Extracellular matrix growth	Direct	Indirect	Indirect
Reduction in healing time	↓	↓↓	↓↓
Cost	↑--↑↑	↑↑↑--↑↑↑↑	↑↑

Table 1.
Advanced wound therapies.

With time more sophisticated dressings are developed. FSG might have superior qualities compare to many cellular therapies available today (**Table 1**). Superior anti-inflammatory properties due to LCPUFAs and unique anti-bacterial properties compete head-to-head with various stem cells, cytokines and growth factors that amniotic membranes and umbilical cord dressings provide. While UM/UC dressings cost hundreds to thousands of dollars, cost of FSG starts at 80 to about 500 dollars on average, depending on the size. Comparing to many SOC products used in pediatrics such as silver, honey or hydrogel creams as well as collagen products, both FSG and UM grafts are more expensive per product application. However, faster and complete wound closure and fewer required applications decreased the cost overall.

7. Conclusion

Advanced cellular therapies for neonatal and pediatric skin have to be safe, effective, easy to apply, and take into consideration the challenging size and location of a wound. While adult patients are commonly taken to an operating suite to apply therapeutic products, neonate transport from the neonatal unit is not advisable. Connection to many invasive devices, tube dislodgement, risk of hypothermia, and side effects of anesthesia provide strong deterrents from the treatments necessitating outside transports. Therapies with prolonged shelf-life, easy application, and bolstering are attractive to neonatal and pediatric providers. Collagen products represent such therapy to me. Multiple easy-to-apply preparations and shortened healing time make sense in many hypercatabolic and critically ill children. The price point is reasonable and most pediatric practitioners can apply these products without the need of sub-specialists. I often think of collagen preparations as standard-of-care for every day, easy application by any practitioner in pediatrics.

As advanced biologic cellular therapies developed amniotic membranes and umbilical cord preparations, I incorporated them into my armamentarium. The proliferative and anti-inflammatory boost these products provide is crucial for stagnant wounds. I found these therapies even more integral in areas where contractures, scars, and disfigurement are potentially life-altering. It has become my "first-choice" therapy in a fresh wound located over a joint, hands, feet, or face. These products are very easy to apply (especially the dehydrated amniotic variety), only need re-application once in 7–10 days and a simple secondary dressing or NPWT is sufficient as an outer dressing.

Finally, as FSG has entered the neonatal and pediatric wound arena I can see its reasonable cost, ease of application, anti-inflammatory and, especially anti-microbial properties, leading to a wide-spread use, especially in patients with nutritional deficiencies, bacterial colonization, and minimal tolerance for hand-on handling.

The safety of these products has been evaluated and shown via available literature and I encourage pediatric practitioners to develop the knowledge and skills necessary to apply these therapies to our fragile patients.

Author details

Vita Boyar[1,2,3]

1 Cohen Children's Medical Center of NY, Northwell Health, New Hyde Park, NY, USA

2 Pediatrics, Neonatal-Perinatal Medicine, New Hyde Park, NY, USA

3 Donald and Barbara Zucker School of Medicine at Hofstra, Northwell, Hempstead, NY, USA

*Address all correspondence to: vboyar@gmail.com

References

[1] Ness M, Davis D, Carey W. Neonatal skin care: A concise review. International Journal of Dermatology. 2013;**52**:14-22

[2] Kusari A, Han A, Virgen A, et al. Evidence-based skin care in preterm infants. Pediatric Dermatology. 2019;**36**:16-23

[3] Metzker A, Brenner S, Merlob P. Iatrogenic cutaneous injuries in the neonate. Archives of Dermatology. 1999;**135**:697-703

[4] Fox M. Wound care in the neonatal intensive care unit. Neonatal Network. 2010;**30**(5):291-302

[5] Johnson D. Extremely preterm infant skin care. Advances in Neonatal Care. 2016;**16**(5S):S26-S32

[6] Telofski A, Morello P, Mack Correa C, Stamatas G. The infant skin barrier: Can we preserve, protect, and enhance the barrier? Dermatology Research and Practice. 2012;**2012**:198789

[7] Amer Y, Bridges C, Marathe K. Epidemiology, pathophysiology and management strategies of neonatal wound care. Neoreview. 2021;**22**(7):e452-e460

[8] Bhatta D, Subramanya S, Hamal D, et al. Bacterial contamination of neonatal intensive care unit: How safe are the neonates? Antimicrobial Resistance & Infection Control. 2021;**26**:1-6

[9] Senn V, Bassler D, Choudhury R, et al. Microbial colonization from fetus to early childhood—A comprehensive review. Frontiers in Cellular and Infectious Microbiology. 2020;**10**:1-12

[10] Visscher M, McKeown K, Nurre M, et al. Skin care for the extremely low-birthweight infant. Neoreview. 2023;**24**(4):229-242

[11] Dao D, Anez-Bustillos L, Cho B, et al. Assessment of micronutrient status in critically ill children: Challenges and opportunities. Nutrients. 2017;**9**:1185

[12] Marino L, Valla F, Beattie R, Verbruggen S. Micronutrient status during pediatric critical illness: A scoping review. Clinical Nutriton. 2020;**39**:3571-3593

[13] Molnar J, Underdown M, Clark W. Nutrition and wounds. Advances in Wound Care. 2014;**3**(11):663-681

[14] Irving S, Berry K, Morgan S, et al. Nutrition associated with skin integrity and pressure injury in critically ill pediatric patients. Nutrition in Clinical Practice. 2023;**38**:S125-S138

[15] Berry K, Seiple S, Stellar J, et al. A scoping review to inform a multi-disciplinary approach for nutrition therapy in critically ill children with pressure injuries. Translational Pediatrics. 2021;**10**(10):2799-2813

[16] Fumarola S, Allaway R, Callaghan R, et al. Overlooked and underestimated: Medical adhesive-related skin injuries. Best practice consensus document on prevention. Journal of Wound Care. 2020;**29**(S3C):S1-S24

[17] Lund C. Medical adhesives in the NICU. Newborn and Infant Nursing Reviews. 2014;**14**:160-165

[18] McNichol L, Lund C, Rosen T, Gray M. Medical adhesives and patient safety: State of the science. Journal of Wound, Ostomy and Continence Nursing. 2013;**40**(4):365-380

[19] Kim M, Jang J, Kim H, et al. Medical adhesives-related skin injury in a pediatric intensive care unit: A single-center observational study. Journal of Wound, Ostomy, and Continence Nursing. 2019;**46**(6):491-496

[20] August D, New K, Ray R, Kandasamy Y. Frequency, location and risk factors of neonatal skin injuries from mechanical forces of pressure, friction, shear and stripping: A systematic literature review. Journal of Neonatal Nursing. 2018;**24**:173-180

[21] Pettit J. Assessment of an infant with a peripheral intravenous device. Advances in Neonatal Care. 2003;**3**(5):230-240

[22] Infusion Nurses Society. Infusion nursing standards of practice. Journal of Infusion Nursing. 2011;**34**:91S, S65-S67

[23] Amjad I, Murphy T, Nylander-Housholder L, et al. A new approach to management of intravenous infiltration in pediatric patients: Pathophysiology, classification and treatment. Journal of Infusion Nursing. 2011;**34**:242-249

[24] Frank L, Hummel D, Connel K, et al. The safety and efficacy of peripheral intravenous catheters in all neonates. Neonatal Network. 2001;**20**:33-38

[25] Baharestani M. An overview of neonatal and pediatric wound care knowledge and considerations. Ostomy Wound Management. 2007;**53**(6):34-40

[26] Baldwin KM. Incidence and prevalence of pressure ulcers in children. Advances in Skin and Wound Care. 2002;**15**(3):121-124

[27] Baharestani M. Pressure ulcers in neonates and children: An NPUAP white paper. Advances in Skin & Wound Care. 2007;**20**(4):208-220

[28] Gefen A. A new consensus on medical-related pressure ulcers. Journal of Wound Care. 2019;**28**:315

[29] Schluer A. Pressure ulcers in maturing skin—A clinical perspective. Journal of Tissue Viability. 2017;**26**:2-5

[30] Stellar J, Hasbani N, Kulik L, et al. Medical device-related pressure injuries in infants and children. Journal of Wound, Ostomy, and Continence Nursing. 2020;**47**:459-469

[31] Schultz G, Davidson J, Kirsner R, et al. Dynamic reciprocity in the wound environment. Wound Repair and Regeneration. 2011;**19**(2):134-148

[32] Gurtner G, Werner S, Barrandon Y, et al. Wound repair and regeneration. Nature. 2008;**453**:314-321

[33] Fleck C, Simman R. Modern collagen dressings: Function and purpose. The Journal of the American College of Certified Wound Specialists. 2010;**2**:50-54

[34] Brett D. A review of collagen and collagen-based wound dressings. Wounds. 2008;**20**(12):347-356

[35] Reinke J, Sorg H. Wound repair and regeneration. European Surgical Research. 2012;**49**:35-43

[36] Chattopadhyay S, Raines R. Collagen-based biomaterials for wound healing. Biopolymers. 2014;**101**(8):821-833

[37] Hochstein A, Bhatia A. Collagen: Its role in wound healing. Podiatry Management. 2014;**8**(103-106):109-110

[38] Schmiedova I, Dembickaja A, Kiselakova L. et al, Using of amniotic

membrane derivatives for the treatment of chronic wounds. Membranes. 2021;**11**:941-955

[39] Singh S, Srivastava N, Ahmed I, et al. Human amniotic membrane usage from bench to bedside in congenital defects and wounds in pediatric surgery: A systematic review. Medical Research Archives. 2023;**11**(2):1-7

[40] Pourmoussa A, Gardner D, Johnson M, Wong A. An update and review of cell-based wound dressings and their integration into clinical practice. Annals of Translational Medicine. 2016;**4**(23):457-467

[41] Acevedo P. Successful treatment of painful chronic wounds with amniotic and umbilical cord tissue: A case series. SAGE Open Medical Case Reports. 2020;**8**:1-6

[42] Koob T, Lim J, Massee M, et al. Properties of dehydrated human amnion/ chorion composite grafts: Implications for wound repair and soft tissue regeneration. Journal of Biomedical Materials Research B: Applied Biomaterials. 2014;**102B**(6):1-10

[43] Zelen C, Snyder R, Serena T, Li W. The use of human amnion/ chorion membrane in the clinical setting for lower extremity repair: A review. Clinics in Podiatric Medicine and Surgery. 2015;**32**:135-146

[44] Branski L, Herndon D, Celis M, et al. Amnion in the treatment of pediatric partial-thickness facial burns. Burns. 2008;**34**:393-399

[45] Tenenhaus M. The use of dehydrated human amnion/chorion membranes in the treatment of burns and complex wounds. Annals of Plastic Surgery. 2017;**78**(1):s11-s13

[46] Kim T, Park J, Jeong H, Wee S. The utility of novel fish-skin derived acellular dermal matrix (keresis) as a wound dressing material. Journal of Wound Management and Research. 2021;**17**(1):39-47

[47] Esmaelli A, Biazar E, Ebrahimi M, et al. Acellular fish skin for wound healing. International Wound Journal. 2023;**20**:2924-2941

[48] Yoon J, Yoon D, Lee H, et al. Wound healing ability of acellular fish skin and bovine collagen grafts for split-thickness donor sites in burn patients: Characterization of acellular grafts and clinical application. International Journal of Biological Macromolecules. 2022;**205**:454-461

[49] Ciprandi G, Kjartansson H, Grussu F, et al. Use of acellular intact fish skin grafts in treating acute pediatric wounds during the COVID-19 pandemic: A case series. Journal of Wound Care. 2022;**31**(10):824-831

[50] Mitri M, Di Carmine A, Thomas E. Fish skin graft: Narrative review and first application for abdominal wall dehiscence in children. PRS Global Open. 2023;**11**(9):e5244-50. DOI: 10.1097?GOX.0000000000005244

[51] Ibrahim M, Ayyoubi H, Alkhairi L, et al. Fish skin grafts versus alternative wound dressings in wound care: A systematic review of the literature. Cureus. 2023;**15**(3):e36348

[52] Kirshner R, Margolis D, Baldursson B, et al. Fish skin grafts compared to human amnion/chorion membrane allografts: A double-blind, prospective, randomized clinical trial of acute wound healing. Wound Repair and Regeneration. 2020;**28**:75-80

[53] Stone R, Saathoff E, Larson D, et al. Accelerated wound closure of deep

partial thickness burns with acellular fish skin graft. International Journal of Molecular Sciences. 2021;**22**:1590

[54] Wallner C, Holtermann J, Drysch M, et al. The use of intact fish skin as a novel treatment method for deep dermal burns following enzymatic debridement: A retrospective case-control study. European Burn Journal. 2022;**3**:43-55

[55] Lima Junior E, De Moraes F, Costa B, et al. Innovative burn treatment using tilapia skin as a xenograft: A phase II randomized controlled trial. Journal of Burn Care & Research. 2020;**41**:585-592

[56] Lullove EJ, Liden B, Winters C, et al. A multicenter, blinded, randomized controlled clinical trial evaluating the effect of omega-3-rich fish skin in the treatment of chronic, nonresponsive diabetic foot ulcers. Wounds. 2021;**33**:169-177